CLINICAL TUMOR IMMUNOLOGY

EORTC Monographs on Cancer

Symposium of

CLINICAL TUMOR IMMUNOLOGY

Edited by

JOSEPH WYBRAN and MAURICE J. STAQUET

Institut Jules Bordet,
Centre des Tumeurs de l'Université Libre de Bruxelles
and
Hôpital Universitaire Saint-Pierre, Bruxelles

Published as a supplement to the *European Journal of Cancer*

Published for the European Organization for Research on Treatment
of Cancer (EORTC)

PERGAMON PRESS

Oxford · New York · Toronto · Paris · Sydney · Frankfurt

U.K.	Pergamon Press Ltd., Headington Hill Hall, Oxford OX3 0BW, England
U.S.A.	Pergamon Press Inc., Maxwell House, Fairview Park, Elmsford, New York 10523, U.S.A.
CANADA	Pergamon of Canada Ltd., P.O. Box 9600, Don Mills M3C 2T9, Ontario, Canada
AUSTRALIA	Pergamon Press (Aust.) Pty. Ltd., 19a Boundary Street, Rushcutters Bay, N.S.W. 2011, Australia
FRANCE	Pergamon Press SARL, 24 rue des Ecoles, 75240 Paris, Cedex 05, France
WEST GERMANY	Pergamon Press GmbH, 6242 Kronberg/Taunus, Pferdstrasse 1, Frankfurt-am-Main, West Germany

First edition 1976

Library of Congress Cataloging in Publication Data

Symposium of Clinical Tumor Immunology, Brussels,
    1975.
    Clinical tumor immunology.
    "Organized jointly be the EORTC and the Depart-
ment of Immunology of the University Hospital of
Brussels."
    1. Cancer—Immunological aspects—Congresses.
2. Immunodiagnosis—Congresses. 3. Immunotherapy—
Congresses. I. Wybran, Joseph. II. Staquet, Maurice.
III. European Organization for Research on Treatment
of Cancer. IV. Brussels. Hôpital Saint-Pierre. Départment
d'immunologie. V. Title. [DNLM: Neoplasms—
Immunology. QZ200 C644]
RC262.S93 1975   616.9'94'079   76–3458
ISBN 0–08–020570–4
ISBN 0–08–021101–1 FLEXI

Typeset by E.W.C. Wilkins Ltd., London and Northampton
Printed in Great Britain by A. Wheaton & Co., Exeter

CONTENTS

Introduction

The Immunological Dream of an Oncologist   xi
J. Wybran and M.J. Staquet

EORTC, Aim, Structure and Activity   xiii
M.J. Staquet and J. Wybran

General Mechanisms in Tumor Immunity

Biological Activities of the Circulating Thymic Hormone   3
Jean-François Bach

Macrophage Secretions Affecting the Growth of Other Cells   9
F.J. Lejeune

Immune Cellular Mechanisms at the Site of the Tumor   19
E.H. Betz and L.J. Simar

Tests in Cancer Patients

T-cell Rosettes in Human Cancer   31
J. Wybran and H.H. Fudenberg

Cell-mediated Cytotoxicity *in vitro*. Mechanisms and Relevance to Tumor
    Immunity   41
J.-C. Cerottini and K.T. Brunner

Function and Evaluation of Human K-cells   47
I.C.M. MacLennan

Lymphocyte Stimulation Test for Detection of Tumor Specific Reactivity in
    Humans   55
F. Vánky, E. Klein and J. Stjernswärd

The Leucocyte Migration Technique in Studies of Tumor-directed Cellular
    Immunity in Malignant Melanoma   69
A.J. Cochran, R.M. Mackie, C.E. Ross, L.J. Ogg and A.M. Jackson

Detection of Cell-mediated Immunity against Tumor-associated Antigens of
    Human Breast Carcinoma by Migration Inhibition and Lymphocyte-
    stimulation Assays   77
J.L. McCoy, J.H. Dean, G.B. Cannon, B.A. Maurer, R.K. Oldham and
    R.B. Herberman

Tumor Antigens

The Use of CEA (Carcinoembryonic Antigen) and Other Carcinofoetal Antigens in
   Human Cancer   89
S. von Kleist

HL-A in Cancer

HL-A and Cancer   107
A. Govaerts

Classification of Leukemias and Lymphomas

Immunological Approaches to the Identification of Leukaemic Cells   115
M.F. Greaves, G. Brown, D. Capellaro, G. Janossy and T. Revesz

Lymphocyte Membrane Markers in B-cell Proliferations and Human
   Non-Hodgkin's Lymphomas   123
J.C. Brouet, J.L. Preud'homme and M. Seligmann

Classification of Leukemias and Hematosarcomas Based on Cell Membrane
   Markers and Scanning Electron Microscopy   131
D. Belpomme, D. Dantchev, R. Joseph, A. Santoro, F. Feuilhade de Chauvin,
   N. Lelarge, D. Grandjon, D. Pontvert and G. Mathé

Immunotherapy

Preclinical Approaches in Tumor Immunochemotherapy   147
A. Goldin and D.P. Houchens

Levamisole in Resectable Human Bronchogenic Carcinoma   159
W. Amery

Mediation of Immune Responses to Human Tumor Antigens with "Immune"
   RNA   169
Y.H. Pilch, D. Fritze and D.H. Kern

Transfer Factor: the Current Picture, with Special Reference to Human Cancer   191
H.H. Fudenberg

New Frontiers of Cancer Active Immunotherapy   207
G. Mathé

The Immunotherapy of Acute Myeloblastic Leukaemia   223
J.M.A. Whitehouse

Immunotherapy of Human Solid Tumors: Prolongation of Disease-free Interval
   and Survival in Malignant Melanoma, Breast and Colorectal Cancer   233
J.U. Gutterman, G.M. Mavligit, M.A. Burgess, J.O. Cardenas, R.C. Reed,
   G.R. Blumenschein, J.A. Gottlieb, C.M. McBride and E.M. Hersh

Abstracts of Papers Presented at the Symposium
J. Bertoglio, A. Bourgoin, K. Gronneberg and J.F. Dore   251

CONTENTS   vii

B.R. Bullen, G.R. Giles and T.G. Brennan   251

N. Carpentier-Bricteux and G. Degiovanni   252

A.L. Claudy, J. Viac, N. Pelletier, N. Fouad-Wassef, A. Alario and J. Thivolet   252

D. Collavo, G. Biasi, A. Colombatti and L. Chieco-Bianchi   253

P. de Baetselier, R. Hooghe, J. Grooten, C. Hamers-Casterman and R. Hamers   253

J.E. de Vries and P. Rümke   254

H.-D. Flad, C. Huber, K. Bremer, U. Fink and H. Huber   254

C.B. Freeman, G.M. Taylor, R. Harris, C.G. Geary, J.E. MacIver and I.W. Delamore   255

M.A. Frost and A.S. Coates   256

A. Hekman   256

K. Krohn, A. Uotila, P. Gröhn, J. Väisänen and K.-M. Hiltunen   257

M. Moore and N. Robinson   257

H.H. Peter, R.F. Eife and J.R. Kalden   258

M.M. Roberts   258

E. Robinson, A. Bartal, Y. Cohen and R. Haasz   259

M.R.G. Robinson, C.C. Rigby, R.B.C. Pugh, R.J. Shearer, D.C. Dumonde and
    L.C. Vaughan   260

G.F. Rowland, G.J. O'Neill and D.A.L. Davies   260

M. Segerling, S.H. Ohanian and T. Borsos   261

B. Serrou, J.B. Dubois and C. Thierry   261

P. Stryckmans   262

G.M. Taylor, R. Harris and C.B. Freeman   262

R.D. Thornes   263

B. Van Camp   263

C. Vennegoor   264

R. Verloes, G. Atassi and L. Kanarek   264

O. Wetter and K.H. Linder   265

Author Index   267
Subject Index   279

INTRODUCTION

THE IMMUNOLOGICAL DREAM OF AN ONCOLOGIST

JOSEPH WYBRAN and MAURICE J. STAQUET

*Department of Immunology, Hôpital Universitaire Saint-Pierre, Brussels and
Institut Jules Bordet, Brussels*

This book is the Proceedings of the Symposium of Clinical Tumor Immunology held in Brussels (May 26–29, 1975) and organized jointly by the EORTC and the Department of Immunology of the University Hospital of Brussels. This Conference was mainly educational and developed in a few days most of the general topics and some special subjects related to this new field of Cancer Medicine.

The importance of immunology is, indeed, growing not only in oncology but in most sectors of medicine. This can easily be explained. First, the basic mechanisms of the immune reactions are better understood and immune phenomenon in diseases appear numerous. Secondly, immunological reactions in biological and medical sciences are widely used. This is mainly due to the fact that they offer both the specificity and the possibility of measuring trace amounts of substances (e.g. radioimmunoassay of hormones, blood proteins). Finally, and therefore, the immunologist has left his ivory tower to join the glorious life of the day to day medicine. Immunology is no more dealing only with animals but has wide human applications. It is frequently possible to determine the specific defect in patients with immunological diseases and sometimes completely correct it. The oncologist asks four basic questions of the immunologist. Their answer should provide a clue to the diagnosis, treatment and prevention of cancer.

(a) Is there an immunological defect in cancer patients? If yes, is it primary or secondary? A primary failure is not easy to determine since only a prospective study of the normal population by a battery of tests could possibly detect those subjects who have perhaps only subtle immune defects and who will develop a malignancy. Also, if this study could theoretically be done, such a defect, if present, may be transient which implies frequent testing. Finally, the tests should be rapid, reliable, reproducible and done on a small blood sample. These are difficult criteria. Nothing, as yet, suggests that this type of test is known. Therefore the question of a primary defect in cancer remains unanswered.

(b) The second question asked of immunologists is to provide a way of making an early diagnosis of cancer. Some hopes, in this field, were raised by the discovery of fetal-linked tumor specific antigens. It appears that their determination is not yet helpful in making a clear-cut diagnosis. This is, quite often, due to their non-specificity, for both the diseased organ and the type of disease. A lot of non-malignant diseases can be associated with measurable levels of these foeto-proteins. Similarly, malignant diseases may not be associated with such foeto-proteins. These antigens are, however, of value in determining the recurrence or the cure of disease. Since this area is being intensively investigated, a good chance exists to find a battery of foeto-antigens, organ and disease specific. For instance, alpha-protein is very interesting. It appears to be a rather specific marker for hepatoma and some testicular carcinoma. Recently, it was discovered that it has immunosuppressive properties. This finding should open a new avenue of investigation and, perhaps, bring some exciting new concepts regarding the question of immune defect in cancer.

(c) A third important question asked of immunologists concerns the field of therapy. According to classical data of cell kinetics, chemotherapy will not kill the last tumor cell. It has been proposed that the role of immunotherapy is to eradicate these last tumor cells. Some preliminary data also suggest that immunotherapy could act in combination with chemotherapy or other forms of classical therapy.

Of interest is that cytotoxic drugs given on an intermittent basis are not, or are less, immunosuppressive than the one given on a chronic basis. Recent data also appear to indicate that immunotherapy can be helpful even in the presence of a relative number of tumor cells. Current clinical applications, fully discussed in this book, indeed suggest that immunotherapy can be a useful adjunct to classical therapy. Finally, since so few tests correlate with the clinical status of the patients, who do or do not respond to therapy, one could heretically think that non-specific immunotherapy works, in fact, through non-immune mechanisms.

(d) The final and more important question concerns the hope of an immune prevention of cancer. For instance, conflicting data suggest that BCG vaccination, in neonates, decreases the incidence of acute leukemia. Active immunization by a vaccine against cancer seems now a dream, but progress in the fields of basic science, virology, immunochemistry and cellular immunology should eventually materialize such a dream and kill the nightmare of cancer.

EORTC, AIM, STRUCTURE AND ACTIVITY

M.J. STAQUET and J. WYBRAN

*Institut Jules Bordet, Brussels, and Department of immunology,
Hôpital Universitaire Saint-Pierre, Brussels*

The aims of the European Organization for Research on Treatment of Cancer (EORTC) are to conduct, develop, coordinate and stimulate research in Europe on the experimental and clinical bases of treatment of cancer and related problems. Extensive and comprehensive research in this wide field is often beyond the means of the individual European laboratories and hospitals and can be best accomplished through the joint efforts of the clinical and basic research groups of several countries.

The organization was founded in 1962 by research workers in the main cancer research institutes of the Common Market countries and Switzerland. It was named "Groupe Européen de Chimiothérapie Anticancéreuse" (GECA). Representatives from Great Britain and from Austria joined the organization in 1966 and 1970 respectively. EORTC has a Council which plans and supervises the activities within the organization. The Administrative Board of the Council prepares the meetings of the Council and handles the daily work involved with administrative and financial matters. Within the EORTC clinical and laboratory research is carried out by clinical cooperative groups, cooperative research project groups, working parties and research information exchange clubs. The Council meets six to eight times per year in the various European institutes associated with EORTC to discuss scientific as well as administrative matters. At regular intervals it receives the results of the drug screening programs and those of the clinical cooperative groups and the research project groups. Cooperative groups, project groups, working parties and clubs meet as often as their activity requires. An annual plenary meeting is organized in June for all members of EORTC on one or more subjects related to the treatment of cancer.

EORTC has initiated four major efforts in the field of cancer treatment:
a screening program of potential anti-cancer agents;
the organization of clinical and preclinical cooperative groups aimed at carrying out controlled clinical trials with new therapeutic agents and regimens;
the organization of collaborative research programs;
the initiation of symposia, courses and publications on the subject of cancer research and treatment.

The clinical cooperative groups have organized themselves under the auspices of EORTC to carry out collaborative work, mostly aimed at the clinical evaluation of new drugs and treatments for cancer. Through this cooperation, data on large numbers of patients treated according to one or more accepted protocols can be collected at a much faster rate than within any of the clinical centers alone. To assist the groups in their administrative and scientific work, the EORTC Coordinating Office was established in 1969 and expanded in a EORTC Coordinating Office and Data Center in 1974. The purpose of the Coordinating and Data Center is to provide central coordination for the activities of the EORTC groups and to make available to the groups a wide range of statistical and data processing expertise, including advice on study design as well as analysis and reporting of results, at a central, and hence economical, location.

EORTC is not a scientific society, but a transnational institution consisting of laboratories and clinical services situated in different countries: 15 laboratories, 1500 research personnel, 200 clinical services and several hundreds of clinicians are associated with EORTC. This structure permits an increasing number of patients to be treated every year, according to the highest international standards and in such a way that the results of the treatment can be evaluated within a short time. It also provides opportunities for the organization and integration of research programs on cancer treatment on a level that could never be attained by individual institutes or services.

Table 1. *EORTC Trials Involving Immunotherapy*

		Trial's secretary
ACUTE MYELOCYTIC	two arms protocol comparing chemo-immuno-therapy to immunotherapy during maintenance	M. HAYAT (Villejuif)
EPIDERMOID BRONCHIAL CARCINOMA	four arms protocol comparing chemo-immuno-therapy to chemotherapy to immunotherapy and to no treatment in postsurgical patients	L. ISRAEL (Paris)
EPIDERMOID BRONCHIAL CARCINOMA	same as above in inoperable irradiated patients	L. ISRAEL (Paris)
MALIGNANT MELANOMA	two arms protocol comparing immunotherapy to no treatment in residual primary melanoma of the skin	J.P. CESARINI (Paris)
MALIGNANT MELANOMA	four arms protocol comparing immunochemotherapy to chemotherapy to immunotherapy and to no treatment in postoperative melanoma of the skin with positive lymph nodes	J.P. CESARINI (Paris)
ACUTE LYMPHOBLASTIC LEUKEMIA	two arms protocol comparing chemotherapy to immunotherapy in maintenance	P. STRYCKMANS (Brussels)

Numerous attempts at modifying the course of cancer by inducing changes of the immunologic response of the host have been tried in the last 10 years. Although a rational approach to the problem is still missing because of the lack of knowledge of fundamental mechanisms, several empirical trials have indicated the possible usefulness of immunological treatment. Many authors have shown that immunotherapy alone is unable to inhibit the progressive growth of a tumor, and that it will be best used in conjunction with surgery, chemotherapy and irradiation. This, in turn, explains the very complex clinical trials involving strict prognosis stratification. Because of the large number of patients which will be necessary to detect small changes in responses to therapy, very few clinical institutions will be able to conduct phase III trials alone. Therefore, they have to resort to multi-center trials and complex statistical techniques. EORTC has initiated six cooperative clinical trials (Table 1) in the field of immunotherapy, all using live BCG.

The symposium reported in this issue is part of a collaborative effort aiming to inform oncologists in the recent developments in cancer research and to increase collaboration between the researchers in the field of immunology.

EORTC is grateful to the chairmen of the sessions and to the lecturers for their collaboration.

GENERAL MECHANISMS IN TUMOR
IMMUNITY

BIOLOGICAL ACTIVITIES OF THE CIRCULATING THYMIC HORMONE

JEAN-FRANÇOIS BACH

Hôpital Necker, 161, rue de Sèvres, 75015 Paris

The mechanisms of T-cell maturation are still a matter of speculation and controversy. There are several arguments in favour of a direct differentiation of stem cells at the contact of the thymic epithelium microenvironment. The seeding of T-cells from the thymus, as proved by experiments using chromosomal markers [1] and the presence itself of large numbers of lymphocytes within the thymus, are among the best of these arguments. Conversely, the restoration of immunocompetence in neonatally thymectomized (NTx) mice by thymus grafts in cell-impermeable Millipore chambers [2], and especially by cell-free thymic extracts, argue in favour of humoral mechanisms [3, 4]. In fact these two theories are not mutually exclusive since, as is known for erythrocytes or granulocytes, there might be a first microenvironmental stage of differentiation followed by a hormone-dependent phase.

Our approach to the problem was perceptibly different from that mentioned above. We had demonstrated that a large percentage of rosette-forming cells (RFC) are thymus-dependent and bear the theta (θ) antigen, specific to T-cells [5–7]. Conversely, other RFC, thymus-independent, do not bear the θ antigen and include both B-cells and T-cell precursors. We first showed that thymic extracts (given by Goldstein and White, and Trainin) induced the appearance of the θ antigen on certain RFC from the bone marrow [6, 8, 9]. Similarly, spleen cells from adult thymectomized (ATx) mice, which had lost the θ antigen [8], recovered their sensitivity to anti-θ serum after *in vivo* or *in vitro* treatment by thymic extracts. These experiments, perhaps more analytical then the previous ones by Goldstein and White, and Trainin, were, however, submitted to the same specificity criticism, even if spleen extracts were essentially inactive. The demonstration that there was a substance in normal mouse serum, with the same activities as thymic extracts, that was absent in the serum of Tx mice brought the definitive proof of the specificity of the phenomenon [10, 11]. Besides the action of the hormone on RFC provided a simple and reproducible bioassay that allowed us to isolate and characterize the serum thymic hormone. The hormone appears to be a peptide with a molecular weight (MW) of about 1000; i.e. 10 times lower than that of the thymosin of Goldstein and White, but also 10 to 1000 times more active for the same molarity. We have temporarily called this peptide "thymic factor" (TF) and not "thymosin" because the thymic factor and thymosin are obviously two distinct entities, even if they may be biochemically related.

I shall not give details, in this article, on TF biochemistry nor on the physiological conditions of its secretion (such as age-dependence, thymectomy and thymus grafting experiments published elsewhere [12]), limiting myself to the TF biological activities. This is a particularly important matter since the assay in which TF has been isolated and characterized is an *in vitro* assay and as such always submitted to a number of possible artefacts and to pharmacological effects of biologically irrelevant substances.

The effects of pig TF have been studied in various *in vivo* and *in vitro* systems. It should be emphasized that all the studies which will be mentioned have been performed with fairly purified preparations, active *in vivo* and *in vitro* at ng levels at variance with experiments reported by other authors, using rather unfractionated preparations (even if purified materials had been made available for biochemical studies) at μg or even mg levels. One should also stress that in *in vivo* studies TF was bound to carboxymethyl-cellulose (CMC) in order to increase its half-life [12].

THETA CONVERSION

Purified TF can induce the appearance of the θ antigen on previously θ-negative RFC. However, with some very active AθS batches, it may be shown that there is in fact some inhibition on the TF-sensitive RFC before TF treatment, as seen in normal bone marrow or in spleen from ATx or nude mice. In that case, TF increases θ antigen expression rather than provokes its appearance [11, 13].

Similar data have been obtained in normal spleen cells at ng levels using a cytotoxic assay after cell fractionation on a BSA gradient, as described by Komuro and Boyse [14]. These results [13] must, however, be interpreted with caution since some θ conversion can be obtained by incubating the cells at 37°C without any added material, suggesting a possible fragilization of cells with small amounts of θ antigen, making them more sensitive to otherwise non-cytotoxic concentrations. This criticism does not apply to the sheep cell rosette assay which does not involve BSA fractionation and long-term incubation.

The mechanism of action of TF on RFC θ conversion has been investigated with regard to the cAMP system. In brief, TF effects are mimicked by low (and physiological) concentrations of cAMP, theophylline and prostaglandins [13]. One can even show a synergy between cAMP and TF, both used at subliminal levels. Lastly, indomethacin, a prostaglandin synthetase inhibitor, blocks TF effect [13] as well; injected into normal mice it decreases transiently the number of θ-positive cells in the spleen (but interestingly not in lymph nodes) [15]. Finally, it appears that θ antigen expression has a rapid turn-over and is probably regulated by agents altering cAMP synthesis, TF possibly acting in this system through stimulation of cAMP synthesis, eventually itself through prosta-glandin stimulation in view of indomethacin data.

MITOGEN RESPONSES

TF has been shown to induce some responsiveness to Concanavalin A (Con A) and, to a lesser degree, to PHA in nude mouse spleen cells and in low density normal spleen cells separated on a Ficoll gradient (P. Hayry and J.F. Bach, in preparation). However, one should emphasize that the increase, although significant, was not dramatic ($\times 2 - \times 4$).

Similarly, a 2-week treatment with TF increases significantly Con A and PHA responses in the spleen of NZB mice at an age when they show decreased mitogen responses. Interestingly, a similar restoration is obtained by grafting a thymus eventually in a Millipore chamber (to be published).

AUTOLOGOUS ROSETTES [16, 17]

A small percentage of normal mouse lymphocytes form rosettes when mixed with autologous (or syngeneic) erythrocytes. These autologous RFC (ARFC) normally predominate in the thymus. Interestingly, their number increases with age and especially after ATx within a few days after the operation, ARFC level reaching its peak 30–45 days after the operation ($\times 20$ increase). TF normalized ARFC level in ATx mice injected *in vivo* or after *in vitro* incubation. ARFC characteristics indicate that they belong to the pool of post-thymic or To cells. The significance of the ARFC phenomenon is still obscure but might have some relevance to autoantigen recognition. Anyhow, autologous rosette formation appears to be a marker of To cells and the effects of TF on this marker can be utilized as a useful TF assay.

ANTIGEN-INDUCED CAPPING

It has been reported that RFC (like radio-labelled antigen-binding cells) redistribute their antigen-binding receptors after 15 min incubation at $37°C$ with the antigen in question. We have shown that such "capping" could be observed at the T-RFC level in the spleen and that ATx depleted the capacity of these T-spleen RFC to cap. Interestingly, *in vitro* treatment with purified TF rapidly restored normal capping characteristics when added to the spleen cells simultaneously with SRBC. Whereas normal mouse serum also showed that effect, serum from ATx mice and nude mice did not exhibit it [18].

STEROID RECEPTORS

Thymocytes include two cell subpopulations, one mainly present in the cortex which is sensitive to the *in vivo* and *in vitro* lytic action of steroids, the other predominant in the thymus medulla which is corticoresistant. It has been reported by Trainin [19] that *in vitro* incubation of thymus cells with the dialysable thymus humoral factor decreased the sensitivity of thymocytes to *in vitro* cortisol-induced lysis. We have investigated this experimental system by studying the receptors for steroids present on the surface of thymocytes in collaboration with D. Duval. These receptors, which are detected by their property of binding triated dexamethasone, are specific for cortisol. They are located in the cell cytosol from which they are extracted. We have examined the effect of *in vitro* TF treatment of thymocytes on the expression of steroid receptors. Purified TF was shown to induce a 70% inhibition of steroid-specific uptake by thymus cells, suggesting that decrease in the number or in the availability of receptors for steroids is one of the mechanisms by which T-cells lose their high steroid sensitivity as they mature. Our experiments also indicate that such changes might be due to TF action (to be published).

SUPPRESSOR T-CELLS

NZB mice show an abnormally high antibody response to polyvinyl pyrrolidone increasing with age, probably due to the loss of suppressor T-cells. *In vivo* TF treatment (500 ng) 3 times weekly for 3 weeks has been shown to normalize anti-PVP antibody responses in 6–9-month-old NZB mice. Interestingly, 1-week treatment had no effect, suggesting that suppressor T-cell maturation takes 2–3 weeks (to be published).

A last and important *in vivo* TF activity concerns the rejection of virus-induced sarcomas (studied in collaboration with J.C. Leclerc and E. Gomard). Thymectomized irradiated bone marrow reconstituted C57B1/6 mice were injected into the thigh with MSV Moloney virus and treated by the purified serum TF (40 ng of TF 4 times a week, bound to CM cellulose, s.c.). The treatment was begun the day of MSV-virus injection and was continued for 25 days. Controls included normal mice and thymectomized irradiated bone marrow reconstituted mice injected with CM cellulose alone. There was a high percentage of sarcoma incidence in normal mice as is well documented, but all the tumors were rejected within 20 days after virus injection. In thymectomized mice treated with CM cellulose alone, there was no rejection and the mice with tumors ultimately died. Conversely, in the TF-treated group of thymectomized mice, 85% of mice had rejected their tumors at day 25 when TF treatment was stopped. However, a large percentage of tumors reappeared 20–40 days after the treatment was stopped, whereas there was no tumor recurrence in normal mice. These data indicate that serum TF enabled the mice to reject the tumors, probably through recruitment of cytotoxic cells, but that this recruitment was reversible. It is interesting to note in this context that thymus grafts also rapidly restore the capacity of thymectomized mice to reject MSV-induced sarcomas more rapidly than they restore the capacity to respond to phytohaemagglutinin or to reject skin grafts (Davies, personal communication).

CONCLUSIONS

TF target cell

Purified TF has been shown to possess several biological activities in addition to the sheep cell assay utilized for its purification. The *in vivo* data obtained at low doses (100–500 ng) indicate a possible physiological role in the periphery. The TF target cell is not definitively known. However, one is struck by the relative easiness with which biological activities are shown in T-cell functions altered by ATx (autologous rosettes, suppressor T-cells). Conversely, it appears to be much more difficult to obtain similar effects in nude mice where 10–20 times higher doses are needed [12]. Moreover, data showing restoration of helper function, *in vivo* GVH or skin-graft-rejecting capacity have not yet been obtained with TF. This may prove a fairly difficult task since it takes several weeks [4–8] to obtain the immunological reconstitution of Tx mice with a fully functional thymus graft [20]. In other words, it will be probably necessary to give chronic long-term TF treatments over several weeks, which has not been easy to achieve so far. Finally, TF target cell could be a To cell, as found in the thymus cortex, pre-thymic cells as found in nude mice needing a direct thymic traffic eventually to find high concentrations of thymic factor [21].

REFERENCES

1. A.J.S. Davies. The thymus and the cellular basis of immunity. *Transpl. Rev.* **1**, 43 (1969).
2. D. Osoba and J.F.A.P. Miller. Evidence for humoral thymus factor responsible for the maturation of immunological faculty. *Nature*, **199**, 653 (1963).
3. A. Goldstein and A. White. Thymosin and other thymic hormones: their nature and roles in the thymic dependency of immunological phenomena. In: *Contemporary Topics in Immunobiology*, edited by A.J.S. Davies and R.L. Carter, Plenum Press, New York, N.Y., 1973.
4. N. Trainin and M. Small. Thymic humoral factors. In: *Contemporary Topics in Immunobiology*, edited by A.J.S. Davies and R.L. Carter, p. 321. Plenum Press, 1973.
5. J.F. Bach and M. Dardenne. Antigen recognition by T-lymphocytes. I. Thymus and bone marrow dependence of spontaneous rosette forming cells in normal and neonatally thymectomized mice. *Cell. Immunol.* **3**, 1 (1972).
6. J.F. Bach and M. Dardenne. Antigen recognition by T-lymphocytes. II. Similar effects of azathioprine, ALS and antitheta serum on rosette forming lymphocytes in normal and neonatally thymectomized mice. *Cell. Immunol.* **35**, 11 (1972).
7. J.F. Bach. Thymus dependency of rosette forming cells. In: *Contemporary Topics in Immunobiology*, edited by A.J.S. Davies and R.L. Carter, 2, 189. Plenum Press, New York, N.Y., 1973.
8. J.F. Bach, M. Dardenne, A. Goldstein, A. Guha and A. White. Appearance of T-cell markers in bone marrow rosette forming cells after incubation with purified thymosin, a thymic hormone. *Proc. Nat. Acad. Sci. U.S.A.* **68**, 2734 (1971).
9. M. Dardenne and J.F. Bach. Studies on thymus products. I. Modification of rosette forming cells by thymic extracts. Determination of the target RFC subpopulation. *Immunology* **25**, 343 (1973).
10. J.F. Bach and M. Dardenne. Thymus dependency of rosette forming cells. Evidence for a circulating thymic hormone. *Trans. Proc.* **4**, 345 (1972).
11. J.F. Bach and M. Dardenne. Studies on thymus products. II. Demonstration and characterization of a circulating thymic hormone. *Immunology* **25**, 353 (1973).
12. J.F. Bach, M. Dardenne, J.M. Pleau and M.A. Bach. Isolation, biochemical characteristics and biological activity of a circulating thymic hormone in the mouse and in the human. *Ann. N.Y. Acad. Sci.* **249**, 186 (1975).
13. M.A. Bach, C. Fournier and J.F. Bach. Regulation of theta antigen expression by agents altering cyclic AMP level and by thymic factor. *Ann. N.Y. Acad. Sci.* **249**, 316 (1975).
14. K. Komuro and E.A. Boyse. *In vitro* demonstration of thymic hormone in the mouse by conversion of precursor cells into T-lymphocytes. *Lancet*, i, 740 (1973).
15. M.A. Bach. Transient loss of theta antigen after indomethacin treatment. *Ann. Immunol.* **125c**, 865 (1974).
16. J. Charreire and J.F. Bach. Self and not self. *Lancet*, **2**, 229 (1974).
17. J. Charreire and J.F. Bach. Binding of autologous erythrocytes to immature T-cells. *Proc. Nat. Acad. Sci. U.S.A.* (1975).
18. J.F. Bach, M.A. Bach and J. Charreire. Variability of the expression of membrane receptors in immature T-cells. The role of cyclic AMP, prostaglandins and thymic hormone. In: *Lymphocyte Membrane Receptors*, M. Seligmann, ed. North-Holland, 1975.
19. N. Trainin, Y. Levo and V. Rotter. A thymic humoral factor increases the hydrocortisone-resistant cell population of the thymus. *Eur. J. Immunol.* **4**, 634 (1974).
20. M.J. Deonhoff and A.J.S. Davies. Reconstitution of the T-cell pool after irradiation of mice. *Cell. Immunol.* **1**, 82 (1971).
21. J.F. Bach. Target cell for thymic hormone. *Lancet*, **9**, 1320 (1973).

MACROPHAGE SECRETIONS AFFECTING THE GROWTH OF OTHER CELLS

FERDY J. LEJEUNE

The Laboratory of Experimental Surgery, Department of Surgery, Institut Jules Bordet,
Rue Héger-Bordet, 1, 1000 Bruxelles, Belgium

ABSTRACT

The author has reviewed evidence for the direct involvement of macrophages in tumour rejection. He presents the arguments for the control of the growth of other cells by macrophages, through the release of soluble products. Finally a summary is given of work showing the secretion by macrophages of cytostatic factors, acting on cultured melanoma cells.

ABBREVIATIONS

SMAF	Specific macrophage arming factor.
C. parvum	*Corynebacterium parvum.*
BCG	Bacille de Calmette et Guérin.
dSRNA	Double-stranded RNA.
$C'3$	Third component of complement.
$H_3 TdR$	Tritiated thymidine.
$I_{125} UdR$	Iodo (I_{125}) deoxyuridine.
HP cells	Harding–Passey melanoma cells.

It is now well established that macrophages (mononuclear phagocytes) play a central role in both primary and secondary immune reactions. In addition, it seems at present unquestionable that macrophages are directly involved in the mechanisms leading to the rejection of tumours [1, 2].

ACTIVE ROLE OF MACROPHAGES IN TUMOUR REJECTION

Tumour rejection mediated by macrophages can be either immunologically specific or non-specific. When it is specific, a lymphocyte–macrophage cooperation is a prerequisite, as it was shown with the SMAF produced by T-lymphocytes [3]. When the mechanisms of tumour rejection are non-specific, they seem to involve a direct macrophase activation. For example, there were several reports on macrophages rendered cytotoxic to tumour cells, after *in vivo* activation by various infections: protozoal infections (Toxoplasma [4], Nitrospongylus [5]) or bacterial vaccines (*C. parvum* [6], BCG [7]). Macrophages could also be rendered cytotoxic after *in vitro* activation by

9

endotoxins [(*Salmonella* [8] or viral d SRNA or by Lipid A [8], or by synthetic poly-nucleotides (Poly I: C [8]).

All the above systems have one major property in common: they absolutely require a cell-to-cell, macrophage-to-target cell contact for the cytotoxic effect to be exerted.

In contrast with these systems, we have had evidence that a strong cytotoxic effect could be produced by macrophages on cultured tumour cells, with no contacts with the target cells and by the release of cytostatic products [9, 10]. This evidence for cytotoxic factors fits very well with the new concept that macrophages are secretory cells.

MACROPHAGE AS A SECRETORY CELL [11]

It seems paradoxical that a cell which was named macrophage by Metchnikoff [12] because of its major property of endocytosis (that is engulfment of materials) appears now as a *secretory cell*.

There are substances which have been reported to be secreted by cultured macro-phages. They were biochemically characterized but their effect on cell growth is still undefined.

It was demonstrated a long time ago [13] that macrophages can release various lysosomal enzymes during phagocytosis. Recently, it was found that macrophages can secrete other enzymes such as lysozyme [14, 15] (which is a potent antibacterial factor and has some cytostatic effect on mammalian cells), a plasminogen activator [16], collagenase [17] and β_{1-c}, a component of $C'3$ [18].

Interferon was demonstrated to be synthesized and released by properly stimulated macrophages [19]. Although we have not assayed macrophage interferon, we found (Lejeune and De Clerck, E., unpublished data) that L-cells interferon exerts a cytostatic effect on cultured melanoma cells, in a similar way as described, in the last paragraph, by macrophages.

SECRETION BY MACROPHAGES OF FACTORS AFFECTING THE GROWTH OF OTHER CELLS

Recently, several workers have had evidence that some substances, released by cultured macrophages can affect the growth of other cells. One can separate them into three groups, according to their biological effect: (a) stimulatory, (b) inhibitory, (c) killing. Table 1 displays the major properties of these factors. It is worthwhile to point out that most of the experiments in the human, involved cultured blood monocytes, which readily transform into macrophages; in mouse and rat, peritoneal macrophages were used.

The factor promoting the blast transformation of lymphocytes, in mixed culture, was the first to be demonstrated [20]. Later, others showed that T-lymphocytes [21] and B-lymphocytes [22] function better when exposed to culture supernatants of macro-phages. An important factor seems to be the CSF which promotes the *in vitro* growth of bone marrow stem cells [23].

Two different laboratories [24, 25] independently, but simultaneously, found that some culture supernatants from mouse peritoneal macrophages could strongly inhibit the thymidine uptake by lymphocytes. In terms of growth of the target cell, this

Table 1. *Factors Released by Macrophages and Affecting the Growth of Other Cells in vitro*

Factor	Method	References
A. Stimulatory		
Conditioned medium reconstituting factor (CMRF)	Promotes blast transformation in mixed lymphocyte culture	20
–	Potentiates T-lymphocytes response to PHA	21
Factor released by cultured human monocytes	Stimulates IgM and IgG response and growth of B murine lymphocytes	22
Colony stimulatory factor (CSF)	Stimulates the growth of bone marrow stem cells	23
B. Inhibitory		
Macrophage dialysable factor (MDF)	Inhibition of H_3 TdR uptake by non-stimulated and antigen stimulated lymphocytes	24
–	Inhibition of H_3 TdR uptake by lymphocytes stimulated with PHA, Con A, endotoxin	25
Macrophage cytostatic factor released by normal macrophages	Inhibition of growth and H_3 TdR uptake by cultured melanoma tumour cells	9, 10
Ditto	Inhibition of H_3 TdR uptake by leukemic cells, fibroblasts and lectin stimulated lymphocytes	30
Released by activated macrophages	Inhibition of ^{125}I UdR. Uptake by allogeneic lymphoma cells	31
C. Killing		
Cytotoxin: factor cytolytic to tumour cells	Factor released by immune macrophages in allogeneic murine system	26
Lysosomal products	Transfer of lysosomal products from BCG activated macrophages to tumour cells	29
Macrophage cytolytic factor (MCF)	Labile substance lysing syngeneic erythrocytes	27
Effect on growth?		
Lysozyme (muramidase)	Antibacterial	14
	Affects growth pattern and morphology of cultured normal and tumour cells	15
Plasminogen activator		16
Collagenase		17
–	C'3 component	18

phenomenon looks exactly the opposite of the first (A in Table 1). Up to now, there are no data showing the presence or the absence of any interrelation of the two factors.

The existence of factors which inhibit the growth of tumour cells will be discussed in the following paragraph.

The existence of a cytolytic factor specifically released by "immune" macrophages was suggested [26] in an allogenic system. A labile substance having a strong lytic effect on erythrocytes was discovered by Melson [27]. Cohn and his collaborators (see review 28) have extensively demonstrated the very active lysosomal system of macrophages. It was shown [29] that macrophages could inject their lysosomal content into tumor cells. Therefore, it was proposed that lysosomal enzymes could be responsible for the subsequent lysis of the target cells.

STUDIES ON A CYTOSTATIC FACTOR RELEASED BY CULTURED NORMAL MACROPHAGES

We found [9, 10] that peritoneal macrophages from unstimulated and apparently non-infected mice, from several strains, produce a growth inhibition of cultured mouse Harding–Passey melanoma cells. This effect was appreciated by a decrease of cell counts and tritiated thymidine uptake (Fig. 1). The growth inhibition was paralleled by a striking morphological alteration of the melanoma cells (Figs. 2 and 3).

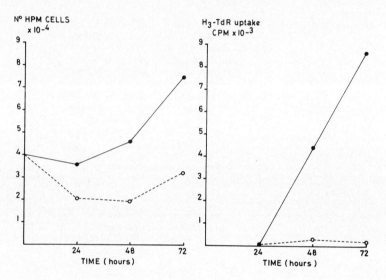

Fig. 1. Effect of normal macrophages on the growth of HP cells in culture. 4×10^4 HP cells were layered at time 0, on top of a loose 10^6 peritoneal macrophages monolayer (normal Balb/c mice). Left: HP cell count. Right: H_3 TdR uptake (CPM) – ●, HP cells cultured alone. ○, HP cells cultured with normal macrophages.

Moreover, it was found [10] that the "normal" mouse macrophages release both enhancing and cytostatic factors in the culture medium. Enhancing factors were found in the early supernatants (1 hour) while cytostatic factors were prominent in the "late" (72 hr) supernatants (Fig. 4). Such "late" supernatants could be diluted and provided a concentration dependent cytostatic effect (Fig. 5). The cytostatic factor was found to be at least partially thermostable, dialysable and reversible [10].

The cytostatic factor released by normal macrophages, which was also found independently from us by others [30], remains to be identified. It might be a substance resulting from the processing of serum factors, present in the culture medium. To support this hypothesis, we found [10] that autologous and various xenogeneic sera (including foetal bovine serum and human AB serum) activate normal macrophages within 72 hr and render their lysates strongly cytostatic (Fig. 6).

The existence of cytostatic factors secreted by activated macrophages against allogeneic

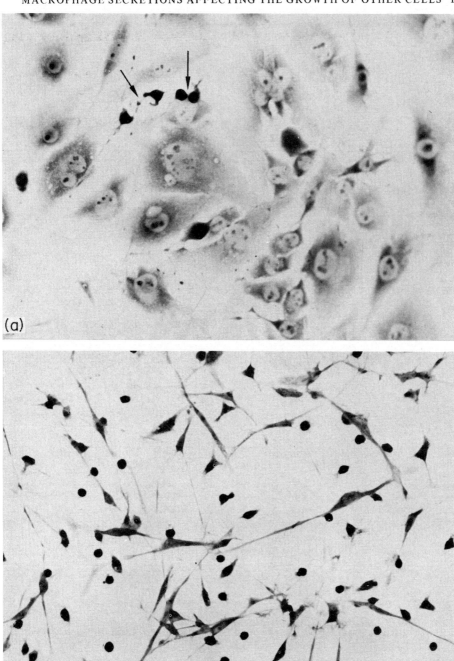

Fig. 2. Effect of normal macrophages on the morphology of HP cells in culture. Same culture conditions as in Fig. 1. Cells fixed and stained at 72 hr. (a) HP cells cultured alone. The monolayer is nearly confluent, the cells are well spread. There are (arrows) two figures of telophasis. (b) HP cells cultured with macrophages. The small dark cells are macrophages, some are in contact with HP cells. The HP cells cytoplasm is shrunken. The density of the monolayer is very loose. Light microscopy: × 340.

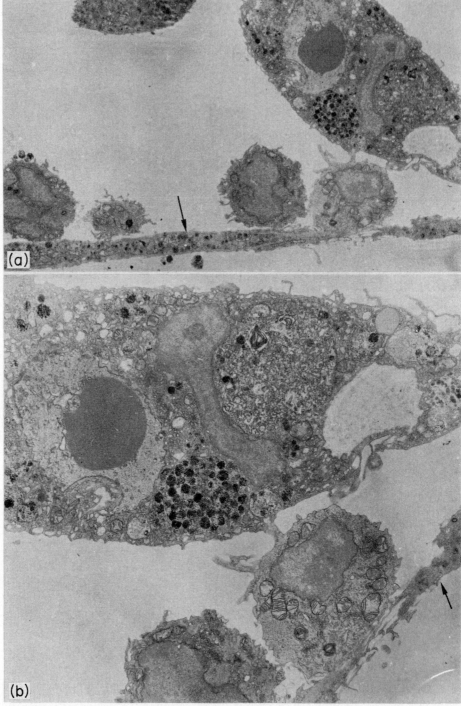

Fig. 3. Same as for Fig. 2b but the culture was processed for electron microscopy by *in situ* fixation, embedding and sectioning. (a) Dendritic process (arrow) of a HP cell in contact with four small mononuclear phagocytes, and one large typical macrophage with engulfed melanin in the vicinity. (b) Higher magnification of a part of the same area. Electron microscopy: (a) × 4200; (b) × 7800.

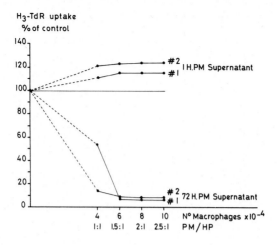

Fig. 4. Effect of "early" (1 hr) and "late" (72 hr) supernatants of macrophage cultures on the growth of HP cells. 4×10^4 HP cells were cultured for 72 hr in all conditions.

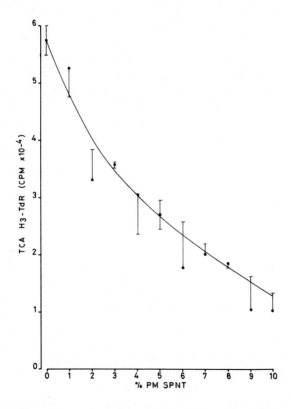

Fig. 5. Effect of dilution on the cytostatic factor of normal macrophages. Dose response curve obtained by diluting the supernatant from 10^6 macrophages. H_3TdR uptake at 72 hr by 4×10^4 HP cells plated at time 0.

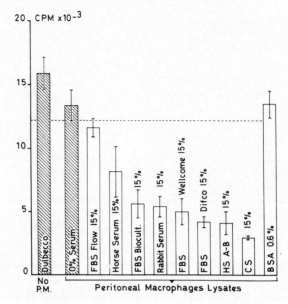

Fig. 6. Activation of normal macrophages by various sera from different species (FBS from different origins). 10^5 macrophages were cultured for 72 hr in the presence of either of the sera or BSA. They were washed and macrophage lysates were made by freezing–thawing. 4×10^4 HP cells were cultured for 72 hr on these lysates. H_3TdR incorporation between 70 and 72 hr after washing.

cells was also reported [31]. These authors confirmed that serum is a prerequisite in the macrophage culture, for a cytostatic effect to be seen.

Mononuclear phagocytes are widespread in melanoma and in close contact with the melanoma cells. This is in contrast to the lymphoid cells which are located on the periphery of the tumor [32]. In addition to the clearing of melanin and cell debris by phagocytosis, tumour macrophages might play a role in the, *in vivo*, tumour growth control. The cytostatic effect is non-specific and does not require an immune sensitization. Therefore, it might play an early role, before an antitumour specific immunity appears.

As far as *in vitro* tumour immunity tests are concerned, one must take into account that most systems using lymphoid cells as effector cells, or tumour cells as target cells are contaminated with macrophages. The results in the literature showing non-specific cytotoxicity might thus be due to the macrophages, i.e. activated by serum factors, and not due to the lymphoid cells.

ACKNOWLEDGEMENTS

Mrs. Y. Garcia and Ms. E. Beaumont are acknowledged for their skilful technical assistance. I thank Prof. Peter Alexander for encouragement and criticism. I am grateful to Prof. Smets, Prof. Henry and Dr. Gerard for their support. Prof. Tagnon, Prof. Drochmans and Dr. Heuson are acknowledged for their help and hospitality.

This work was supported by the grants 20.200 and 3.45.45.75 of the FRSM (Fonds de la Recherche Scientifique Médicale) in Belgium.

REFERENCES

1. P. Alexander, The role of macrophages in tumour immunity. *J. Clin. Path.* **27**, *Suppl. Roy. Coll. Path.* **7**, 77 (1974).
2. F. Lejeune, Role of macrophages in immunity, with special reference to tumour immunology. A review. *Biomedicine,* **22,** 25 (1975).
3. R. Evans and P. Alexander, Mechanism of immunologically specific killing of tumour cells by macrophages. *Nature,* **236**, 168 (1972).
4. J.B. Hibbs, L.H. Lambert and J.S. Remington, Possible role of macrophage-mediated non-specific cytotoxicity in tumour resistance. *Nature New Biol.* **235**, 48 (1972).
5. R. Keller, Cytostatic elimination of syngeneic rat tumour cells *in vitro* by non-specifically activated macrophages. *J. Exp. Med.* **138**, 625 (1973).
6. M. Olivotto and R. Bomford, *In vitro* inhibition of tumour cell growth and DNA synthesis by peritoneal and lung macrophages from mice injected with *Corynebacterium parvum. Int. J. Cancer,* **13**, 478 (1974).
7. D. Juy, C. Bona and L. Chedid, Effet anti-tumoral de macrophages péritonéaux activés par un adjuvant hydrosoluble d'origine mycobactérienne. *C.R. Acad. Sci. Paris,* t. 278, série D, p. 2859 (1974).
8. P. Alexander and R. Evans, Endotoxin and double-stranded RNA render macrophages cytotoxic. *Nature New Biol.* **232**, 76 (1971).
9. F. Lejeune and R. Regnier, Studies on a non-specific and non-cytolytic cytostatic factor produced by macrophages (abstract). *Br. J. Cancer* **30**, 181 (1974).
10. F. Lejeune and R. Regnier, Foetal bovine serum (FBS) induced cytostatic effect of peritoneal macrophages against mouse melanoma. *Proc. Int. Symp. Immunological Reactions to Melanoma Antigens. Behring Inst. Mitt.* **56**, 28 (1975).
11. Z.A. Cohn, *Recent Studies on the Physiology of Cultivated Macrophages in the Phagocytic Cell in Host Resistance,* edited by Bellanti and Dayton, p. 15, North Holland Publ., 1975.
12. E. Metchnikoff, Sur la lutte des cellules de l'organisme contre l'invasion des microbes (théorie des phagocytes). *Ann. Inst. Pasteur* **7**, 321 (1887).
13. Z.A. Cohn and E. Weiner, The particulate hydrolases of macrophages. II. Biochemical and morphological response to particle ingestion. *J. Exp. Med.* **118**, 1009 (1963).
14. S. Gordon, J. Todd and Z.A. Cohn, In vitro synthesis and secretion of lysozyme by mononuclear phagocytes. *J. Exp. Med.* **139**, 1228 (1974).
15. E.F. Osserman, M. Klockars, J. Halper and R.E. Fischer, Effects of lysozyme on normal and transformed mammalian cells. *Nature,* **243**, 331 (1973).
16. J.C. Unkeless, S. Gordon and F. Reich, Secretion of plasminogen activator by stimulated macrophages. *J. Exp. Med.* **139**, 834 (1974).
17. L.M. Wahl, S.M. Wahl, S.E. Mergen-Hagen and G.R. Martin, Collagenase production by endotoxin activated macrophages. *Proc. Nat. Acad. Sci. USA* **71**, 3598 (1974).
18. V.J. Stecher and G.J. Thorbecke, Sites of synthesis in serum proteins. I. Serum proteins produced by macrophages *in vitro. J. Immunol.* **99**, 643 (1967).
19. T.J. Smith and R.R. Wagner, Rabbit macrophage interferons. II. Some physicochemical properties and estimations of molecular weights. *J. Exp. Med.* **125**, 579 (1967).
20. F.H. Bach, B.J. Alter, S. Solliday, D. Zoschke and M. Janis, Lymphocyte reactivity *in vitro.* II. Soluble reconstituting factor permitting response of purified lymphocytes. *Cell. Immunol.* **I**, 219 (1970).
21. I. Gery and B.H. Waksman, Potentiation of the T-lymphocyte response to mitogens. II. The cellular source of potentiating mediators, *J. Exp. Med.* **136**, 143 (1972).
22. D. Wood and P. Cameron, Studies on the mechanism of stimulation of the humoral response of murine spleen cultures by culture fluids from human monocytes. *J. Immunol.* **114**, 1094 (1975).
23. P. Chervenick and A.F. Lobuglio, Human blood monocytes: stimulators of granulocyte and mononuclear colony formation *in vitro. Science,* **178**, 164 (1972).
24. S.R. Waldman and A.A. Gottlieb, Macrophage regulation of DNA synthesis on lymphoid cells: effects of a soluble factor from macrophages. *Cell. Immunol.* **9**, 142 (1973).
25. D.S. Nelson, Production by stimulated macrophages of factors depressing lymphocyte transformation. *Nature,* **246**, 306 (1973).
26. K. McIvor and R.S. Weiser, Mechanisms of target cell destruction by alloimmune peritoneal macrophages. II. Release of a specific cytotoxin from interacting cells. *Immunology,* **20**, 315 (1971).
27. H. Melson, G. Kearny, S. Gruca and R. Seljelid, Evidence for a cytolytic factor released by macrophages. *J. Exp. Med.* **140**, 1085 (1974).
28. Z.A. Cohn, Lysosomes in mononuclear phagocytes. In: *Mononuclear Phagocytes,* edited by Van Furth, p. 50, Blackwell Publ., London, 1970.

29. J.B. Hibbs, Heterocytolysis by macrophages activated by BCG: lysosome exocytosis into tumour cells. *Science,* 184, 468 (1974).
30. J. Calderon, R. Williams and E. Unanue, An inhibitor of cell proliferation released by cultures of macrophages. *Proc. Nat. Acad. Sci. USA* 71, 4273 (1974).
31. M.D. Boyle and M.G. Ormerod, The destruction of tumour cells by alloimmune peritoneal cells: mechanism of action of activated macrophages *in vitro. J. Reticulo-endothel. Soc.* 17, 73 (1975).
32. F.J. Lejeune, Harding–Passey melanoma in the Balb/c mouse as a model for studying the interactions between host macrophages and tumour cells. Proc. Conf. Pigment Cell. Biol. Jan. 73, Yale University. *Yale J. Biol. Med.* 28, 80 (1973).

IMMUNE CELLULAR MECHANISMS AT THE SITE OF THE TUMOR

E.H. BETZ and L.J. SIMAR

Department of Pathology, University of Liège, 1, rue des Bonnes Villes,
B-4000 Liège (Belgium)

ABSTRACT

Grafts of chemically induced syngeneic sarcomas are infiltrated by mononucleated cell population containing monocytes, lymphocytes, immunoblasts and macrophages. The proportion of these cells as compared to tumor cells increases during the two first weeks following grafting and decreases later on; monocytes are the most frequent cell type infiltrating these tumor grafts. Very close contacts exist between tumor cells and various types of infiltrating cells. In this regard, no difference could be found between immunoblasts, lymphocytes and monocytes. On the contrary, "debris" loaded macrophages never show these contacts with tumor cells. When growth of the tumor progresses, the frequency of contacts between cells decreases. On the basis of these observations and of previous studies on the morphological changes in lymphnodes, a hypothesis is proposed.

It is suggested that as the tumor graft grows, the production of sensitized cells tends to decrease whereas factors appear which prevent the infiltrating cells to attack the target tumor cells.

INTRODUCTION

In syngeneic systems, cancer cells possess special tumor antigens which are different from the antigens of the corresponding normal cells. The specificity of these antigens may vary according to the etiological agent responsible for the neoplastic cell transformation. In the present paper, we shall exclusively deal with chemically induced cancers.

Numerous experiments have shown that tumors produced by chemical carcinogens are immunogenic when grafted in syngeneic hosts [1–4]. In such *in vivo* systems, the main immunological response is the development of a transplantation immunity directed against antigens which are specific for each single tumor [4–5]. In addition to this cell bound response, tumor antigens are also able to induce an immune reaction of the humoral type [6].

The influence of these immunological responses on the behavior of the tumor cells appears to be a very complicated phenomenon. In the present work, an attempt has been made to study certain morphological changes occurring in tumors in relation to the cell-bound immunological processes. In the cell mediated immunological responses, sensitized lymphoid cells are released in the lymph and the blood gets in contact with the antigenic target cells [7–8]. The accumulation of mononucleated cells in allogenic grafts of normal tissue has been described in various systems, and is thought to be responsible for the rejection of these grafts. Among this mononucleated cell population, several cell types are found as shown by ultrastructural investigations. This heterogeneous population contains besides small lymphocytes, immunoblasts and a few plasma cells, a fourth cell type which is characterized by the presence of a large number of lysosomes [9–11]. There has been some controversy about the exact nature of the latter cell type; it is very likely that these cells belong to the monocyte group.

The presence of mononucleated cell infiltrates in many tumor tissues has often been ascribed to an immunological response induced by the tumor antigens. In the present work, our aim was:

1. to study the ultrastructure of mononucleated cells infiltrating syngeneic chemically induced tumors and to investigate the connections between these cells and the tumor cells;
2. to follow the qualitative and quantitative changes occurring in the mononucleated cell population during the growth of the tumor;
3. to see if any relationship exists between the number and the type of mono-nucleated cells and the growth rate of the tumor.

MATERIAL AND METHODS

Sarcomas were induced in C57 B1 mice by implanting methylcholanthrene pellets in the muscle tissue of the right leg. The tumors obtained were serially grafted in syngeneic hosts. Among the tumors produced in this manner, two were selected owing to their very different growth rate. The first of these sarcomas (T9) grows very slowly since 50% of the animals still survive 96 days after grafting. The second tumor (T10) grows faster and kills 50% of mice before day 65.

Histological procedures

The tumor-bearing mice were killed at various delays (8 to 60 days) after grafting. Pieces of tumors were fixed during 45 min in phosphate buffered 1% osmium tetroxide. After dehydration, the blocks were embedded in Epon. Ultra-thin sections were stained with lead citrate and uranyl acetate, and then examined with an electron microscope (Siemens 101 or Philips 301).

Quantitative analysis

The stereological methods according to the procedures previously proposed by Weibel [12–13] were used. At each delay and for each tumor, fifteen blocks chosen at random were cut into ultra-thin sections. Only one section on each block was used to take micro-graphs at the primary magnification of 2800.

First the number of mononucleated and tumor cells per unit volume of tumor (numerical density N_V) was measured. Knowing the volume of the tumor, it is possible to calculate the absolute number of these two kinds of cells per tumor.

The numerical density N_V is obtained using the formula of De Hoff and Rhines [14] :

$$N_V = \frac{NA}{D}$$

in which NA represents the number of structure profiles per unit area of a section and D the mean diameter of the structure. As this formula can only be used for the analysis of spherical particles, we have in practice measured the numerical density of the nuclei. Indeed the shape of the studied cells was irregular whereas the nuclei were reasonably spherical.

(a) *Determination of NA* The number of nucleus profiles of tumoral and mono-nucleated cells has been measured on the sections for each animal at each delay for both tumors T9 and T10.

(b) *Determination of D* The profile size distribution of the nuclei of mononucleated and tumor cells is obtained by direct measurements on the micrographs. The size distribution of nuclei and the nuclear diameter were derived by applying the semi-graphic method described by Giger and Riedwyl [15].

(c) *Determination of the nucleus and cell volume* From the mean nuclear diameter, the nuclear volume (V_n) was calculated. The cell volume was obtained by applying the formula:

$$V_{cel} = \frac{V_n}{V_{Vn}}$$

where V_{Vn} is the part of the cell volume which is occupied by the nucleus (volume density of nucleus). To obtain this volume density, we have superimposed on the micrographs a multipurpose test grid containing 84 lines and 168 points representing the end points of the lines. We have determined the number of points falling on the nucleus Pn and on the cytoplasm Pc and obtained V_{Vn} by applying the formula:

$$V_{Vn} = \frac{P_n}{Pc + Pn}$$

The mean diameter D of the cell has been derived from the value of its volume.

(d) *Determination of tumor volume* The volume of the total tumor has been obtained from its mean diameter D_m by applying the formula:

$$D_m = \sqrt[3]{d^2 \cdot D}$$

in which d is the lesser diameter and D the larger diameter perpendicular to the first one.

RESULTS

1. Qualitative study

Already 8 days after grafting, both tumors are infiltrated by mononucleated cells which can be distributed in four categories according to their ultrastructural aspect. Few of them are *immunoblasts* characterized by a large amount of ribosomes grouped in

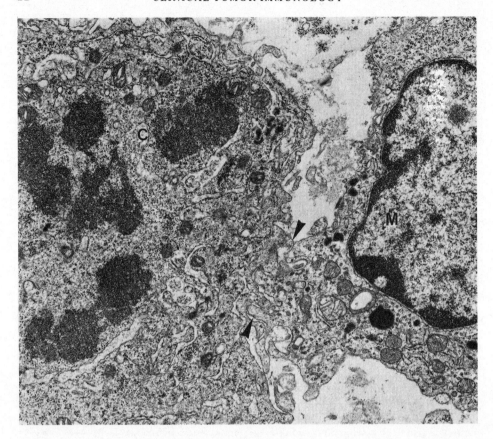

Fig. 1. Interlocking (arrows) between a monocyte (M) and a cancer cell (C) which is in mitosis.
×13,600

rosettes uniformly distributed throughout the cytoplasm. The sacks of the ergastoplasmic reticulum are flat and lined by a small number of ribosomes. The Golgi zone is moderately developed and its vesicles do not contain any dense material. A second cell type is represented by the small *lymphocytes*, the ultrastructure of which is well known and does not need to be described here. Some *macrophages* containing a large amount of phagocytized "debris" are also scattered throughout the tumor. The most frequent cell type infiltrating the tumor tissues corresponds probably to *monocytes*. These cells are larger than the small lymphocytes; their nucleus is irregular in shape with deep indentations of the nuclear membrane and contains small blocks of dense chromatin (Fig. 1). In the cytoplasm, the ribosomes are free or grouped in small clusters but never in spiral-shaped polysomes. Flat sacks of rough ergastoplasm are always present and often located at a pole of the cell. The Golgi zone is usually well developed. This cell type contains lysosome like dense bodies which may be present in large amount, but does not contain either phagosomes nor phagocytized material. These four types of infiltrating cells may be grouped in small foci without any preferential location inside the tumor.

    Very close connections may exist between the infiltrating cells and the tumor cells. Sometimes the cytoplasmic membranes of both cells are arranged in parallel and get in

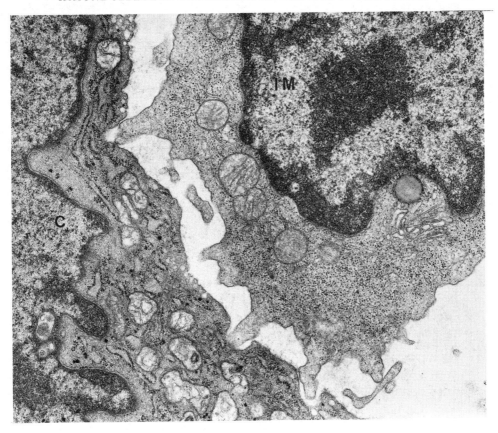

Fig. 2. Cytoplasmic expansions of an immunoblast (IM) penetrating into invaginations of the cytoplasmic membrane of a cancer cell (C). ×20,000.

close contact on a certain distance; at this level, the two cell membranes are only a few Å
apart. In other places, digit-like cytoplasmic expansions of the infiltrating cells penetrate
deeply into invaginations of the cytoplasmic membrane of the tumor elements (Fig. 2).
Sometimes a real interlocking of the two cells may take place (Fig. 1).

2. Quantitative analysis

(a) *Number of cells* The measurements indicate that the tumor cells are smaller in T9
than in T10. Therefore, the number of cells per volume unit is greater in T9. This number
decreases slowly when growth of T9 progresses and when an increasing amount of
collagen fibers is produced in the tumor.

The number of infiltrating cells per volume unit of tissue increases in both tumors up
to day 15 after grafting (Fig. 3). Later on, this "numerical density" of infiltrating cells
drops rapidly. On the basis of the previous data, it is possible to calculate the percentage
of infiltrating cells present in the tumor tissue. This figure which is higher in T10 than in
T9 also decreases rapidly after the 15th day.

Knowing the tumor volume, it is possible to calculate the variation of the absolute

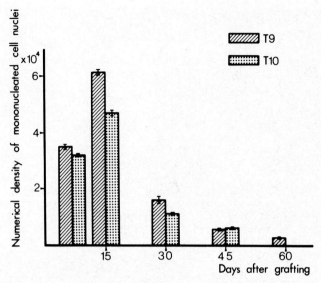

Fig. 3. Variation of the number of mononucleated cells per mm³ of tumor tissue (numerical density).
This parameter increases in T9 and T10 up to day 15 after grafting and decreases rapidly later on.

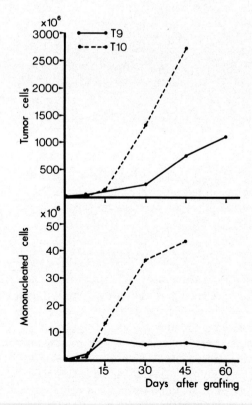

Fig. 4. Variation of the absolute number of cancer and mononucleated cells per tumor. The number of
mononucleated cells rises progressively in T10 whereas it reaches rapidly a plateau in T9.

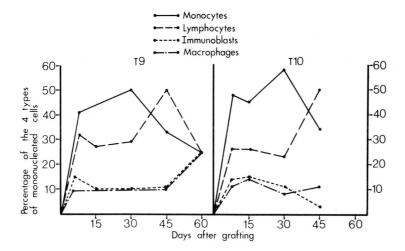

Fig. 5. Relative frequency of the four types composing infiltrating cell population and its variation during tumor growth.

number of tumor and infiltrating cells per tumor during the whole growth period. Figure 4 confirms that T10 grows much more rapidly than T9 and it shows also that the evolution of the absolute number of infiltrating cells is very different in both tumors. In T9 this value reaches its maximum 15 days after grafting and remains constant later on. In fact, the decrease of the percentage of infiltrating cells previously reported is due to the fact that the number of cancer cells increases. In T10 the infiltrating cells increase progressively until the death of the animal but as the number of cancer cells increases still more rapidly, the percentage of infiltrating cells drops also after the 15th day.

(b) *Variations of the infiltrating cell types* The above-mentioned four cell types making up the infiltrating cell population are present in very different proportions. In both tumors, immunoblasts and "debris" loaded macrophages represent each about 10% of the total amount of the infiltrating cells (Fig. 5). This value does not show any significant change during the growth period. Up to day 15, monocytes form the majority of infiltrating cells representing about 50% of the whole population. This value drops after the 15th day. Small lymphocytes are also frequently encountered. After the 15th day they become the most important group of infiltrating cells.

(c) *Frequency of contacts between infiltrating and tumor cells* Examining directly the specimens under the electron microscope, it is possible to count the contacts between infiltrating cells and tumor cells and to calculate their frequency. The results are expressed as the percentage of cells of a given type showing the contacts previously described.

The results indicate that lymphocytes, immunoblasts and monocytes get in contact with tumor cells. This is not the case for macrophages containing phagocytized material. The frequency of these contacts varies during the growth period (Fig. 6). It is clear that the connections between cells are most frequent during the two first weeks after grafting and then decrease. As far as cell contacts are concerned no difference could be found between T9 and T10.

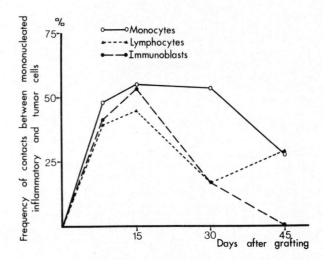

Fig. 6. Frequency of contacts between cancer cells and infiltrating cells during the growth of tumor graft.

DISCUSSION

Our results demonstrate that grafts of chemically induced syngeneic sarcomas are infiltrated by a mononucleated cell population which contains monocytes, lymphocytes, immunoblasts and macrophages. Such infiltrates are very similar to those found in allogeneic grafts of normal tissues before and during their rejection. Similar infiltrates are never found in syngeneic grafts of normal tissues. It is likely that the occurrence of these infiltrates is in the tumor graft related to the immune reactions induced by the cancer cells. This hypothesis is further supported by the presence in the graft of a certain number of typical immunoblasts.

Alexander *et al.* [16] have claimed that during the immunization against 3–4-benzpyrene induced sarcoma, immunoblasts do not leave the lymphnodes as long as the tumor tissue is present. According to these authors, immunoblasts would be released from the nodes after removal of the tumor. In our system, immunoblasts reach the graft and their number increases rapidly during the two first weeks after grafting. Simultaneously, large numbers of monocytes and lymphocytes accumulate in the tumor tissue. It is generally thought that sensitized cells are distributed at random through the body and retained where they get in contact with the antigen [17]. Very little is known about the factors which are responsible for the accumulation of other mononucleated cells; it is likely that substances released by lymphoid cells (lymphokines and MIF) play a role in this phenomenon [18].

We have shown that the proportion of infiltrating cells as compared to tumor cells decreases after the 15th day. This could be due to the fact either that less mononucleated cells reach and/or are retained in the tumor tissue or that the number of tumor cells increases at a faster rate than that of mononucleated cells. Our calculations show that the situation is somewhat different for the two tumors we have investigated. Whereas the total number of cells infiltrating the graft of T10 increases steadily, it increases up to the 15th day and then remains constant in T9. This indicates that at least in T9, less cells reach or are retained in the graft. On the other hand, there is some evidence that the number of sensitized cells produced in the lymphnodes decreases after the 15th day following grafting. In previous investigations, we have shown that the paracortical area, i.e. the area of the nodes where sensitized cells are produced, undergoes a depletion and later on a real atrophy. These structural changes are the same whether the nodes drain T9 or T10. However, this does not rule out the possibility that the retention of cells inside the tumor also decreases. Nothing is known about the traffic of these cells in and out of the tumor.

It is tempting to assume that the contacts between tumor cells and infiltrating cells are the morphological expression of an attack of target cells by the host cells and are a prerequisite for a cytotoxic effect. We have seen that such contacts exist between tumor cells and various types of infiltrating cells. In this regard, there is no significant difference between immunoblasts, lymphocytes and monocytes.

The use of various models *in vitro* has shown that several categories of cells may be involved in cytotoxicity: T-cells, B-cells, monocytes, macrophages. Their relative participation in the cytotoxic effect may vary according to the model system used, namely the nature of target cells, the presence of antibody, etc. How the data derived from the studies of *in vitro* system correlate to the *in vivo* phenomena is difficult to say. On the basis of experiments performed in relation to allografts rejection, one may expect T-cells to be the most important killer cells [19]. In the tumor system, however, it is possible that non-T-cells may also act as killer cells [20].

According to other reports, "macrophages" could be predominant killer cells *in vitro* and even more so *in vivo* [21–23]. The killing activity of macrophages could be specific when these cells are "armed" by cytophilic antibodies or cytophilic factors produced by T-cells arriving in contact with antigen [24]. Macrophages activated by a variety of unspecific procedures can also become cytotoxic for tumor cells [25]. In our system, monocytes are the most frequent cell type infiltrating the tumors; they get frequently in contact with tumor cells whereas macrophages loaded with phagocytized material never do so. With our tumors, we could not confirm the observations made by Evans [26] claiming that the tumors that grow slowly are more infiltrated by macrophages than tumors with a fast growth.

When growth progresses, the number of contacts between cells decreases and this suggests that the possibility for infiltrating cells to exert their cytotoxic activity is impaired. It is tempting to assume that at that time, factors have appeared which prevent these contacts. The possible role of blocking factors such as antibodies, excess of antigen or antigen–antibody complexes may be thought of. In this regard, we should recall that at the same time the lymphnodes show morphological changes suggesting a strong immune reaction of the humoral type. This could strongly influence the relation between target cells and killer cells.

As a pure hypothesis, it might be proposed that as the tumor graft grows, the production of specifically sensitized cells tends to decrease whereas factors appear which prevent the remaining cells to attack the target tumor cells.

REFERENCES

1. E.J. Foley, Antigenic properties of methylcholanthrene-induced tumors in mice of the strain of origin. *Cancer Res.* **13**, 835 (1953).
2. R.T. Prehn and J.M. Main, Immunity to methylcholanthrene-induced sarcomas. *J. Nat. Cancer*

Inst. **18**, 769 (1957).

3. L. Revesz, Detection of antigenic differences in isologous host-tumor systems by pretreatment with heavily irradiated tumor cells. *Cancer Res.* **20**, 443 (1960).

4. G. Klein, H.O. Sjögren, E. Klein and K.E. Hellström, Demonstration of resistance against methylcholanthrene-induced sarcomas in the primary autochtonous host. *Cancer Res.* **20**, 1561 (1960).

5. P. Alexander, D.I. Connell and Z.B. Mikulska, Treatment of a murine leukaemia with spleen cells or sera from allogeneic mice immunized against the tumor. *Cancer Res.* **26**, 1508 (1966).

6. H.F. Jeejeebhoy, E.J. Delorme and P. Alexander, The anti-tumor effect of lymphoid cells placed in millipore diffusion chambers. *Transplantation*, **4**, 397 (1966).

7. J.G. Hall and B. Morris, The output of cells from the popliteal lymph node of sheep. *Q.J. Expt. Physiol.* **47**, 360 (1962).

8. J.G. Hall, Studies on the cells in the afferent and efferent lymph of lymph node draining the site of skin homografts. *J. Exp. Med.* **125**, 737 (1967).

9. J. Weiner, R.G. Lattes and J.S. Pearl, Vascular permeability and leukocyte emigration in allograft rejection. *Am. J. Path.* **55**, 295 (1969).

10. L.J. Simar and E.H. Betz, Ultrastructural investigations on the inflammatory response in skin allografts. *Path. Europaea*, **5**, 131 (1970).

11. L.J. Simar, Modifications structurales des ganglions drainant un greffon allogénique. Relations avec la réaction inflammatoire du greffon. *Arch. Anat. Path.* **21**, 13 (1973).

12. E.R. Weibel, G.S. Kistler and W.F. Scherle, Practical stereologic methods for morphometric cytology. *J. Cell Biol.* **30**, 23 (1966).

13. E.R. Weibel, Stereological principles for morphometry in electron microscopic cytology. *Int. Rev. Cytol.* **26**, 235 (1969).

14. R.T. De Hoff and F.N. Rhines, *Quantitative Microscopy*, McGraw Hill, New York, 1968.

15. H. Giger and H. Riedwyl, Bestimmung der Grössenverteilung vom Kugem aus Schnittkresradien. *Biometr. Ztschr.* **12**, 156 (1970).

16. P. Alexander, J. Rensted, E.J. Delorme, J.G. Hall and J. Hadgett, The cellular immune response to primary sarcoma in rats. II. Abnormal response of nodes draining tumor. *Proc. Roy. Soc.* B, **174**, 237 (1969).

17. R.A. Prendergast, Cellular specificity in the homograft reaction. *J. Expt. Med.* **119**, 377 (1964).

18. D. Vaillier, M. Donner, J. Vaillier and C. Burg, Release of lymphotoxins by spleen cells sensitized against mouse tumor associated antigens. *Cell. Immunol.* **6**, 466 (1973).

19. J.C. Cerottini and K.T. Brunner, Cell-mediated cytotoxicity, allograft rejection, and tumor immunity. In: *Advances in Immunology*, vol. 18, edited by F.J. Dixon and M.G. Kunkel. Academic Press, New York and London, 1974.

20. E.W. Lamon, H. Wigzell, E. Klein, B. Andersson and H.M. Skurzak, The lymphocyte response to primary Moloney sarcoma virus tumors in BALB/C mice. *J. Exp. Med.* **137**, 1472 (1973).

21. W. Den Otter, R. Evans and P. Alexander, Cytotoxicity of murine peritoneal macrophages in tumor allograft immunity. *Transplantation*, **14**, 220 (1972).

22. G.A. Granger and R.S. Weiser, Homograft target cells. Specific destruction in vitro by contact interaction with immune macrophages. *Science*, **145**, 1427 (1964).

23. R. Evans and P. Alexander, Cooperation of immune lymphoid cells with macrophages in tumor immunity. *Nature (Lond.)*, **228**, 620 (1970).

24. R. Evans and P. Alexander, Rendering macrophages specifically cytotoxic by a factor released from immune lymphoid cells. *Transplantation*, **12**, 227 (1970).

25. J.B. Hibbs, L.M. Lambert and J.S. Remington, Control of carcinogenesis: a possible role for the activated macrophage. *Science*, **177**, 998 (1973).

26. R. Evans and P. Alexander, Role of macrophage tumor immunity. I. Co-operation between macrophages and lymphoid cells in syngeneic tumor immunity. *Immunology*, **23**, 615 (1972).

TESTS IN CANCER PATIENTS

T-CELL ROSETTES IN HUMAN CANCER

JOSEPH WYBRAN and H. HUGH FUDENBERG

Service d'Immunologie, Hôpital Universitaire Saint-Pierre, Brussels

and

Department of Clinical and Basic Immunology and Microbiology,
Medical University of South Carolina, Charleston, S.C.

ABSTRACT

Human lymphocytes that bind to normal sheep red blood cells, *in vitro*, in a rosette formation are T-cells. This is based on findings in human fetuses, in immunodeficient patients and on the absence of B-cell markers on these rosette-forming cells. We have described the active T-rosette test detecting a subpopulation of T-lymphocytes and the total T-rosette test detecting all of them. Cancer patients, depending on the sheep used, will have decreased blood active T-lymphocytes whereas the total T-lymphocytes are in the normal range. Since these active T-rosette-forming cells correlate with the immune status in immunodeficient patients and also increase after the induction of immune functions in various diseases, we propose that the subpopulation of blood active T-rosette-forming cells, present in cancer patients, is an index of their cellular immunocompetence and a reflection of their system of immunosurveillance.

INTRODUCTION

According to the present concept of immunology, lymphocytes are divided into T- and B-cells. The T-lymphocytes are basically involved in cellular immunity whereas B-lymphocytes will be responsible for the humoral immunity. This strict concept can, however, be challenged since B-cells synthesize also a mediator of cellular immunity like macrophage inhibitory factor. Furthermore, in the field of tumor immunology, it is readily apparent that cellular cytoxicity against tumor cells cannot only be mediated by T-lymphocytes but also by non-T-cells. It remains, however, very important to be able to differentiate between T- and B-lymphocytes since this should lead to a better comprehension of the basic mechanisms of immunity. As yet, morphology has not been very helpful since the usual microscopical techniques do not allow the differentiation between T- and B-lymphocytes. Sophisticated techniques like scanning electron microscopy should be considered with much caution when applied to the differentiation of T- and B-cells [1, 2].

Fortunately, these lymphocytes can be distinguished on the basis of surface markers. In this paper, we will address ourselves only to the problem of blood human T-cells in cancer using as a tool the specific T-cell rosette formation obtained, *in vitro*, in the presence of sheep red blood cells (SRBC) [3, 4]. This marker is the one most used for

31

identifying human T-lymphocytes. The two techniques that we have used throughout the various studies should be briefly summarized here. The first, termed the active rosette test, requires a short contact between the lymphocytes, previously preincubated in heat-inactivated calf serum at 37°C, and the SRBC. In fact, these cells are in contact only during the 5 min of a low-speed centrifugation [5, 6]. This test investigates only (a) sub-population(s) of all T-cells, perhaps the one with the highest affinity receptors for SRBC [7]. The second test, termed the total rosettes test, investigates all T-cells. Technically, it is done by a fast centrifugation of SRBC and lymphocytes in the presence of fetal calf serum [8]. The cells will remain in contact for at least 1 hr before evaluating the percentage of rosette-forming cells (RFC). In both tests and by definition, an RFC is a lymphocyte with at least three SRBC surrounding it. Usually, in the active test, a lymphocyte is surrounded by three or more SRBC while in the total test the lymphocyte is completely surrounded by the SRBC. The active RFC (TEa) is not stable and should be read immediately, while the total RFC (TEt) is more stable. The percentage of blood TEa is 27 ± 6.5% and the lower values of the normal is 15%; the blood TEt percentage is 64 ± 6.5% and the lower values of the normal is 51%.

ROSETTE FORMING CELLS ARE T-CELLS

The evidence that these RFC are indeed T-cells stems from various sources. First, we have demonstrated that, in human fetuses, RFC are already present in the thymus when few or no RFC are present in the other lymphoid organs or in the blood [3, 4, 9]. In older fetuses, an increase in RFC outside the thymus has been observed. It is interesting to note that the percentage of TEa in the thymus will decrease after the 15th week of gestation while, at the same period, almost all the thymocytes are TEt, and this percentage remains stable in older fetuses [10]. Since it is also around this time that the cortex of the thymus enlarges, one can speculate that the TEa are present in the medulla rather than in the cortex. This is of importance since, in the mouse, it appears that the immunocompetent T-cells are in the medulla and not in the cortex. Secondly, RFC do not possess specific B-cell markers [11]. This is the general rule although a small percentage of lymphocytes appear to have both T- and B-markers (e.g. receptor for SRBC and surface immunoglobulins detected by immunofluorescence). The meaning of this population is unclear (uncommitted stem cell? activated T-cell?) [12]. In sharp contrast is the presence, in human peripheral blood, of null lymphocytes which cannot be characterized by any known markers. The meaning of these cells, perhaps increased in diseases like lupus erythematosus diffusis, is also unknown. These two exceptions, probably not accounting for more than 7% of peripheral blood lymphocytes, being rapidly mentioned, the other lymphocytes can be classified as T-cell or B-cell. We will not discuss here the problem of the K-cells, presented elsewhere in this volume. Thirdly, the distribution of B- and T-cells in patients with immunodeficiencies usually fits well with their defective functions. For instance, patients with thymus hypoplasia have very low percentage of RFC [5]. Also, in chronic lymphatic leukemia of B-cell type, only very few T-cells are found [8]. On the basis of these arguments, it seems reasonable to accept the rosette formation as a specific marker for human T-cells.

The phenomenon remains, however, to be explained. The receptor for SRBC has not yet been clearly identified. The nature of the binding between T-lymphocytes and SRBC is still to be elucidated. It appears highly unlikely that immunological mechanisms like antigen recognition play a role in the binding. The distribution of the electrostatic surface charges of both T-cells and SRBC clearly influences the rosette formation. Finally, it may be stressed that, also in animals, T-cells can bind to erythrocytes in a rosette formation. This is the case for guinea pig T-lymphocytes with rabbit erythrocytes, dog T-lymphocytes with human erythrocytes and pig T-lymphocytes with human erythrocytes [13, 14]. In view of these already numerous examples, it is likely that the list of erythrocytes binding specifically to T-lymphocytes can only grow, provided that the right techniques are used. The system autologous red cell and T-lymphocytes is another example of a rosette formation that involves only a subpopulation of T-cells [15]. Why T-lymphocytes should bind to erythrocytes is certainly puzzling. Could this phenomenon play a role in some autoimmune mechanisms like hemolytic anemia? The difficulties in understanding the system, the fact that no rational explanation can be proposed for it should, however, not discourage the workers in this field. It is always very frustrating not to be able to answer simple questions like "how?" and "why?". Finally, in cancer patients the rosette system, which already requires very precise techniques, is highly dependent on the SRBC used.

HUMAN CANCER

The importance of the immune system should hardly be stressed although the intimate mechanisms are still unclear. Unfortunately, most of the *in vitro* tests poorly correlate with the clinical status or evolution of the patients. Nevertheless, it remains important to investigate these patients further in order to determine their specific and non-specific immune status. This should give a better rationale to our current methods of immunotherapy and provide new immunotherapeutic approaches. Oncology may thus benefit from a better knowledge of B- and T-cells in cancer patients. One should, however, be aware that this determination in the blood provides only an indirect measurement. It is obvious that the determination of the type and function immune cells present in the tumor and also in the adjacent lymph nodes are a more direct approach to the understanding of the immune mechanisms. Some observations indicate that T-cells can be present in the tumor itself. It is not known whether these cells are capable of killing the malignant cells. Furthermore, this killing could, *in vivo*, be inhibited by the presence of blocking factors. Peripheral blood lymphocytes of cancer patients can kill, *in vitro*, tumor cells of the same type as the patient's tumor although the specificity of this phenomenon is not clear. This killing can be inhibited by the serum of the patient. The cells responsible for the action belong to the non-T and T-cells [16, 17]. It has, for instance, been shown that bladder tumor cells are killed, *in vitro*, by non-T cells of cancer patients bearing a bladder carcinoma [16]. In melanoma, both non-T and T-cells have been shown to be capable of such killing properties. It is possible that, during the evolution of the disease in the same patient, T- and non-T cells can, in turn or together, be killer cells. Indeed, we have demonstrated this to be the case in osteosarcoma patients [18]. Since suppressor cells can be present in the isolated T- and non-T cell populations, they may decrease or inhibit the properties of the killing cells; this indicates the complexity of the phenomenon.

All these studies clearly point out that the determination of the immune cells in cancer patients is important. We will thus describe the results of our studies done in cancer patients using the blood T-rosettes-forming cell as a tool. In general, both the active T-test and total T-test were used. However, since we first described the active rosettes test, and later on the total T-test, some patients have been studied only for their TEa.

Presently, we have studied more than 500 patients with various types of solid tumor [6] . About 100 of them had their TEa measured early in the disease, at the time of diagnosis and when it was not metastatic. Approximately 65% of them have low TEa while only 5% have decreased TEt. However, before further describing our results, we want to re-emphasize again the importance of the sheep used in the study. Indeed, in a separate study using different sheep, we did not detect any differences between cancer patients and the normal population. This result completely contradicted our previous published work. Trying to understand the reasons of these surprising results, we realized that only the red cells of one sheep out of six could discriminate between the lymphocytes of cancer patients and normal individuals (Table 1). Other groups have confirmed

Table 1. *Influence of Different Sheep on the Percentage of Active and Total T-rosette-forming Cells*

	Sheep number					
	1	2	3	4	5	6
Cancer patients						
Bone cancer (4)	8–64	17–65	20–64	23–68	19–67	21–66
Breast cancer (5)	11–63	19 –63	24–65	22–67	24–68	21–67
Melanoma cancer (5)	7–69	20–68	19–70	24–67	23–72	24 -68
Colon cancer (4)	10–68	21–66	18–65	21–66	20–66	22–67
Normal controls						
Subject A	22–65	25–64	21–64	22–66	24–63	25–67
Subject B	27–64	30–65	28–66	29–62	27–66	30–68
Subject C	20–69	25–65	23–64	22–63	21–64	25–66
Subject D	24–62	22–61	25–59	25–60	22–59	24–63

The first number is the mean TEa percentage; the second the mean TEt percentage. In this example, only the SRBC of sheep number 1 indicates low TEa values for cancer patients. The TEt are always normal. In parentheses are indicated the number of patients investigated.

this observation which obviously explains some contradictory results found in the literature regarding the blood T-lymphocytes in cancer patients. Unfortunately, it is not yet possible to determine which sheep should be used in the test. We have, however, found that it is not related to the blood group of these sheep [19] . Thus, the only way, as yet, of knowing which sheep should be used is to test a number of them with the lymphocytes of cancer subjects and normal controls. This allows the selection of sheep whose red blood cells can discriminate, in the active test, between the lymphocytes from cancer and normal individuals. Once the sheep has been selected, it should always be used. Usually, we store the SRBC for 2 weeks in Alsever's solution at 4°C. The sheep is thus bled every 2 weeks. In all our studies reported in this paper, we have only used sheep that have empirically been tested and found to be discriminatory [6] . Patients newly diagnosed and with metastatic diseases usually have lower TEa than the group of patients with localized tumor. The TEt are decreased in about 25% of them. We have also tested patients who were either cured or in remission (at least 2 years after treatment and without any signs of tumor). These patients present normal values of both TEa and TEt. The group of patients presenting a localized recurrence show decreased TEa in about 60% of the cases and usually normal TEt. This group of patients did not receive any therapy for the last 2 years. When the recurrence is metastatic the values of the TEa are, once again, decreased in about 70% of the cases. The TEt are decreased in about 25% of the cases. Usually the TEa values are also lower in the metastatic patients than in those with localized disease.

It is not clear yet whether the low TEa values are more frequent in some types of cancer than in others. Indeed some authors have reported, using still another method for detecting T-cell rosettes, a very high incidence of low blood T-cells in localized lung cancer [20]. It is important to mention that their test, like the TEa, also does not detect all T-cells. Other investigators, using a modified active rosette assay, have also found decreased T-cell rosettes in about 90% of patients with various localized or metastatic carcinoma [21]. Thus, all these data clearly indicate that cancer patients present T-lymphocytes defective in their rosetting property. It may reflect a pure T-cell defect or an absence of some T-cell subpopulation(s).

Repeated testing in the same cancer patients has yielded interesting data. Both in osteosarcoma patients treated with specific transfer factor and in some untreated melanoma patients, we and others have observed that a fall in TEa, without necessarily a simultaneous decrease in TEt, was usually followed in the next weeks or months by the clinical detections of new lesions [6, 22, 23]. The spread of the disease was heralded by a drop in TEa. This decrease may be followed by an unexpected and unexplained return to normal values. The drop usually lasts 3 to 6 weeks. It can thus remain undetected if frequent testings are not performed. Some cautionary note should, however, be mentioned here regarding intercurrent viral infections. We have observed, and it has been repeatedly confirmed, that viral infections will transiently lower the TEa, and quite often the TEt, values [6]. Thus, each patient before being tested should be checked for a viral infection. The T-cells usually will return to normal values in a few days, but low values can persist for several weeks. Cancer patients, with an intermittent viral disease, also show such a drop. Follow-up of more than 1 year of these patients, who remained in remission, clearly indicated that the decrease was due to the viral infection and not to a relapse of their disease.

THE FUNCTIONAL MEANING OF ACTIVE T-ROSETTES FORMING CELL

All these observations suggest that cancer patients, even with localized disease, have a non-specific defect in their T-cells. It may not be quantitative but rather qualitative since usually the TEt are normal. The hypothesis of a qualitative defect is raised by the observations of ourselves and others in patients with immunodeficiencies [5, 24]. In the Wiskott—Aldrich syndrome and in chronic mucocutaneous candidiasis, the patients exhibit a defective cell-mediated immunity. About 50% of the Wiskott—Aldrich patients can benefit from transfer factor therapy. These responding patients will remain free of disease for a period of approximately 6 months and their immune defects will be partially corrected. These patients, before therapy, have low TEa. The responders will, very rapidly, increase their TEa but not their TEt and simultaneously the other immune defects improve. The chronic mucocutaneous candidiasis patients studied had a defect in cell

Table 2. *Percentage of Blood Active and Total T-rosette in Various Conditions*

	Active T-rosettes	Total T-rosettes
Cancer	Usually decreased	Usually normal
Lupus erythematosus diffusis	Usually decreased	Decreased or normal
Wiskott–Aldrich syndrome	Decreased	Decreased or normal
Chronic mucocutaneous candidiasis	Usually decreased	Usually normal
Lepromatous leprosy	Decreased	Decreased or normal
Post-transfer factor therapy	Increased	Unchanged
Post-BCG therapy	Increased	Usually unchanged
Old age	Usually decreased	Normal
Thymosin, *in vitro*	Increased	Unchanged

mediated immunity. Their TEa were decreased while their TEt were normal. These two examples clearly indicate the existence of a correlation between the status of cellular immunity and the TEa percentage. Other diseases, with known defects in cell mediated immunity, may also exhibit low blood TEa and normal blood TEt percentages (Table 2) [25–26].

Finally, we have recently investigated the influence of age [27]. There is a significant decrease in TEa while the TEt remain normal in the older normal subjects (more than 70 years old). It was also confirmed that this group of old people have a decreased lymphocyte response to non-specific mitogens. Thus, in humans as in animals, cellular immunity decreases with age. The qualitative defect is correlated with the decreased TEa. The normal TEt, once again, should be considered as a marker for the presence of T-cells, whose deficient function is reflected by the decreased TEa. On the basis of these observations, we interpret the low TEa in cancer patients, even with localized disease, as a qualitative defect in non-specific cell mediated immunity. Alternatively, it may reflect the absence of a population of immunocompetent T-cells. There is general agreement that patients with widespread metastatic disease exhibit decreased cell mediated immunity. For instance, their skin tests are usually weak, their lymphocytes poorly react to mitogens and in mixed leucocyte culture. In melanoma, a lack of dinitrochlorobenzene sensitization is associated with a poor prognosis. However, in the case of localized disease and thus a small tumor burden, these tests usually do not show any abnormalities. The fact that 60% of the patients, according to our data or 90% of patients according to other data, have decreased T-cell rosette in localized disease suggests that a non-specific T-cell defect can be detected even with a small lesion. However, when the patients are first seen they already have numerous tumor cells, which may be non-specifically immuno-suppressive and also immunostimulant by inducing specific mechanisms against the tumor. This in turn or perhaps simultaneously, could boost non-specific immune defenses. Therefore, one should expect that not all patients, when first seen by the physician, will have low TEa or detectable non-specific immune defects.

There are some arguments suggesting a link between defective cellular immunity as measured by low TEa, and the development of malignancies. For instance, a patient with acquired hypogammaglobulinemia and low TEa developed a lung cancer 2 years after being tested for his T-cell rosettes (case number 9 of reference 5). The same observation has been made in a patient with idiopathic thrombopenic purpura who developed a kidney tumor [6]. Perhaps more intriguing and less anecdotal is the observation that in the healthy members of families with high incidence of cancer, the percentage of subjects with low TEa is high. These subjects are followed for the possible development of malignancies [6]. The drop in TEa before the detection of new lesion may also be due to defective non-specific mechanisms allowing the growth of new cells which may, in turn, boost specific and non-specific immunity and thus raise the TEa to normal values.

Before pursuing the discussion about the meaning of decreased TEa in cancer patients, we will summarize two types of data in the field of immunotherapy. First, melanoma patients with skin metastases who had received intralesional BCG showed a rapid increase in their blood TEa associated with a regression of the nodules [28]. The TEt can or cannot raise after BCG therapy. Similar data have been observed by other investigators [29]. In the non-responders, TEa did or did not increase. At the same time, other immunologic tests, such as lymphocyte proliferation or production of leucocyte inhibitory factor, were induced or increased [30]. Once again, the TEa are closely associated with changes of the immune status. A second type of data comes from the osteosarcoma patients treated with specific transfer factor. Quite often, after the injection of transfer factor, their TEa will increase. This is usually associated with an increase in cell-mediated cytotoxicity of the patient's lymphocytes against osteosarcoma tumor cells. Interestingly, the TEa will increase only in the patients who have an apparent response to therapy, some being free of disease for more than 24 months [22]. Thus, in this circumstance as well as in the Wiskott—Aldrich syndrome, the TEa determination closely correlates the clinical and immune changes induced by transfer factor therapy.

A rather striking point, observed in both the BCG or transfer factor therapy, is the rapid increase in peripheral blood TEa. Several hypotheses could explain this phenomenon. The most likely explanation for the BCG is that this adjuvant, or perhaps products (tumor antigens, enzymes) released by its injection, will directly activate the T-cells, as reflected by the increase in TEa but rarely in TEt. The target cell of transfer factor is not known. Transfer factor confers to the recipient the specific immunity of the donor. It may also boost the non-specific immunity of the recipient. Many speculations regarding its mode of action have been made. We wish to add a new hypothesis to this already crowded world of endless discussions. We have previously shown that thymosin, an extract of calf thymus, can increase, *in vitro*, the percentage of TEa but not TEt [31]. We have also provided some evidence that the target cell may be a non-active T-cell. This fits with some observations regarding an increase in mitogen responsiveness or in mixed leucocyte culture, in the presence of thymosin [32]. This effect is apparently non-specific. Since transfer factor sometimes induced non-specific immunity [33] we propose that the transfer factor induces the synthesis of thymic factor by the thymus epithelium. This might explain the non-specific effects of the transfer factor and the rapid raise of TEa, a non-specific T-cell index. This hypothesis does not, however, fully explain the instances where transfer factor has induced only specific immunity in the recipient.

Let us now turn to another aspect of malignancies. We have studied and followed more than 100 melanoma patients [34]. The period of observation was up to 3 years for some of them. Many of these patients had low TEa values. It is mainly in the group of subjects with low TEa that progression of the disease, and sometimes death, was recorded. Thus, here too, the TEa appears a helpful test and a bad prognostic factor if they are low. No correlation with TEt was found.

CONCLUSIONS

In this paper, we have always considered the TEa as reflecting immunocompetent cells, actively and mainly involved in T-cell mediated immune mechanisms. It remains possible that soluble factors interfere with the test. We have discussed this problem elsewhere [5]. For instance, during the spread of the disease, soluble factor(s) released or induced by the tumor are in the circulation and could hinder the receptors for SRBC detected in the TEa test. This could decrease the TEa. Antigen—antibody complexes can be present in cancer patients. They can theoretically hinder the rosette formation since activated T-cells appear to have a receptor for the free Fc of the complex. Similarly, anti-T factor, synthesized perhaps by the cancer lymphocytes, could also block the rosette formation. A metabolic modulation of the expressivity of receptor, through abnormal or low thymic factors or through some other factor(s) present in cancer serum, could possibly affect the TEa test.

In conclusion, we have briefly reviewed some problems regarding T-cells in cancer patients. On the basis of these observations and for the following reasons, we propose that TEa reflect T-cell competence and indirectly immuno-surveillance.

1. TEa are at their highest percentage in the fetal thymus when the medulla (containing immunocompetent cells in the mouse) is the largest in this organ. The percentage of TEt does not decrease with the enlargement of the cortical area.
2. Low TEa, in the presence of normal TEt, can be found in various immunologic disorders with cellular defects as well as with old age.
3. The increase of TEa, without a concomitant rise in TEt, after transfer factor therapy or BCG therapy, is associated with the induction or the increase of cell mediated mechanisms.
4. There is a correlation between low TEa but not TEt with poor prognosis in melanoma patients.
5. Thymosin, *in vitro,* increases the percentage of TEa without affecting the TEt. It can also increase cellular immune reactivity.

In view of all these observations and the low TEa values found in healthy members of families with high incidence of cancer, the development of cancer in some subjects with low TEa, the drop of TEa before the clinical detection of new lesions, we propose that the low blood TEa of cancer patients reflect a defect in their immune surveillance apparatus.

ACKNOWLEDGEMENTS

Part of this work has been supported in part by grants of the Belgian Fonds de la Recherche Scientifique et Médicale, the NIH (AI 09145-14) and the American Cancer Society (IM 16I).

REFERENCES

1. M.M. Kay, B. Belohradsky, K. Yee, J. Vogel, D. Butcher, J. Wybran and H.H. Fudenberg, Cellular interactions: scanning electron microscopy of human thymus-derived rosette-forming lympho-cytes. *Clin. Immunol. Immunopathol.* **2**, 301 (1974).
2. E.L. Alexander and B. Wetzel, Human lymphocytes: similarity of B and T cell surface morphology. *Science,* **188**, 732 (1975).
3. J. Wybran and H.H. Fudenberg, Rosette formation, a test for cellular immunity. *Trans. Ass. Am. Phys.* **84**, 239 (1971).

4. J. Wybran, M.C. Carr and H.H. Fudenberg, The human rosette forming cell as a marker of a population of thymus-derived cells. *J. Clin. Invest.* **51**, 2537 (1972).
5. J. Wybran, A.S. Levin, L.E. Spitler and H.H. Fudenberg, Rosette forming cells, immunological diseases and transfer factor. *New Eng. J. Med.* **288**, 710 (1973).
6. J. Wybran and H.H. Fudenberg, Thymus-derived rosette forming cells in human disease state: cancer, lymphomas, viral and bacterial infections, and other diseases. *J. Clin. Invest.* **52**, 1026 (1973).
7. J. Wybran and H.H. Fudenberg, Thymus-derived rosette forming cells. *New Engl. J. Med.* **288**, 1072 (1973).
8. J. Wybran, S. Chantler and H.H. Fudenberg, Isolation of normal T cells in chronic lymphatic leukemia. *Lancet,* **1**, 126 (1973).
9. J. Wybran, M.C. Carr and H.H. Fudenberg, Effect of serum on human rosette forming cells in fetuses and adult blood. *Clin. Immunol. Immunopathol.* **1**, 408 (1973).
10. A. W. Hayward and G. Ezer, Development of lymphocyte populations in the human foetal thymus and spleen. *Clin. Exp. Immunol.* **17**, 169 (1974).
11. M. Jondal, G. Holm and H. Wigzell, Surface markers on human T and B lymphocytes. I. A large population of lymphocytes forming nonimmune rosettes with sheep red blood cells. *J. Exp. Med.* **136**, 207 (1972).
12. H.B. Dickler, Jr., N.F. Adkinson and W.D. Terry, Evidence for individual human peripheral blood lymphocytes bearing both B and T cell markers. *Nature,* **247**, 213 (1974).
13. C. Bowles, G.S. White and D. Lucas, Rosette formation by canine peripheral blood lymphocytes. *J. Immunol.* **114**, 399 (1975).
14. M.J. Stadecker, G. Bishop and H.H. Wortis, Rosette formation by guinea pig thymocytes and thymus derived lymphocytes with rabbit red blood cells. *J. Immunol.* **111**, 1834 (1973).
15. G. Baxley, G.B. Bishop, A.G. Cooper and H.H. Wortis, Rosetting of human red blood cells to thymus-derived cells. *Clin. Exp. Immunol.* **15**, 385 (1973).
16. C. O'Toole, P. Perlmann, H. Wigzell, B. Unsgaard and C.G. Zetterlund, Lymphocyte cytotoxicity in bladder cancer. No requirement for thymus derived effective cells. *Lancet,* **1**, 1085 (1973).
17. J. Wybran, I. Hellström, K.E. Hellström and H.H. Fudenberg, Cytotoxicity of human rosette-forming blood lymphocytes on cultivated human tumor cells. *Int. J. Cancer,* **13**, 515 (1974).
18. J. Wybran, V. Byers, A.S. Levin and H.H. Fudenberg, unpublished results.
19. J. Wybran, D. Robbins, B. Rasmussen and H.H. Fudenberg, unpublished results.
20. R.L. Gross, A. Latty, E.A. Williams and P.M. Newberne, Abnormal spontaneous rosette formation and rosette inhibition in lung carcinoma. *New Engl. J. Med.* **292**, 439 (1975).
21. J. Djeu, J.L. McCoy and R.B. Herberman, personal communication.
22. A.S. Levin, V.S. Byers, H.H. Fudenberg, J. Wybran, A.J. Hackett and J.O. Johnston, Osteogenic sarcoma. Immunologic parameters before and during immunotherapy with tumor-specific transfer factor. *J. Clin. Invest.* **55**, 487 (1975).
23. A.L. Claudy, J. Viac, N. Pelletier, N. Fouad-Wassef, A. Alario and J. Thivolet, Prognostic correlations in malignant melanoma (abstract). This volume, pp. 252–253.
24. R. Hong and S. Horowitz, Thymosin therapy creates a "Hassal". *New Engl. J. Med.* **292**, 104 (1975).
25. D.T. Yu, P.J. Clements, J.B. Peter, J. Levy, H.E. Paulus and E.V. Barnett, Lymphocyte characteristics in rheumatic patients and the effect of azathioprine therapy. *Arthritis Rheum.* **17**, 37 (1974).
26. I. Nath, J. Curtis, L.K. Bhutani and G.P. Talwar, Reduction of a subpopulation of T lymphocytes in lepromatous leprosy. *Clin. Exp. Immunol.* **18**, 81 (1974).
27. J. Wybran and A. Govaerts, unpublished results.
28. J. Wybran, L.E. Spitler, R. Lieberman and H.H. Fudenberg, Active T-cell rosettes and total T-rosettes in patients with melanoma following intratumoral inoculation of BCG: a clue to the mechanism of action of bacillus Calmette-Guérin? *Cancer Immunol. Immunother.* (in press).
29. J. Bertoglio, A. Bourgoin, K. Gronneberg and J.F. Dore, Active rosettes in BCG-treated melanoma patients and untreated leukaemic children (abstract). This volume, p. 251.
30. R. Lieberman, J. Wybran and W. Epstein, The immunologic and histopathologic changes of BCG mediated tumor regression in patients with malignant melanoma. *Cancer* **35**, 756 (1975).
31. J. Wybran, A.S. Levin, H.H. Fudenberg and A.L. Goldstein, Thymosin: effects on normal human blood T cells. *Ann. N.Y. Acad. Sci.* **249**, 300 (1975).
32. G.H. Cooper, J.A. Hooper and A.L. Goldstein, Thymosin. Induced differentiation of murine thymocytes in allogeneic mixed lymphocyte cultures. *Ann. N.Y. Acad. Sci.* **249**, 145 (1975).
33. C. Griscelli, J.P. Revillard, H. Betuel, C. Herzog and J.L. Touraine, Transfer factor therapy in immunodeficiencies, *Biomedicine* **18**, 220 (1973).

34. J. Wybran, L.E. Spitler and H.H. Fudenberg, Rosette forming cells and melanoma. *Clin. Res.* **21**, 655 (1973).
35. J. Wybran and H.H. Fudenberg, Human thymus derived rosette forming cells. Their role in immunocompetence and immunosurveillance. In: *Lymphocytes and their Interactions: Recent Observations*, edited by R.C. Williams, Jr., Raven Press, New York, pp. 113–132, 1975.

CELL-MEDIATED CYTOTOXICITY *IN VITRO*. MECHANISMS AND RELEVANCE TO TUMOR IMMUNITY

J.-C. CEROTTINI and K.T. BRUNNER

Department of Immunology, Swiss Institute for Experimental Cancer Research and Lausanne Unit of Human Cancer Immunology, Ludwig Institute for Cancer Research, in conjunction with Policlinique Médicale Universitaire, Lausanne, Switzerland

INTRODUCTION

During the last 5 years, several authors have reported the occurrence, in blood of cancer patients, of leukocytes which exerted a toxic effect *in vitro* on cultured syngeneic or allogeneic tumor cells (for references, see Hellström and Hellström [1]). Concomitantly, studies in experimental tumor model systems have shown that cytotoxic effector cells appeared in blood and lymphoid tissues during the development of tumor immunity. Based on these results, it has been assumed that the *in vitro* cytotoxic activity of peripheral blood leukocytes from cancer patients was a direct manifestation of a state of cell-mediated immunity to tumor-associated antigens.

Recently, this concept has been seriously challenged. With the development of different assay methods and of refined cell separation techniques, it has become clear that (a) cell-mediated cytotoxicity (CMC) *in vitro* encompasses various effects of lymphocytes or other cell types, acting alone or in combination, and (b) CMC does not necessarily reflect the activity of effector cells *in vivo*.

Since CMC *in vitro* is commonly used in studies of human tumor immunology, it seems important to assess the relevance of the *in vitro* reactions to protective immunity in the cancer patient. However, in view of the complexity of the *in vitro* reactions themselves, it is necessary first to define the parameters measured in the different CMC assay systems, to characterize the possible effector cells and to analyze the mechanism of target cell destruction. In the present report, we shall briefly discuss some recent data concerning the mechanism of CMC *in vitro*. Further details can be found in recently published review articles or books [1–5].

ASSAY SYSTEMS

The first source of difficulty in the interpretation of CMC results concerns the complex nature of the effects which are measured in the various assay systems in common use [5–6]. In the microcytotoxicity assay according to Takasugi and Klein [7], lymphoid cells from cancer patients are incubated with attached tumor cells for 48 hr. The number of attached tumor cells remaining at the end of the incubation period is determined by visual counting. Obviously, this number may be influenced by several factors related to immunological cell-mediated reactions, such as direct lysis, growth inhibition and/or loss of adherence of tumor cells, but also to spontaneous cell death and growth stimulation by the lymphoid cell population. In contrast, only direct lysis of tumor cells is measured in the ^{51}Cr release assay, and direct lysis and/or detachment of tumor cells from a surface in the ^{3}H-proline assay described by Bean and collaborators [8]. Because of the differences it is likely, as reported by Plata *et al.* [9] in the Moloney sarcoma virus (MSV) system, that different results may be obtained when the activity of the same lymphoid cell population is tested using two different assay methods. This subject has been reviewed recently [5].

At present, there is no assay allowing the detection of effector cells at the single-cell level. It is thus impossible to determine the number of effector cells present in a given cell population. In some instances, however, an estimation of the relative frequency of effector cells can be obtained provided there is a single dose–response relationship, i.e. the cytotoxic activity varies proportionally with the number of lymphoid cells added. Titration curves, using varying numbers of lymphoid cells added to a constant number of target cells, are therefore essential to evaluate the significance of positive reactions.

In order to avoid deleterious culture conditions, it appears important to keep the number of lymphoid cells to be added to tumor cells within a certain limit. In general, ratios of lymphoid to target cells above 200 cannot be used. As the frequency of effector cells in a given lymphoid cell population has to reach a certain value before lytic activity can be detected, negative findings, i.e. the lack of significant target cell lysis and/or growth inhibition by a given cell population, cannot be interpreted as indicating the absence of effector cells in that population. In cases where the physical or immunological properties of the effector cells are different from that of the bulk of the lymphoid cells, cell-separation techniques can be applied to obtain cell populations enriched in effector cells. An example of the usefulness of such techniques for the detection of low numbers of effector cells has been recently reported by Vasudevan *et al.* [10]. However, the general applicability of these techniques to the detection of effector cells in blood from cancer patients remains to be determined.

NATURE OF EFFECTOR CELLS

Analysis of the mechanisms underlying CMC *in vitro* has revealed the existence of several pathways involving the participation of different effector cells. This subject has been reviewed recently [2]. In brief, three model systems have been described: (a) lysis of tumor cells by cytolytic T-lymphocytes (CTL) which are specifically sensitized against tumor-associated membrane bound antigens; (b) lysis of tumor cells coated with IgG antibody by "killer" (K) mononuclear cells which possess surface receptors for the Fc portion of IgG molecules; and (c) lysis of tumor cells by "armed" or "activated" macrophages.

The present knowledge of the biolological properties of these different effector cell types is still fragmentary. For example, the fate of CTL generated *in vivo* is unknown. In the model systems where the presence of CTL has been followed as a function of time, it has been a common finding that CTL appear early in the immune response and reach peak levels after 1–2 weeks. Thereafter, CTL activity declines progressively, so that lymphoid cells collected 2 months after the onset of the immune response generally have no detectable lytic activity mediated by thymus-derived effector cells. Recent studies, however, indicate that this lack of CTL activity does not necessarily reflect the absence of CTL in immune lymphoid cell populations. As demonstrated by Plata *et al.* [11], spleens of mice resistant to MSV challenge, although they contained no detectable CTL, appeared to have an increased number of CTL precursor cells which rapidly differentiated into highly lytic effector cells following *in vitro* exposure to the relevant antigens. As discussed elsewhere in detail [12], there is indirect evidence that CTL are not necessarily end cells, but may become "memory" cells, i.e. small T-lymphocytes, with no direct lytic activity, but capable of differentiating into active effector cells within 24 hr following exposure to the relevant antigenic stimulus. Although further work is needed to establish the validity of this concept, the findings of an increased generation of CTL in murine mixed leukocyte tumor cell reactions containing immune lymphoid cells may stimulate similar studies in man.

The three types of effector cells mentioned above have been demonstrated in well-defined experimental systems using the ^{51}Cr release assay. In cancer patients, there is as yet no direct evidence of the presence of CTL in circulating blood. On the other hand, human peripheral blood appears to be the best source of K-cells. *In vitro* activation of human peripheral blood monocytes into non-specific cytolytic macrophages has been recently achieved by Noerjasin and Stjernswärd (personal communication). The nature of the effector cells detected in peripheral blood of cancer patients by the microcytotoxicity assay is unknown in most cases. In the work of O'Toole *et al.* [13] on CMC of peripheral blood lymphocytes from cancer patients with bladder carcinoma, the effector cell population reactive against bladder carcinoma cell lines was found in the non-T-cell fraction. The exact nature of these effector cells and the possible participation of antibody in the effect detected in the microcytotoxicity test remain to be determined.

SPONTANEOUS LYTIC ACTIVITY OF NORMAL PERIPHERAL BLOOD

In the microcytotoxicity assay, the activity of blood lymphoid cells from cancer patients is expressed as the percentage reduction in the number of attached tumor cells as compared to the controls, i.e. microplates containing tumor cells incubated with lymphoid cells from normal donors. With the development of the ^{51}Cr release assay, it has been possible to use as controls labeled tumor cells incubated in medium alone. This has led to the detection of a direct lytic activity of the peripheral blood lymphoid cell population of normal individuals against some human lymphoid cell lines [14].

These findings have been confirmed in our laboratory. Blood was obtained from twelve healthy individuals, and a lymphocyte-enriched population was obtained after treatment with carbonyl iron and separation on Ficoll-sodium metrizoate. The lytic activity of each individual cell population was tested on ^{51}Cr-labeled MOLT-4 target cells, as presumably T-cell lymphoid cell line, using a 6 h incubation period. In order to get a quantitative comparison of the lytic activity in the individual cell populations, dose–response curves were established from the results obtained at varying lymphocyte-target cell ratios. The data are represented in Table 1. It can be seen that lymphocyte preparations from all twelve normal donors showed lytic activity against the MOLT-4 target cells, even at lymphocyte ratios as low as 1:1. When the different dose–response curves were

Table 1. *Cytolytic Activity of PBL*[a] *from Normal Individuals on*
^{51}Cr Labeled MOLT-4 Lymphoid Cell Line

Donor	% specific ^{51}Cr release[b]					Ratio at 30% lysis
	PBL-target cell ratio					
	100	30	10	3	1	
1	55	38	23	9	4	150
2	47	27	13	6	2	33
3	39	28	21	12	4	34
4	35	25	21	10	2	75
5	64	47	27	18	7	12
6	58	35	22	10	7	20
7	31	17	8	3	1	100
8	25	15	9	3	0	150
9	39	25	16	11	4	43
10	65	46	36	24	15	6

[a] After carbonyl iron and Ficoll-sodium metrizoate.
[b] Incubation time: 6 hr.

compared, it became evident that the lytic activity varied from one population to another, with up to a 30-fold difference in the number of lymphocytes needed to achieve the same level of lysis. Recently, a spontaneous cytotoxic activity of lymphoid cells from normal rats and mice against some rat or mouse lymphoma cell lines has been reported by several groups [15–17]. According to Herberman and collaborators [15], this spontaneous activity appears to be directed against antigens associated with endogenous C-type viruses. That the lytic activity displayed by peripheral blood lymphocytes from normal human donors might also be directed against virus associated antigens is an intriguing possibility.

There is also evidence that peripheral blood lymphocytes from normal individuals has a lytic activity against some human non-lymphoid tumor cell lines (for references see papers by de Vries, Moore and Peter in this issue). In Table 2, the results of assays of the lytic activity of blood lymphocyte-enriched cell populations from six normal donors on ^{51}Cr labeled IgR-3 melanoma target cells, an adherent cell line, are presented. It can be seen that the percentage of the total incorporated ^{51}Cr released with 6 hr is slightly higher in cultures containing lymphocytes rather than medium alone. By 24 hr, the lytic activity of the lymphoid cell populations is evident, with more than twice as much ^{51}Cr released by the target cells in the presence of lymphoid cells as compared to controls.

RELEVANCE TO TUMOR IMMUNITY

The relevance of CMC reactions to protective immunity is by no means clear. From the variety of mechanisms just described, it is obvious that the demonstration of a cytotoxic effect *in vitro* using unseparated lymphoid cell populations gives little information about the type of effector cell involved. Similarly, the results obtained in tumor model systems using transfer of lymphoid cells from immune animals give no clue as far as the mechanism of protection is concerned. Even the demonstration that a purified population of immune T-cells is able to confer protection to normal animals does not necessarily indicate that the actual effector cells are thymus-derived. In addition to CTL,

Table 2. *Cytolytic Activity of PBL*[a] *from Normal Individuals on*
^{51}Cr Labeled IgR-3 Melanoma Cell Line

Incubation time (hr)	Target cells alone	% total ^{51}Cr release (range)		
		PBL-target cell ratio		
		10	15	100
6	10 (9–12)	13[b] (10–19)	15 (11–20)	18 (13–29)
24	22 (20–24)	31 (26–46)	37 (32–50)	46 (39–65)

[a] After carbonyl iron and Ficoll-sodium metrizoate.
[b] Mean values of six individual donors.

the immune T-cell population may contain helper cells which are required for the differentiation of IgG antibody-forming cells and/or cells which produce macrophage activating factors. The possibility thus exists that K-cells and/or macrophages may be involved in the protective effect observed *in vivo* following transfer of a purified T-cell population.

Due to the complexities inherent to the methodology used, to the nature of the effector cells involved, to the biochemical characterization of tumor-associated antigens, and to our ignorance of the mechanisms of tumor immunity, the clinical interpretation of a positive CMC is still very difficult. Extensive experimental studies are thus needed to resolve some of these complexities. Also, careful studies in cancer patients, combining cell-separation techniques and culture reactions to immunochemical characterization of tumor-associated antigens, may be helpful for a better assessment of the value of CMC in clinical tumor immunology.

REFERENCES

1. K.E. Hellström and I. Hellström, Lymphocyte-mediated cytotoxicity and blocking serum activity to tumor antigens. In: *Advances in Immunology*, edited by F.J. Dixon and H.G. Kunkel, Vol. 18, p. 209. Academic Press, New York, 1974.
2. J.-C. Cerottini and K.T. Brunner, Cell-mediated cytotoxicity, allograft rejection, and tumor immunity. In: *Advances in Immunology*, edited by F.J. Dixon and H.G. Kunkel, Vol. 18, p. 67. Academic Press, New York, 1974.
3. R.B. Herberman, Cell-mediated immunity to tumor cells. In: *Advances in Cancer Research*, edited by G. Klein and S. Weinhouse, Vol. 19, p. 207. Academic Press, New York, 1974.
4. G.A. Currie, Cancer and the immune response. In: *Current Topics in Immunology*, edited by J. Turk, Vol. 2, p. 1. Edward Arnold, London, 1974.
5. *Immunobiology of the Tumor–Host Relationship*, edited by R.T. Smith and M. Landy, Academic Press, New York, 1975.
6. J.-C. Cerottini, Lymphocyte-mediated cytotoxicity and tumor immunity. In: *Recent Results in Cancer Research*, edited by G. Mathé and R. Weiner, Vol. 47, p. 118. Springer-Verlag, Berlin, 1974.
7. M. Takasugi and E. Klein, A microassay for cell-mediated immunity. *Transplantation* 9, 219 (1970).
8. M.A. Bean, H. Pees, G. Rosen and H.F. Oettgen, Prelabeling target cells with ^{3}H-proline as a method for studying lymphocyte cytotoxicity. *Nat. Cancer Inst. Monograph* 37, 41 (1973).
9. F. Plata, E. Gomard, J.-C. Leclerc and J.-P. Levy, Comparative *in vitro* studies on effector cell diversity in the cellular immune response to murine sarcoma virus (MSV)-induced tumors in mice. *J. Immunol.* 112, 1477 (1974).

10. D.M. Vasudevan, K.T. Brunner and J.-C. Cerottini, Detection of cytotoxic T lymphocytes in the EL4 mouse leukemia system: increased activity of immune spleen and peritoneal cells following preincubation and cell fractionation procedures. *Int. J. Cancer*, **14**, 301 (1974).
11. F. Plata, J.-C. Cerottini and K.T. Brunner, Primary and secondary in vitro generation of cytolytic T lymphocytes in the murine sarcoma virus system. *Eur. J. Immunol.* **5**, 227 (1975).
12. J.-C. Cerottini, H.R. Macdonald, H.D. Engers and K.T. Brunner, Differentiation pathway of cytolytic T lymphocytes: *in vitro* and *in vivo* studies. In: *Progress in Immunology II*, edited by L. Brent and J. Holborow, Vol. 3, p. 153. North-Holland, Amsterdam, 1974.
13. C. O'Toole, V. Stejskal, P. Perlmann and M. Karlsson, Lymphoid cells mediating tumor specific cytotoxicity to carcinoma of the urinary bladder. Separation of the effector population using a surface marker. Manuscript submitted for publication.
14. E.B. Rosenberg, J.L. McCoy, S.S. Green, F.C. Donnelly, D.F. Siwarski, P.H. Levine and R.B. Herberman, Destruction of human lymphoid tissue culture cell lines by human peripheral lymphocytes in ^{51}Cr-release cellular cytotoxicity assays. *J. Nat. Cancer Inst.* **52**, 345 (1974).
15. R.B. Herberman, C.C. Ting, H. Kirchner, H.T. Holden, M. Glaser, G.D. Bonnard and D. Lavrin, Effector mechanisms in tumor immunity. *Proc. 9th Int. Cancer Congress*, edited by P. Bucalossi, U. Veronesi and N. Cascinelli, Vol. 1, p. 258. Excerpta Medica, Amsterdam, 1975.
16. R. Kiessling, E. Klein and H. Wigzell, "Natural" killer cells in the mouse. I. Cytotoxic cells with specificity for mouse Moloney leukemia cells. Specificity and distribution according to genotype. *Eur. J. Immunol.* **5**, 112 (1975).
17. R. Kiessling, E. Klein, H. Pross and H. Wigzell, "Natural" killer cells in the mouse. II. Cytotoxic cells with specificity for mouse Moloney leukemia cells. Characteristics of the killer cell. *Eur. J. Immunol.* **5**, 117 (1975).

FUNCTION AND EVALUATION OF HUMAN K-CELLS

I.C.M. MacLENNAN

Nuffield Department of Clinical Medicine,
Radcliffe Infirmary, Oxford OX2 6HE, U.K.

SUMMARY

K-cells are a distinct population of lymphoid cell which can kill target cells by using IgG as a specific sensitizing agent. The lack of glass-adherence and phagocytic properties distinguishes these cells from other cell types showing antibody-dependent cell-mediated cytotoxicity. Other data are presented to show that K-cell development is not thymus dependent and that K-cells are not directly involved in antibody production. The K-cell system is particularly well developed in man and its possible role in human neoplastic diseases is discussed.

INTRODUCTION

There are a number of cell types which can kill target cells by using IgG as a specific sensitizing agent. These include granulocytes [1, 2], macrophages [1, 2] and B-cells [3] as well as K-cells [4–10]. However, K-cells can be clearly distinguished from these other cell types on the basis of physical properties, distribution, sensitivity to agents used in cancer therapy and the target cells which they are able to kill. Some of the evidence which identifies K-cells as a distinct cell type will be given later but at this point it is sufficient to say that they are: non-phagocytic, non-glass adherent cells which have the morphological appearance of lymphocytes but do not show the characteristics of any class of immunologically competent cell. K-cells can kill a wide range of nucleated target cells but are unable to kill certain targets such as human erythrocytes which are vulnerable to lysis by phagocytic cells (Table 1).

Clearly the possibility of this activity being directed against tumor associated antigens in man is a cause for interest by oncologists. For, this interesting possibility would apply not only to direct patient resistance to tumours but also to the use of passively transferred antibodies. As yet these are no more than interesting possibilities. However, interest in K-cells in the field of cancer treatment may extend to infections occurring in association with combination therapy [11]. Some information without precise effector cell characterization is now available to show that cell-mediated damage to herpes virus-infected cells can be specifically induced by antiviral antibody [12] and that damage to parasites may be caused by leukocytes and specific antibody [13].

Table 1. *Effector Cells Active in Different Antibody-sensitized Target Cell Systems*

Target	Antibody	References
Predominant K-cell activity		
Chang cells	Human, rabbit	4, 7
Human lymphoblastoid line	Human	10
Human peripheral blood lymphocytes	Human	6, 9
DBA2 mastocytoma	Rabbit	2
Mixed K-cell monocyte and B-cell		
Chicken red blood cell	Rabbit	2, 5, 8
Monocyte and neutrophil		
Human group A red cells	Human	1, 2

QUANTITATION OF CYTOTOXIC CELLS

Accurate quantitation of K-cell activity is essential if studies are to be made of the nature of K-cells, their numbers and the effect treatment has on them. Firstly, a target cell should be used which is more or less exclusively damaged by K-cells when antibody is added and not by monocytes or granulocytes (Table 1).

The most convenient, accurate way for quantitation is by measuring the number of lymphoid cells required to kill a fixed number of target cells under standard culture conditions. The actual number of target cells used must be stated, as different absolute numbers in the same lymphocyte to target cell ratio can give markedly different results [10]. In our laboratory we have measured K-cell activity using Chang cells as a target [4, 7]. The Chang cells are labelled with ^{51}Cr chromate and the release of the isotope is

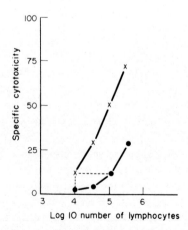

Fig. 1. Cytotoxicity against 10^4 ^{51}Cr labelled Chang cells, mediated by different numbers of human peripheral blood lymphocytes; X————X in the presence of 1:10,000 rabbit anti-Chang antibody, •————• in culture medium alone. The dotted lines indicate that 10^5 lymphocytes produce a spontaneous cytotoxic effect equal to the effect produced by 10^4 lymphocytes in the presence of antibody. Full explanation of the correction for spontaneous cytotoxicity is given in the text.

a measure of number of target cells lysed. Percent specific cytotoxicity is calculated taking the difference between spontaneous ^{51}Cr release and maximum release to be 100%. Figure 1 shows a typical experiment where 10^4 Chang cells, with and without sensitizing antibody, are exposed to different numbers of human peripheral blood lymphocytes. It will be seen that there is cytotoxicity even in the absence of antibody. The mechanism of this spontaneous cytotoxicity is not known; however, it can be blocked with aggregated IgG [4, 14]. The cells responsible for spontaneous cytotoxicity are not separable in our hands from K-cells by physical means. However, spontaneous cytotoxicity may not be due to K-cells, for it can vary independently of antibody-induced cytotoxic activity.

Spontaneous cytotoxicity occurs against many cell types [4] and is undoubtedly responsible for some of the cytotoxic effect seen against tumour cells cultured with human lymphocytes [15, 16]. K-cell assays can be performed on cell lines which are not susceptible to spontaneous cytotoxicity in the presence of human lymphocytes. We have found this applies to the mouse lymphoma line AKR–A. The P815 DBA$_2$ mastocytoma has similar resistance to spontaneous lysis [2]. The contribution of spontaneous cytotoxicity to the K-cell lysis is usually small. For example, in Fig. 1 the spontaneous cytotoxicity when 10^5 lymphoid cells are added is equal to that produced by 10^4 cells in the presence of antibody. In other words, if spontaneous cytotoxicity was mediated by cells other than K-cells, then the number of K-cells required to produce 50% lysis would be $10^4 + 10^5$ and not 10^5. Obviously if spontaneous cytotoxicity is mediated by K-cells then no correction should be made.

Under the conditions of the experiment shown in Fig. 1 increase in cytotoxicity is sigmoid with log increase in the number of lymphocytes added. By constructing a standard curve one can estimate the number of lymphocytes which would be required to produce 50% target cell lysis by extrapolation from a single point. The details of this have been reported previously [7, 17]. We have called the $\log^{10}$ number of lymphoid cells which are required to produce 50% lysis of target cells, SC_{50}. SC_{50}, therefore, increases inversely in relation to K-cell activity. By subtracting SC_{50} from the log number of peripheral blood lymphocytes per ml of blood we obtain a measure of cytotoxic capacity of 1 ml of blood. More recently we have found that K-cell activity can be measured using whole blood [18]. In this case $100\,\mu l$ of blood is added to 10^4 Chang cells in 1 ml of culture. This method gives essentially the same result as that obtained with purified lymphocytes providing there is no serum inhibitory factor such as immune complex [19, 20]. In this case the activity is that of a given volume of blood. As before cytotoxicity follows a sigmoid distribution with log increase in blood volume added. The percentage specific cytotoxicity p can be linearized using the calculation: $\log [p/(1-p)]$.

One source of error in this sort of assay is that some cells may act as inhibitors of K-cell cytotoxicity. This is particularly apparent when large numbers of leukocytes are added to cultures. If these inhibitory cells are removed cytotoxicity will increase to a greater extent than would be anticipated by the enrichment of effector cells as the result of neutral cell removal. Figure 2 gives an example of increased cytotoxicity where inhibitory cells are removed. In comparison Fig. 3 shows a 3-fold difference in cytotoxic activity of two different lymphocyte preparations, not showing inhibitory activity. Some inhibitory cell activity is removable by adherence columns which extract granulocytes, macrophages and B-cells. Presumably these cells can compete with K-cells

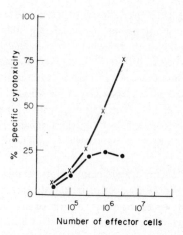

Fig. 2. Cytotoxic effect of rat peritoneal exudate cells on 2×10^4 ^{51}Cr labelled Chang cells in the presence of rat anti-Chang antibody: ×————× after separation of glass-adherent cells; ●———● before separation of glass-adherent cells. This experiment shows that increase in cytotoxicity cannot always be explained by enrichment of K-cells but sometimes, as in this case, by removal of inhibitory cells.

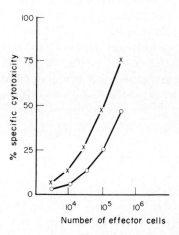

Fig. 3. Cytotoxic activity of human peripheral blood lymphocytes from two donors, ×————× (a) and ●———● (b), towards antibody-sensitized Chang cells. Donor (a) has 3 times as much K-cell activity per unit number of lymphocytes as donor (b). The SC_{50} of (a) is 5.0, that of (b) is 4.5. SC_{50} is the $\log_{10}$ number of lymphocytes required to produce 50% lysis of 10^4 sensitized target cells in 20-hr culture.

for Fc on target cells even though they are not, in themselves, cytotoxic against the target cell. Red cells produce relatively little inhibition of K-cell activity. Under the culture conditions used in our laboratory [17, 18] little or no inhibition occurs when fewer than 10^5 human peripheral blood lymphocytes or 100 μl of whole blood is used. These quantities for healthy controls are near the mean required to produce 50% specific cytotoxicity in 20-hr cultures using 10^4 Chang cells, sensitized with 1:10,000 rabbit anti-Chang antibody.

NATURE OF K-CELLS AND THEIR DISSOCIATION FROM OTHER LEUKOCYTES

Some of the main physical properties of K-cells are listed in Table 2. The property which most easily enables K-cells to be separated from other cells which show antibody dependent cytotoxic activity is that of glass and plastic adherence [1, 2, 5, 6, 7, 10].

Table 2. *Physical Properties of K-cells*

Intermediate-sized lymphocytes
Non-adherent to glass or plastic
Non-phagocytic
Have receptors for Fc of IgG
Probably do not rosette with sheep red cells

Nylon fibre columns which effectively remove B-cells enrich K-cell activity. K-cells can also be dissociated from immunoglobulin bearing cells by the use of immunoabsorbant columns. For instance, in one representative experiment, rat splenic lymphocytes were incubated with ^{125}I rabbit-F(ab$'$)$_2$ anti-rat Fab. Forty-three per cent of the cells were shown to have surface immunoglobulin by autoradiography. When this preparation was passed down a degalan bead column coated with horse anti-rabbit immunoglobulin only 4% of the cells in the effluent had surface immunoglobulin. However, the number of splenic lymphocytes in the pre- and post-column samples required to produce 50% lysis of 2×10^4 sensitized Chang cells with rabbit antibody fell from 1,020,000 to 700,000. This shows that most B-cells but no K-cells had been removed (A. Williams and I. MacLennan, unpublished experiments). The presence of F(ab$'$)$_2$ anti-Fab did not in itself effect cytotoxicity. Whole rabbit anti-rat immunoglobulin does block K-cell activity presumably by forming competitive complexes on B-cell surfaces as described by Halloran and Festenstein [21]. Dissociation of K-cell activity from antibody production has been shown in a number of cases of hypogammaglobulinaemia who have normal K-cell function.

Immunoabsorbent columns which remove cells with Fc receptors can totally remove K-cell activity from human blood lymphocytes. As nearly all the cells passing through such columns are E rosetting cells it may be concluded that most T-cells do not have K-cell activity. Removal of E rosetting cells by gradient centrifugation also fails to deplete K-cell activity (C. Waller and I. MacLennan, unpublished results). Other less direct evidence suggests that at least the majority of T-cells do not have K-cell activity. This includes the fact that K-cell activity is very low in thoracic duct lymph [22, 23], indicating that K-cells are not part of the recirculating pool of lymphocytes. Dissociation of K-cell activity and T-cell numbers is seen following X irradiation. Both populations are similarly depleted during irradiation but K-cell activity returns to normal levels within weeks, while a proportion of T-cells returns very slowly if at all [24, 25]. This only tells us that some of the long-lived T-cells are not K-cells for a proportion of E rosetting and PHA responsive cells return rapidly following irradiation. Similar dissociations are seen after prolonged treatment with azathioprine where there is marked selective loss of K-cells with relatively little effect on circulating immunoglobulin staining cell numbers and PHA responsiveness [26].

The redistribution of different leukocyte types during prednisolone therapy shows particularly interesting dissociations. Neutrophil counts rise markedly as the result of mobilization from the bone marrow and prolongation of blood transit time. The proportion of immunoglobulin staining cells in the blood also rises. K-cell activity is unchanged or slightly depressed while T-cell numbers are grossly reduced [27]. These steroid effects are largely if not entirely temporary for they reverse within a few days even if treatment is continued. Experimental depletion of T-cells with retention of K-cell activity in animals has provided more complete evidence to show that K-cells are not a minority T-cell population [24, 28].

Elegant experiments with transformed human lymphocytes by Trinchieri and his colleagues [10] have shown that while K-cell survival *in vitro* is enhanced by cultures stimulated with allogeneic lymphoid cells, K-cell activity is not found in transformed blasts but remains in the intermediate lymphocyte fraction on size separation. These data tend to argue against the possibility that T-blasts, which may have Fc receptors, can mimic K-cell activity.

The data presented above clearly indicate K-cells to be an independent cell type, whose range of cytotoxic activity is different from that of other cells with cytotoxic potential. The K-cell system seems to be particularly well developed in man, both as regards range of cells that can be killed and the number of K-cells present. Human blood lymphocytes, for example, have approximately 10 times as much cytotoxic activity towards antibody sensitized Chang cells as an equal number of rat spleen cells [29]. It is striking that H_2 differences of mice have only occasionally been shown to induce weak K-cell cytotoxicity, while the HLA differences induce strong and consistent K-cell cytotoxicity in man [30]. The possibility that this system could be important in rejection of human neoplastic cells exists and this possibility is not so remote that we should ignore the chance of using K-cells to therapeutic advantage.

REFERENCES

1. G. Holm, Lysis of antibody treated human erythrocytes by human leukocytes and macrophages in tissue culture. *Int. Arch. Allergy*, **43**, 671 (1972).
2. H.R. Macdonald, A.D. Bonnar, B. Sordat and S.A. Zawodnik, Antibody-dependent cell; mediated cytotoxicity. Heterogeneity of effector cells in human peripheral blood. *Scand. J. Immunol.* (in press).
3. L. Chess, R.P. McDermott, P.M. Sondel and S.F. Schlossman, Isolation and characterisation of cells involved in human cellular hypersensitivity. *Progress in Immunology II*, **3**, 125 (1974).
4. I.C.M. MacLennan, G. Loewi and A. Howard, A human serum immunoglobulin with specificity for certain homologous target cells which induces target cell damage by normal human lymphocytes. *Immunology*, **17**, 887 (1969).
5. P. Perlmann and H. Perlmann, Contactual lysis of antibody-coated chicken-erythrocytes by purified lymphocytes. *Cell. Immunol.* **1**, 300 (1970).
6. J.R. Wunderlich, E.B. Rosenberg and J.M. Connolly, Human lymphocyte-dependent cytotoxic antibody and mechanisms of target cell destruction *in vitro. Progress in Immunology I*, 473 (1971).
7. I.C.M. MacLennan, Antibody in the induction and inhibition of lymphocyte cytotoxicity. *Transpl. Rev.* **13**, 67 (1972).
8. P. Perlmann, H. Perlmann and H. Wigzell, Lymphocyte mediated cytotoxicity *in vitro.* Induction and inhibition by humoral antibody and nature of effector cells. *Transpl. Rev.* **13**, 91 (1972).
9. G. Trinchieri, M. De Marchi, W. May, N. Savi and R. Ceppellini, Lymphocyte antibody lymphocytolytic interaction (LALI) with special emphasis on HL-A. *Transpl. Proc.* **5**, 1631 (1973).

10. G. Trinchieri, P. Baumann, M. De Marchi and Z. Tokes, Effector cell of antibody-dependent cell-mediated cytotoxicity. *J. Immunol.* (in press).
11. J.V. Simone, E. Holland and W. Johnson, Fatalities during remission of childhood leukaemia. *Blood,* **39,** 759 (1972).
12. B. Rager-Zisman and B. Bloom, Immunological destruction of Herpes Simplex virus I infection. *Nature,* **251,** 542 (1974).
13. A.E. Butterworth, R.F. Sturrock, V. Houba and P.H. Rees, Antibody-dependent cell-mediated damage to Schistosomula *in vitro. Nature,* **252,** 503 (1974).
14. I.C.M. MacLennan, The cytotoxic effect of lymphocytes on cells in tissue culture: a study in relation to inflammatory joint disease. University of London Thesis 1970.
15. J. Parie-Fisher, F.M. Kourilsky, F. Picard, P. Banzer and A. Puissant, Cytotoxicity of lymphocytes from healthy subjects and melanoma patients against cultured melanoma cells. *Clin. Exp. Immunol.* (in press).
16. M. Takasugi, H. Lynch and P.I. Terasaki, Histocompatibility and immune responsiveness in human cancer, *XIth International Cancer Congress Abstracts,* p. 390 (1974).
17. D.G. Gale and I.C.M. MacLellan, A method for measuring antibody and phytohaemagglutin-induced lymphocyte-dependent cytotoxicity using whole blood. *Clin. Exp. Immunol.* (submitted).
18. A.C. Campbell, Catherine Waller, Janet Wood, A. Aynsley-Green and V. Yu, Lymphocyte subpopulations in the blood of newborn infants. *Clin. Exp. Immunol.* **18,** 469 (1974).
19. I.C.M. MacLennan, Competition for receptors for immunoglobulin on cytotoxic lymphocytes, *Clin. Exp. Immunol.* **10,** 275 (1972).
20. D.P. Jewell and I.C.M. MacLennan, Circulating immune complexes in inflammatory bowel disease. *Clin. Exp. Immunol.* **14,** 219 (1973).
21. P. Halloran and H. Festenstein, Inhibition of cell dependent cytotoxicity as an assay for mouse allo-antibody. *Nature,* **250,** 52 (1974).
22. I.C.M. MacLennan and B. Harding, Failure of certain cytotoxic lymphocytes to respond mitotically to phytohaemagglutinin. *Nature,* **227,** 5264 (1970).
23. G. Holm, C. Frankson, A.C. Campbell and I.C.M. MacLennan, The cytotoxic activity of lymphocytes from human lymph *in vitro. Clin. Exp. Immunol.* **17,** 361 (1974).
24. B. Harding, D.J. Fudifin, F. Gotch and I.C.M. MacLennan, Cytotoxic lymphocytes from rats depleted of thymus processed cells. *Nature (New Biology),* **232,** 80 (1971).
25. A.C. Campbell, G. Wiernik, J. Wood, P. Hersy, C.A. Waller and I.C.M. MacLellan, Characteristics of lymphopenia induced by radiotherapy. *Clin. Exp. Immunol.* (submitted).
26. A.C. Campbell, J.M. Skinner, P. Hersy, P. Roberts-Thomson, I.C.M. MacLellan and S.C. Truelove, Immunosuppression in the treatment of inflammatory bowel disease. I. Changes in lymphoid sub-populations in the blood and rectal mucosa following cessation of treatment with azathioprine. *Clin. Exp. Immunol.* **16,** 521 (1974).
27. A.C. Campbell, J. Skinner, C.A. Waller, S. Truelove and I.C.M. MacLennan (in preparation).
28. J.A. Van Boxel, J.D. Stobo, W.E. Paul and I. Gren, Antibody dependent lymphoid cell-mediated cytotoxicity: no requirement for thymus derived lymphocytes. *Science,* **175,** 194 (1972).
29. I.C.M. MacLellan, Cytotoxic cells. In: *Contemporary Topics in Immunology,* edited by A.J.S. Davies and R.L. Carter, Vol. 2, p. 175, Plenum Press, New York–London, 1974.
30. P. Hersy, Phillipa Cullen and I.C.M. MacLellan, Lymphocyte-dependent cytotoxic antibody activity against human transplantation antigens. *Transplantation,* **16,** 9 (1973).

LYMPHOCYTE STIMULATION TEST FOR DETECTION OF TUMOR SPECIFIC REACTIVITY IN HUMANS

F. VÁNKY,*† E. KLEIN* and J. STJERNSWÄRD‡

Several methods have been devised to ascertain whether tumor specific immune response occurs in tumor-bearing hosts. Application of these for humans still involves considerable problems. In the majority of the published work attention is mainly focused on the cellular response, as cellular immunity is known to be the main instrument in graft rejection. The presence of antibodies may even be — at least in certain stages — adverse for the host—tumor interaction. The demonstration of antibodies, however, is indicative for the immune response and therefore should not be neglected. There are only a few studies in which tumor specific antibodies in humans are demonstrated. On the other hand, serum factors which can block lymphocyte mediated effects have been documented in several human tumor systems [1–9].

Autologous tumor biopsy cells have been found to stimulate *in vitro* the DNA synthesis of lymphocytes (ATS = autologous tumor stimulation) [7–13]. In our studies, the majority of such tests have been performed on patients with sarcomas, but astrocytomas, chordomas and carcinomas have also been studied.

Sixty of 197 tumors induced statistically significant blastogenesis. The frequency varied, depending upon the tumor group tested. Thirty-nine of the 117 sarcomas, 12 of 39 carcinomas and 9 of 38 brain tumor cases were stimulatory. None of the three myelomas showed the effect.

While the phenomenon may indicate an immunological recognition of the tumor cells, its significance for the *in vivo* situation is unknown.

METHODOLOGICAL CONSIDERATIONS

The advantage of the test is that biopsy material can be used and therefore the antigen source is not subjected to the modification and selective conditions of tissue culture. Its main disadvantage is the variability of the quality and the quantitative limitation of the tumor cell suspension obtained from solid tumor biopsies. Cell viability can vary between 10–90%. The quality of cell suspension was improved in later studies by sedimentation through fetal calf serum for 30 min at 37°C. In this way

*Department of Tumor Biology, Karolinska Institutet, S-104 01 Stockholm 60, Sweden.
†Radiumhemmet, Karolinska Hospital, S-104 01 Stockholm 60, Sweden.
‡Ludwig Institute for Cancer Research (Lausanne Branch), Swiss Institute for Experimental Cancer Research, 1005 Lausanne, Switzerland.

the sediment usually contained more than 50% viable cells. The number of cases which we studied with this type of cell suspension is low and simultaneous tests are necessary to ascertain whether the test results are improved.

Table 1. *Experimental Protocol of a Lymphocyte Stimulation Test Performed with an Osteosarcoma Patient*[a]

Stimulators (MMC-treated)	Cell number	cpm ± SD[b]		RI[c]
–		863 ± 18		
Identical lymphocytes	10^6	897 ± 57	(227 ± 21)	1.00
Autologous tumor cells	10^5	626 ± 28	(115 ± 30)	0.69
Autologous tumor cells	5×10^5	3394 ± 310		3.78**
Autologous tumor cells	10^6	11084 ± 139	(150 ± 13)	12.35**
Autologous tumor cells	5×10^6	7758 ± 351	(538 ± 42)	8.64**
Autologous tumor cells	10^7	2779 ± 513		3.09*
Autologous muscle cells	10^5	512 ± 37	(327 ± 17)	0.57*
Autologous muscle cells	5×10^5	664 ± 58		0.74*
Autologous muscle cells	10^6	844 ± 113	(390 ± 29)	0.94
Autologous muscle cells	5×10^6	1293 ± 307	(818 ± 113)	1.45
Allogeneic lymphocytes	10^6	72972 ± 1147	(227 ± 20)	81.35**
PHA [1]/1000		97874 ± 3027		113.43**

[a] 10^6 responder lymphocytes/culture, culture volume 2 ml.
[b] Values of cpm without responder lymphocytes are given in parentheses.
[c] RI significance $p < 0.001$ **; $p < 0.005$ *.

Meaningful evaluation of the test is only possible if adequate negative and positive controls are introduced. Among other factors cell concentration is known to influence the DNA synthesis of lymphocytes *in vitro* (crowding effect). Therefore with each lymphocyte suspension we use to set up the following cultures in triplicate: lymphocytes admixed to mitomycin treated identical lymphocytes (as control for the cell concentration), and to suspensions of normal tissues (if possible); as positive controls, PHA stimulation (with 1/1000 dilution) and confrontation with allogeneic lymphocytes serve. Each stimulator cell suspension is controlled for incorporation of ^{3}H-thymidine. The details of our procedure are given in the original publications [7, 8]. An example for the experimental protocol is given in Table 1.

The experiments are evaluated by calculating a reactivity index which is the ratio between the isotope uptake (cpm) in the test sample and the isotope uptake in the control samples where identical MMC-treated lymphocytes were added.

$$RI = \frac{(Lymphocytes + "X" \ stimulator_m) - ("X" \ stimulator_m)}{(Lymphocytes + "X" \ identical \ lymphocytes_m) - ("X" \ identical \ lymphocytes_m)},$$

"X" = number of cells,

m = MMC-treated.

By introducing the reactivity index, comparison of different experiments is possible. However, for judging the conditions of test, net cpm values have also to be considered.

When the ^{3}H incorporation in the presence of stimulator tumor cells is increased by at least 100%, the test is considered positive. Thus, RI $\geqslant$ 2.0 is regarded as a positive ATS.

REPRODUCIBILITY

In order to perform repeat tests it is necessary to store the biopsy material. We have compared therefore the stimulatory effect of fresh and frozen-and-thawed biopsies in twenty-six cases.

The tumor suspensions were frozen in 3 parts MEM glucose − 20% glucose in Eagle's minimum essential medium − and 2 parts DMSO. Three parts of a suspension containing 10×10^6 tumor cells in 1 ml of heat inactivated human AB+ serum was carefully mixed with 1 part of the DMSO solution at 4°C, distributed in Dram screw-cap vials (size 11.5×36.5). The vials were kept at 0°C for at least 1 hr followed by 1 hr at −80°C. Thereafter they were stored in liquid nitrogen.

For use the vials were thawed by agitation in 42°C water bath. The cells were transferred to a 16×100-mm centrifuge tube, kept on ice. Five ml MEM with 10% human AB+ serum was added and the cells were sedimented at 400 g for 15 min. The pellet was resuspended in MEM + 10% human serum and the viability and cell number assessed. The proportion of viable cells showed only minor changes (1−5%) compared to the original suspension. With eight of ten tumors, the stimulating property of biopsy cells was retained after freezing. Sixteen biopsies were not stimulatory and thirteen remained so after freezing. The correspondence was thus fairly good and we can conclude that frozen biopsy material can be used in the test.

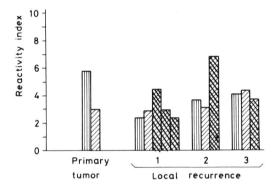

Fig. 1. Comparison of ATS from repeated biopsies with fresh and frozen tumor suspensions. At each occasion fresh (▥) and frozen−thawed (▨) cells were used as stimulator. The frozen material from the recurrences was tested also after storage (▩) with lymphocytes sampled later in tumor-free periods.

In a few cases we could perform repeat tests both with fresh and frozen cell suspensions as the tumor recurred. An example of this is given in Fig. 1. Fresh and frozen osteosarcoma cells from the primary tumor and three recurrencies were used as stimulators for the autologous lymphocytes, both at the time when the tumors were biopsied and also during tumor-free periods. On all occasions the test was positive though it varied somewhat in strength. We do not contribute to this variation biological significance, as according to our experience the ATS can only be judged qualitatively.

DOSE−RESPONSE RELATIONSHIPS

In vitro stimulation of lymphocytes by allogeneic lymphocytes, soluble HL−A antigens, bacteria, viruses shows an antigen concentration dependent optimum [14–18].

Similar dose–response relationship was seen in the ATS system. In several experiments, increasing numbers of tumor or non-malignant cells were admixed to a constant number of lymphocytes. Figure 2 demonstrates the results for twelve tumors, including both sarcomas, astrocytomas and carcinomas. In ten cases, non-malignant cells from the same tissue compartment could be included. The optimal ATS has been found at approximate lymphocyte:tumor cell ratios 1:1 and 2:1 – one fibroliposarcoma (no. 120) had an optimal ratio at 1:10. In none of these tests did non-malignant cells stimulate to a RI above 2.0. Three negative cases are also shown (tumors 124, 348, and 123).

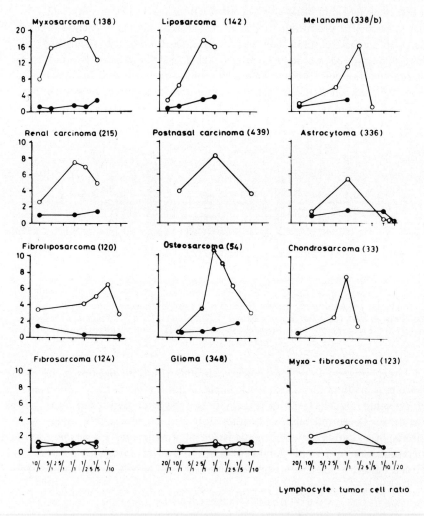

Fig. 2. ATS at different lymphocyte–tumor cell ratios. o—o = Lymphocytes + tumor cells; •—• = Lymphocytes + non-malignant cells, of non-lymphoid tissue origin.

THE STRENGTH OF REACTIVITY AND THE FREQUENCY OF ATS POSITIVE HUMAN TUMORS

The distribution of RI values obtained with eighty-five tumors and fifty-one normal tissue biopsies is shown in Fig. 3 and Fig. 4.

Non-malignant tissue stimulated only in three of fifty-one cases. In two of the

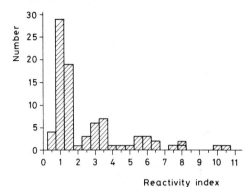

Fig. 3. Lymphocyte stimulation by tumor biopsies.

Tumor type	No. positive / No. tested
Sarcoma[a]	20/44
Astrocytoma	6/29
Carcinoma[b]	5/9
Myeloma	0/3

[a] Sarcomas = osteo-, chondro-, fibro-, lipo-, neurofibro-, synovial-, reticulum-cell-sarcoma and melanoma.

[b] Mammary-, thyroid-, liver- and kidney-carcinomas.

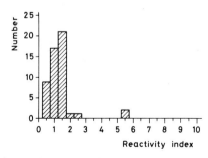

Fig. 4. Lymphocyte stimulation by non-malignant tissue.

Tissue of origin	No. positive / No. tested
Brain	2/23
Connective tissue	0/13
Muscle	0/10
Cartilage (homogenized)	1/3
Thyroid	0/1
Kidney	0/1

cases, the normal tissue was taken from brain tumor patients. One of the two patients had an astrocytoma, where contamination with tumor cells could not be excluded.

The frequency of ATS positive cases varied between different tumor categories. Summarizing the sarcomas, twenty out of forty-four (45%) were positive, while brain tumors stimulated less frequently (21%).

The reactivity is usually rather weak though in two cases the increase of ^{3}H thymidine incorporation was 10-fold.

USE OF SOLID TUMOR EXTRACTS AS ANTIGEN

Soluble tumor extracts have been used as antigens [18, 19] both in humans and in animal systems. We have tested tumor-bearing patients for skin responses to their own tumor extract in parallel with ATS using both the extract and the suspension of biopsy tissue [20]. The extracts were prepared with 3MKCL. A good correlation was found both when the stimulatory effect of the biopsy cells and extract were compared and also when the *in vitro* tests were compared with the outcome of the skin tests (Fig. 5 and Table 2).

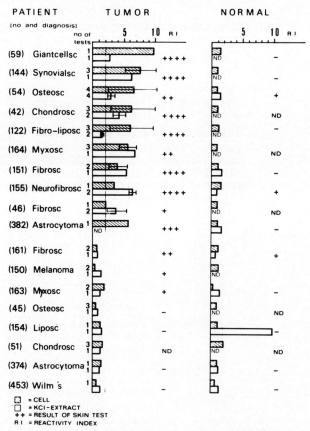

Fig. 5. Lymphocyte stimulation by autologous human tumor cells and KCl extracts and skin tests with KCl extracts. Reactivity indices obtained with tumor and non-malignant tissue using 10^6 lymphocytes and 10^6 stimulator cells or 100–200 μg/ml protein concentration of the KCl extract. Where several tests were performed the standard deviation is indicated.

Similarly to the experiments with biopsy tissue the dose–response curve showed that the KCL extract induced optimal blastogenesis with a certain concentration, beyond which the activity declined (Fig. 6).

Table 2. *Cellular Immunity Against Autochthonous Tumors: Comparison Between* in vivo *and* in vitro *Reactivity*

		KCl-extracts					
		Lymphocyte stimulation			Skin test		
		Pos.	Neg.	N.D.[a]	Pos.	Neg.	N.D.
Tumor cells							
Lymphocyte stimulation	Pos. 10	8	1	1	10	–	–
	Neg. 8	–	8	–	3	4	1
	N.D. 2	–	2	–	–	2	–
Non-malignant tissue cells							
Lymphocyte stimulation	Pos. 1	–	–	1	–	–	1
	Neg. 17	1	8	8	3	9	5
	N.D. 2	–	1	1	–	1	1

[a] N.D. = not done.

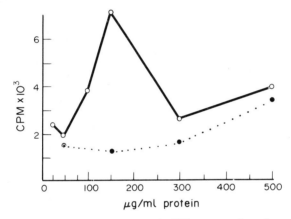

Fig. 6. Dose-dependence of lymphocyte stimulation by KCl extracts of autologous tumor (○) and non-malignant (●) tissue biopsy cells; 10^6 lymphocytes were confronted with different concentrations of KCl extracts.

THE EFFECT OF AUTOLOGOUS SERUM IN THE ATS SYSTEM

Early in the investigation of the autologous tumor cell stimulation the influence of the patients' own serum was included. It was found that if the stimulator biopsy cells were preincubated in autologous serum and then washed prior to the test, their stimulatory capacity was decreased or abolished. Two series of experiments were published from our laboratory, including fifteen tumor cases [7, 8]. With one patient, the ATS test could be repeated 9 times. Preincubation of the stimulator cells with autologous serum invariably reduced the reactivity index by more than 50%. Apart from autologous sera from non-tumor patients (fractures, etc.), sera from patients with the same and other histological type of tumors were also tested for detection of possible cross-reactivity. Among four sera from patients with sarcomas, two were inhibitory (in repeat tests), while sera from carcinoma patients or healthy sera did not reduce the RI.

Except for one patient, all ATS were inhibited by autologous serum. Fourteen of the twenty-five sarcoma sera inhibited in at least one allogeneic ATS test (Table 3), indicating a certain degree of cross-reactivity. Preincubation with control sera inhibited only in five out of the thirty-three tests.

Table 3. *Preincubation of the Stimulated Cells with Autologous and Allogeneic Sarcoma Sera*

Serum donor[a]		ATS system, patient										Inhibitory sera in at least one ATS system
Patient no.	Diagnosis	120	122	116	103	10	13	20	23	29	123[b]	
120	Lipo-fibro-sc	*9/9[c]*					3/3				0/2	
122	Fibro-sc		*2/2*							0/1	0/1	
116	Neurofibro-sc	2/2		*2/2*								
103	Neurofibro-sc		1/1		*2/2*							
10	Lipo-sc	0/1				*0/1*						
13	Chondro-sc	0/2					*4/4*					6/12
20	Chondro-sc						1/1	*1/1*				
23	Chondro-sc	0/1							*0/1*			
29	Osteo-sc									*1/1*		
101	Synovial-sc							1/1				
106	Fibro-sc	1/1									0/1	
108	Myxo-sc	1/1				0/1					0/1	
119	Fibro-sc	0/1								0/1		
121	Fibro-sc	1/1								1/1		
28	Fibro-sc	1/2										
3	Osteo-sc	1/1										
4	Osteo-sc											
6	Osteo-sc									1/1		8/13
25	Osteo-sc	0/2								1/1		
22	Chondro-sc		1/1									
27	Chondro-sc											
18	Lipo-sc	2/2										
113	Neurofibro-sc	1/1	0/1									
8	Myxo-fibro-sc									1/1		
117	Synovial-sc										0/1	

(a) Patients 120–108 and ATS pos. tests; patients 119–117 were ATS neg.
(b) Myxosarcoma.
(c) Number of tests in which the serum inhibited ATS/number of tests performed. Tests with autologous serum in italic figures.

The nature of the inhibition is not known. The fact that inhibition occurred when the stimulator tumor cells were incubated and washed prior to the test may indicate that antibodies could be involved.

In a third series, the question was investigated whether the inhibition is specific for ATS. Therefore, parallel with the ATS test, MLC and PHA stimulation were performed in the presence of allogeneic and autologous serum with thirty patients. In these tests the sera were present through the entire culture period [21].

Evaluation of these experiments is complicated by the possible effect of the autologous serum of the control value, i.e. incorporation when identical lymphocytes were admixed. The details of two experiments are given in Tables 4 and 5. For patient no. 122 (Table 4) this control value is lower in the autologous serum. This leads to a higher RI for MLC in the autologous serum in spite of the decreased net cpm. The rather strong ATS effect disappeared in the autologous serum. However, whether this is due to a specific effect on ATS cannot be decided as the net cpm's were lower also to the MLC and PHA test. In other cases, like patient no. 165, the results are more easily interpreted as the control value did not change in the same direction (Table 5), and this effect on

Table 4. *Lymphocyte Stimulation in Allogeneic and Autologous Serum (Patient 122)*

	Allogeneic control		Autologous	
	cpm	(RI)	cpm	(RI)
IL[(a)]	1424		707	
PHA	257678	(181)	82397	(116)
MLC	126833	(101)	103986	(147)
ATS	15043	(11)	1214	(2)

[(a)] IL = identical lymphocytes.

Table 5. *Lymphocyte Stimulation in Allogeneic and Autologous Serum (Patient 165)*

	Allogeneic control		Autologous	
	cpm	(RI)	cpm	(RI)
IL[(a)]	1547		1891	
NT[(b)]	1388		1601	(1)
PHA	77342	(50)	117483	(62)
MLC	100678	(65)	113100	(60)
ATS	18957	(12)	8364	(4)

[(a)] IL = identical lymphocytes.
[(b)] NT = non-malignant tissue cells.

ATS may be regarded as specific. Such cases strengthen the finding that the presence of autologous serum specifically inhibits ATS.

Table 6 summarizes the results obtained with thirty cases. The number of cases which show significant differences when samples in the presence of the two types of sera are compared is given. The effect of autologous serum on control values and on the lymphocyte–non-malignant tissue cell mixture was random. The former decreased in 13%

and increased in 7% of the cases. The latter decreased in 15% and increased in 20% of the cases. PHA and allogeneic lymphocyte stimulation were expressed somewhat better in the presence of autologous serum, significant cpm increase was observed in 36, respectively, 24% of the tests, and decrease in 14%, respectively, in 10% of the tests. In the lymphocyte–tumor cell cultures, the cpm values decreased in 50% of the tests and increased in 7%. In this evaluation the new cpm values are compared. Among the thirty cultures, fifteen were ATS positive. The RI values of these fifteen were reduced in five and eight tests became negative. Among the two cases representing the 7% with significantly increased cpm values in autologous serum, only one was ATS positive

Table 6. *The Effect of Autologous Serum on Various Lymphocyte Stimulation Tests*

Test type	Number of cases	Number of cases (%) in which thymidine incorporation in autologous serum was		
		lower	higher	unchanged
		compared with allogeneic control serum[a]		
IL[b]	30	4 (13)	2 (7)	14 (80)
NT[c]	20	4 (20)	3 (15)	13 (65)
PHA	28	4 (14)	10 (36)	14 (50)
MLC	21	2 (10)	5 (24)	14 (66)
ATS	30[d]	15 (50)	2 (7)	13 (43)

[a] The categories are selected on the basis of significant differences between cpm values in allogeneic and autologous serum.
[b] Identical lymphocytes.
[c] Non-malignant tissue biopsy cells.
[d] 15/30 had RI ≥ 2.0, i.e. where ATS pos.

(RI over 2.0); however, with this lymphocyte preparation stronger reponses were seen in the other tests also in autologous serum. When individual tests were carefully evaluated we could select five cases in which only the ATS was inhibited while the effects of other stimulators were either unaffected or enhanced. The opposite constellation — lowering the others but increase or no effect of ATS — has never been observed. Analyzing the overall results and the individual cases, we can confidently conclude that, whatever the mechanism might be, blastogenesis induced by autologous tumor cells is often lower in autologous serum as compared to allogeneic normal serum.

On the basis of this finding one may question the relevance of ATS. If ATS detected in the presence of fetal calf serum [7] or allogeneic control serum [8] represent a real tumor specific phenomenon that is inhibited by autologous serum this tumor–lymphocyte interaction may not occur *in vivo*. The fact still remains, however, that ATS may be indicative for a tumor specific host response. If, on the other hand, the foreign sera are instrumental in bringing about the reactivity of the lymphocytes, the definition of the autologous serum effect as inhibitory could be inadequate. This is unlikely, however, because ATS has been demonstrated both in FCS and several batches of human serum.

TUMOR-BOUND IMMUNOGLOBULIN

If tumor specific immune response is present in the patient, it is conceivable that the tumor cells carry bound antibodies. Immunoglobulins in human biopsies were indeed demonstrated [22, 23]. Presence of Ig—assumed to be bound to the tumor cell surface—was related to the degree of malignancy inasmuch as a high proportion of the histologically and clinically defined high malignant tumors were among the positive ones [23]. This fact led the authors to conclude that the immunoglobulins may represent specific antibodies and their presence may affect the tumor—host relationship in favor of the tumor, possibly through the enhancement mechanism. Similarly, Thunold *et al.* [24] detected IgG in all twenty human tumors tested and their analysis suggested that the Ig is firmly and actively bound to the cells.

We selected a radioiodine labeled antibody elution (RIE) test for immunoglobulin

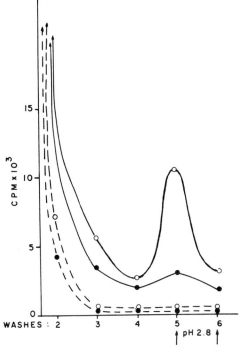

Fig. 7. Radiodine labeled antibody elution (RIE) test with osteosarcoma (○) and muscle (●) biopsy from patient no. 71, reacted with ^{125}I-labeled anti-human IgG and ^{131}I-labeled anti-BSA reagents. [125]I (———) and [131]I (- - - - -) counts in the washing fluids and acid eluates.

detection because its evaluation seems to be independent from non-specific binding of reagent. The method is based on the assumption that specifically bound antibody molecules are not released by washing in the cold at neutral pH but are eluted with low pH treatment at 37°C. Figure 7 gives the details of an experiment performed with an osteosarcoma biopsy.

Two million cells per tube were washed twice with ice-cold PBS, incubated at +4°C for 1 hr with 0.05 ml of the labeled reagents (with activity about 5×10^5 cpm) followed by several washes at room temperature with MEM containing 10% FCS. The radioactivity of each washing fluid is indicated. After four washes, the activity of the washing fluid was low. Then the cells were treated with 0.5 ml of pH 2.8, 0.1 M glycine-HCl buffer for 30 min at 37°C. After centrifugation, the pellet was washed once with the same buffer. The activity of the acid eluates and the residual activity on the cell pellet were measured.

From the cells pretreated with anti-Ig reagent acid treatment releases radioactivity indicating that IgG is present in this biopsy. In the evaluation of the tests the acid eluted counts (AEC) are expressed as a percentage of the total removed activity (present in all the washes except the first and eluates).

Fifty biopsies (derived from forty-four patients) were tested. The results were highly variable. In Fig. 8 the cases are grouped according to the value of AEC, which varied between 0 and 42.4% of the total removed counts. The range for non-malignant tissue in parallel experiments was 0–19%. The mean values were 16.0 for the tumor and 7.0 for the non-malignant cells. Eighteen tumor biopsies were judged as immunoglobulin positive

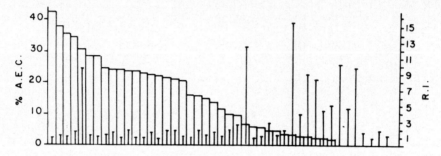

Fig. 8. Binding of anti-Ig reagent and stimulating ability of the tumor biopsies. AEC = Acid eluted counts are expressed as percentage of the total counts removed (excluding the first wash) (□).
RI = Reactivity index (T). Each bar represents one patient.

ones, i.e. after reaction with anti-human IgG conjugate the AEC were higher than 20% of the removed counts. The AEC was higher than 30% for five and between 20 and 30% for thirteen cases. Differentiated tumors were mainly in the group with low or no AEC.

Aliquots of the tumor biopsy suspensions were also tested in the lymphocyte stimulation test. In thirteen of forty-four patients stimulation occurred, with RI varying between 2.0 and 15.5. Among the stimulatory biopsies only one bound the anti-Ig reagent as judged by the AEC (32%). Among the twenty-eight IgG negative tumors, twelve were ATS positive. Summary of the results is given in Table 7.

The results thus indicate the presence of immunoglobulins in a number of tumor biopsies. Correlation was found between the differentiation grade and detectable immunoglobulins in the cell suspension, inasmuch as the differentiated tumors were among those which had no or low amounts of Ig. Otherwise neither the type of the tumor, the quality of the tumor cell suspension as judged by the percentage of viable cells, the clinical history of the case, nor the percentage of infiltrating lymphocytes gave any correlation. Our results correspond well with those reported by Izsak *et al.* [23]. As mentioned

Table 7. *Stimulation of Autologous Lymphocytes Correlated to the Reactivity of the Biopsy with Anti-IgG Reagent*

Ig (AEC)	Lymphocyte stimulation	
	Pos. [a]	Neg.
Pos. [b]	1 (6%)	17 (94%)
Neg.	12 (46%)	14 (54%)

[a] RI higher than 2.0 are considered as positive.
[b] Acid eluted counts higher than 20% of the total removed cpm are considered as positive.

previously in their studies on human tumors, highly malignant ones—as defined by histology and by the clinical history—were among the cases which contained immuno-globulin.

Obviously, the results are not providing evidence for specific antibodies present on the tumor cells. Part of the immunoglobulin detected may be bound to the cell suspension due to the presence of cells with receptors for the FC part of the immunoglobulin molecule.

GENERAL CONCLUSIONS

After an initial enthusiasm concerning the experimental results aimed to prove that tumor specific immune response prevails in tumor patients, objections are raised on the basis of the accumulating data.

The main obstacle in this type of experimentation seems to be that the tumor material is either used as it is collected from the patient—then the quality, purity and possibly modifying factors influence the results, or used after cultivation, then the representativeness and modification of the culture condition may have an effect. On the part of the immune factors, certain compartments of the lymphocyte population may exert non-specific effects on the target cells which might be judged as tumor specific, while in fact they even may blur specific reactions.

The autologous lymphocyte stimulation test was on the scene on the human tumor research since several years. Positive cases were obtained which indicated that the tumor cells may carry antigens which are recognized *in vitro* by the patient's lymphocytes. The effect of serum on the ATS strengthens the possibility that the assay indeed measures a tumor specific response. During the years of our experience, performing the test with solid tumors, it became clear, however, that the test in its present form does not allow to conclude about the clinical condition and prognosis of the patient. Furthermore, it has serious limitations. This is connected mainly with the scarcity of the material and therefore follow up of the patient is only possible in exceptional cases. Much would be gained if a well-defined antigen extract could be used. The amount of blood needed to perform a well-controlled test is high and as the proportion of cases showing a positive ATS is relatively low, many experiments have to be performed blindly when new factors are studied.

The justification of the method lies in its well-defined theoretical basis, the relatively simple procedure which reduces possible artefacts present in other assays.

ACKNOWLEDGEMENTS

The work reported or referred to was supported by the Swedish Cancer Society, and Contract No. NCI-CB-43921-31 with the Division of Cancer Biology and Diagnosis, National Cancer Institute, Department of Health, Education and Welfare.

REFERENCES

1. G.A. Currie and C. Basham, Serum mediated inhibition of the immunological reactions of the patients to his own tumour. A possible role for circulating antigens. *Br. J. Cancer*, **26**, 427 (1972).
2. W.J. Halliday, A. Maluish and W.H. Isbister, Detection of anti-tumor cell-mediated immunity and serum blocking factors in cancer patients by the leukocyte adherence inhibition test. *Br. J. Cancer*, **29**, 31 (1974).

3. I. Hellström, H.O. Sjögren, G. Warner and K.E. Hellström, Blocking of cell-mediated tumor immunity by sera from patient with growing neoplasms. *Int. J. Cancer*, 7, 226 (1971).
4. D.G. Jose and F. Skvaril, Serum inhibitors of cellular immunity in human neuroblastoma. IgG subclass of blocking activity. *Int. J. Cancer*, 13, 173 (1974).
5. M.R. Martin-Chandon, F. Vánky, C. Carnaud and E. Klein, *In vitro* education on autologous human sarcoma generates nonspecific killer cells. *Int. J. Cancer*, 15, 342 (1975).
6. H.O. Sjögren, I. Hellström, S.C. Bansal and K.E. Hellström, Suggestive evidence that the blocking "antibodies" of tumor bearing individuals may be antigen–antibody complexes. *Proc. Nat. Acad. Sci. USA* 68, 1372 (1971).
7. F. Vánky, J. Stjernswärd, G. Klein and U. Nilsonne, Serum-mediated inhibition of lymphocyte stimulation by autochthonous human tumors. *J. Nat. Cancer Inst.* 47, 95 (1971).
8. F. Vánky, J. Stjernswärd, G. Klein, L. Steiner and L. Lindberg, Tumor-associated specificity of serum mediated inhibition of lymphocyte stimulation by autochthonous human tumors. *J. Nat. Cancer Inst.* 51, 25 (1973).
9. J.U. Gutterman, E.M. Hersh, K.B. McCredie *et al.*, Lymphocyte blastogenesis to human leukemia cells and their relationship to serum factors, immunocompetence and prognosis. *Cancer Res.* 32, 2524 (1972).
10. J. Stjernswärd, P. Clifford, S. Singh and E. Svedmyr, Indications of cellular immunological reactions against autochthonous tumor in cancer patients studied *in vitro*. *E. Afr. Med. J.* 45, 484 (1968).
11. F. Vánky and J. Stjernswärd, Tumor distinctive cellular immunity to human sarcoma and carcinoma. *Isr. J. Med. Sci.* 7, 211 (1971).
12. E. Watkins Jr., Y. Ogata, L.L. Anderson, E. Watkins III and M.F. Waters, Activation of host lymphocytes cultured with cancer cells treated with neuraminidase. *Nature (New Biol.)* 231, 83 (1971).
13. G.M. Mavligit, J.U. Gutterman, C.M. McBride and E.M. Hersh, Cell-mediated immunity to human solid tumors. *In vitro* detection by lymphocyte blastogenic response to cell-associated and solubilized tumor antigens. *Nat. Cancer Inst. Monogr.* 37, 167 (1973).
14. D.C. Viza, O. Degani, J. Dausset and D.A.L. Davies, Lymphocyte stimulation by soluble human HL-A transplantation antigens. *Nature*, 219, 709 (1968).
15. D.B. Wilson, Quantitative studies on the mixed lymphocyte interaction in rats. I. Conditions and parameters of response. *J. Exp. Med.* 126, 625 (1967).
16. S.F. Sørensen, V. Andersen and J. Giese, Studies on the quantitation of lymphocyte response *in vitro*. *Acta Path. Microbiol. Scand.* 76, 259 (1969).
17. G.L. Rosenberg, P.A. Farber and A.L. Notkins, *In vitro* stimulation of sensitized lymphocytes by herpes simplex virus and vaccinia virus. *Proc. Nat. Acad. Sci. USA*, 69, 756 (1972).
18. G. Mavligit, J.U. Gutterman, C.M. McBride and E.M. Hersh, Multifaced evaluation of human tumor immunity using a salt extracted colon carcinoma antigen. *Proc. Soc. Exp. Biol. Med.* 140, 1240 (1972).
19. B.H. Littman, M.S. Meltzer, R.P. Cleveland, B. Zbar and H.J. Rapp, Tumor-specific, cell-mediated immunity in guinea pigs with tumors. *J. Nat. Cancer Inst.* 51, 1627 (1973).
20. F. Vánky, E. Klein, J. Stjernswärd and U. Nilsonne, Cellular immunity against tumor-associated antigens in humans: Lymphocyte stimulation and skin reaction. *Int. J. Cancer*, 14, 277 (1974).
21. F. Vánky, E. Klein, J. Stjernswärd and G. Trempe, Human tumor–lymphocyte interaction *in vitro*. Blastogenesis in the presence of autologous or allogeneic serum. Submitted for publication to *Int. J. Cancer*.
22. P.I. Witz, The biological significance of tumor-bound immunoglobulins. In: *Current Topics in Microbiology and Immunology*, Vol. 61, pp. 157, Springer-Verlag, 1973.
23. F.C. Izsak, H.J. Brenner, E. Landes, M. Ran and P.I. Witz, Correlation between clinico-pathological features of malignant tumors and cell surface immunoglobulins. *Isr. J. Med. Sci.* 10, 642 (1974).
24. S. Thunold, O. Tönder and O. Larsen, Immunoglobulins in eluates of malignant human tumors. *Acta Path. Microbiol. Scand. 1973*, Sec. A Suppl., 236, 97 (1973).

THE LEUCOCYTE MIGRATION TECHNIQUE IN STUDIES OF TUMOR-DIRECTED CELLULAR IMMUNITY IN MALIGNANT MELANOMA

ALISTAIR J. COCHRAN, RONA M. MACKIE, CATHERINE E. ROSS,
LINDSAY J. OGG and ALAN M. JACKSON

*University Departments of Pathology and Dermatology, The Western Infirmary,
Glasgow G11 6NT, Great Britain*

INTRODUCTION

We have employed various modifications of the leucocyte migration inhibition technique [1] in studies of tumour-directed cellular immunity in patients with malignant melanoma during the past 5 years. This paper gives an account of the methods employed, compares their advantages and disadvantages and records some recent results obtained from patients during BCG immune-stimulation.

PATIENTS

All melanoma patients had the diagnosis confirmed histologically. They were attending the Karolinska Hospital, Stockholm, The Western Infirmary, Glasgow, Gartnaval General Hospital, Glasgow, or Canniesburn Hospital, Glasgow. Control leucocytes were obtained from normal individuals and patients attending hospital for other forms of cancer or for minor conditions not related to the pigmentary system.

METHODS

These are described in detail in the following papers [2–4] but certain general comments must be made.

1. In study A [2] we were fortunate in obtaining a sample of cyst fluid derived from a secondary melanoma. This material had previously been shown preferentially to transform the lymphocytes of melanoma patients [5].

2. In group B studies [3, 6–8] we employed the centrifuged supernatants of homogenized tumour as antigen and introduced a period of preincubation of leucocytes and antigen prior to their placement in the capillaries. In the section on preparation of the antigenic extracts in the first paper in this group [3] we erroneously stated that the homogenate was spun at 1500 g. This should in fact read 15,000 g.

3. In the early stages of our studies we used capillaries of extreme precision (20-μl micropets—Clay-Adams Inc., U.S.A) but, once the technique was established, were able to change to slightly less precise (but cheaper) capillaries (haematocrit tubes—Hawksley, U.K.) without loss of detectable reactivity.

4. Dissatisfaction with the homogenate-supernatant antigen centred on the low absolute amounts of leucocyte migration inhibition obtained, the lack of good repeatable dose–response curves and the heterogeneous cell components included in such material. We currently employ formalin-fixed intact tumour cells which to some extent answer these problems [4, 9].

5. We assess the significance of tumour cell contact mediated variations from leucocyte migration in medium alone or medium plus foetal calf serum by the ranking test of Mann-Whitney and Wilcoxon rather than by acceptance of arbitrary cut-off points at, say, 0.80 and 1.20.

6. Initially we were interested only in migration inhibition but the less frequent occurrence of a significant increase in leucocyte migration after exposure to tumour materials seems a real phenomenon of some interest and this is now recorded.

RESULTS

1. A comparison of melanoma patients with control donors (Table 1)

Melanoma patients' leucocytes were affected by the various tumour preparations to a significantly greater extent than any of the control groups. Control reactions were infrequent whether the leucocyte donors were normal individuals, patients with nonmalignant conditions or individuals with cancers other than malignant melanoma. The

Table 1. *The Frequency of Leucocyte Migration Inhibition and Enhancement in Melanoma Patients and Control Donors. A comparison of the effect of different types of tumour-derived materials*

Tumour material	Melanoma[a] patients	Control[a] individuals	Breast cancer[a] patients
Fluid from cystic secondary melanoma	11/22 (50)	2/16 (13)	NT[b]
Low molecular weight Sephadex G-100 fraction of above	5/10 (50)	1/9 (11)	NT
Supernatant of tumour homogenate	33/55 (60)	9/63 (14)	1/11 (9)
Formalin-fixed tumour cells	99/120 (83)	9/61 (15)	5/30 (17)

[a] Results given as number of individuals whose leucocyte migration, after exposure to tumour material, was significantly inhibited or enhanced by comparison with migration in medium with foetal calf serum alone, over the total number of individuals tested. Figures in brackets are percentages.

[b] NT means not tested.

highest activity was seen with the formalin-fixed cells and in the study cited such cells were no more active against control donors than were the other tumour preparations.

2. A comparison of reactions induced by autologous and homologous combinations of leucocytes and tumour material from melanomas, breast carcinomas and mouse melanomas (Table 2)

Reactions were observed about as frequently with homologous combinations of leucocytes and tumour material as with autologous combinations. Melanoma patients' leucocytes reacted infrequently with materials derived from human breast carcinoma or mouse melanoma. Reactions were also infrequent with formalinized homologous human liver cells.

Table 2. *The Frequency of Leucocyte Migration Inhibition and Enhancement in Tests with Autologous and Homologous Materials from Melanomas and Other Tumours*

Tumour material	Leucocytes[a] + autologous melanoma "antigens"	Leucocytes[a] + homologous melanoma "antigens"	Leucocytes[a] + homologous antigen from other tumours
Supernatant of tumour homogenate	8/10 (80)	33/55 (60)	1/12 (8)[b]
Formalin-fixed tumour cells	12/15 (80)	87/105 (83)	10/33 (30)[c]

[a] Results given as number of individuals whose leucocyte migration, after exposure to tumour material, was significantly inhibited or enhanced by comparison with migration in medium with foetal calf serum alone, over the total number of individuals tested. Figures in brackets are percentages.

[b] Breast carcinoma extracts.

[c] Cells from five human breast carcinomas and two mouse melanomas.

Table 3. *Variations in the Frequency of Leucocyte Migration Inhibition and Enhancement with Clinical Stage*

	Fluid from[a] cystic secondary melanoma	Sephadex[a] G-100 fraction of column 1	Supernatant[a] of tumour homogenate	Formalin-[a] fixed tumour cells
Primary disease	10/16 (63)	4/6 (67)	24/37 (65)	16/19 (84)
Metastatic disease	1/6 (17)	1/4 (25)	7/21 (33)	41/49 (84)
Nodal secondaries	NA[b]	NA	7/15 (47)	21/21 (100)
Visceral secondaries	NA	NA	0/6 (0)	5/9 (56)
Visceral secondaries treated with BCG	NA	NA	NA	12/12 (100)
Local recurrences	NA	NA	NA	7/7 (100)
Regressing tumour	NA	NA	NA	3/3 (100)

[a] Results given as number of individuals whose leucocyte migration, after exposure to tumour material, was significantly inhibited or enhanced by comparison with migration in medium and foetal calf serum alone, over the total number of individual tests. Figures in brackets are percentages.

[b] NA. Breakdown of figures in this manner not available.

3. Variations in the frequency of reactions with clinical stage (Table 3)

There was a clear decline in reaction frequency with advancing clinical stage in the studies employing the cyst fluid, its low molecular weight fraction and the homogenate supernatants. This difference was markedly less clear in the study employing formalinized cells, but the situation is complicated by the fact that some of the patients with metastatic disease received BCG stimulation which affects the migration (and other) results.

All patients who had local recurrences in the absence of visceral metastases and those whose tumours showed evidence of spontaneous regression were reactive.

4. The effect of treatment on the results of the migration assay

(a) *Surgery* (Table 4). Following a surgical operation there is a transient loss of reactivity in patients who were positive preoperatively. This deficit lasts for about 10 days but may be as short as 5 days or as long as 22 days.

Table 4. *The Frequency of Positive and Negative Leucocyte-migration Tests in Patients with Malignant Melanoma Examined Before and After Surgical Treatment*[a]

Patients tested in						Time to return of reactivity (days)	
Preoperative period		Immediate post-operative period[b]		Later post-operative period			
+ ve	− ve	+ ve	− ve	+ ve	− ve	mean	range
12/16	4/16	1/22	21/22	15/19	4/19	10.6	5–22

[a] Patients with positive or negative reactions/total patients tested at each stage.
[b] Days 1–4 after operation.

Table 5. *Variations in* in vivo *and* in vitro *Immunological Reactions During Immune-stimulation by BCG*

	− to + or increased value	No change		+ to − or decreased value	Inconstant
		+ to +	− to −		
Leucocyte migration (autologous)	5/9 (56)	2/9 (22)	0/9 (0)	1/9 (11)	1/9 (11)
Leucocyte migration (homologous)	5/14 (36)	1/14 (7)	1/14 (7)	3/14 (21)	4/14 (29)
PHA transformation	13/14 (93)	0/14 (0)	0/14 (0)	3/14[a] (21)	1/14 (7)
PPD transformation	5/11 (46)	0/11 (0)	3/11 (27)	0/11 (0)	3/11 (27)
Indirect membrane immunofluorescence	2/7 (29)	3/7 (43)	0/7 (0)	2/7 (29)	0/7 (0)
Lymphocytotoxicity	6/12 (50)	3/12 (25)	0/12 (0)	3/12 (25)	0/12 (0)
Mantoux test	7/10 (70)	0/10 (0)	3/10 (30)	0/10 (0)	0/10 (0)
Other recall skin tests	0/9 (0)	4/9 (44)	5/9 (56)	0/9 (0)	0/9 (0)

[a] Declined terminally.

(b) *Radiotherapy and chemotherapy.* The number of patients in whom this was studied is small, but patients tested during a course of radiotherapy rarely, if ever, reacted positively. The majority of patients tested during chemotherapy were non-reactive but positive reactivity returned relatively rapidly in the period between courses of therapy.

(c) *BCG immune-stimulation.* Table 5 gives a summary of the alterations seen in ·various laboratory tests including the leucocyte migration assay during BCG immune-stimulation. Conversion of a negative reaction to positivity in the autologous situation was seen in 5/9 patients so tested but positive conversion in the homologous situation was less frequent (5/14). Other patients maintained an initially positive reaction against advancing disease but reactions became negative terminally in four of the twenty-three patients. Reactions were quite inconstant in five patients.

The results of the other techniques are included for comparison purposes. PHA induced transformation was increased in almost all patients. PPD transformation also increased in some patients but such an increase was not observed in all seven patients who converted from Mantoux negativity to positivity during BCG administration.

Membrane reactive antibodies developed in two of seven patients tested during BCG stimulation and lymphocytes cytotoxic for cultured melanoma cells were detected in six of twelve previously non-reactive patients at this time. Mantoux conversion was the rule but anamnestic conversion of reactions to other recall skin tests (*Candida, T. rubrum,* mumps, streptokinase-streptodornase) was not seen.

5. *Follow-up status and serial studies* (Table 6)

(a) *Short-term follow up.* The great majority of patients who are tumour-free and examined within 2 years of surgical removal of a primary melanoma are reactive and maintain this reaction during serial tests.

(b) *Long-term follow up.* Patients who are tumour-free and examined at periods beyond the second anniversary of their primary surgery are less likely to give a positive reaction and the frequency of reaction declines progressively with lengthening tumour freedom.

Table 6. *The Frequency of Leucocyte Migration Inhibition and Enhancement in Melanoma Patients, Related to the Period of Tumour Freedom After Operation*

	Total	Reactive	% reactive
Tumour-free < 2 years after surgery	25	23	92
Tumour-free > 2 years after surgery	38	22	58

DISCUSSION

Tumour-directed cell-mediated immunity (TCI) seems likely to be an important means of destruction of tumour cells *in vivo.* This view has been held, with shifts of emphasis, for many years despite the absence of any really convincing evidence that established laboratory phenomena such as direct contact lymphocytotoxicity, macrophage-mediated cell killing, antibody-dependent lymphocytotoxicity and antibody mediated complement dependent cytotoxicity have a real and significant existence and effect *in vivo.* Slow progress in the elucidation of the role of such events in tumour biology is, at least in part, due to the lack of simple repeatable tests to measure tumour-directed immune reactivity. In fact the technology of tumour immunology lags sadly behind the philosophy of the subject.

Three basic techniques exist to examine TCI. The most widely used techniques have investigated the capacity of lymphocytes from tumour-bearing individuals to kill tumour target cells or delay their replication [15–17]. These studies are presently bedevilled by a most discouraging lack of tumour-specificity and it seems that "normal" lymphocytes and lymphocytes from tumour patients show a wide range of apparently spontaneous killing capacity for cultured tumour cells which, in turn, show a wide range of suscepti-bility to lymphocyte-mediated killing. Studies in progress using highly purified lympho-cyte sub-populations and the use of short-term cultures as target cells may restore some degree of tumour specificity to the test, but at present lymphocytotoxicity seems unsuited to routine use.

A second group of tests employs the observation that antigen will cause blast trans-formation of lymphocytes presensitized to that antigen [18, 19]. These tests are similar to the mixed lymphocyte reaction (MLR) except that tumour cells or materials provide the stimulator component of the cultures and the level of transformation observed is usually considerably lower than that observed in the MLR. Some workers have reported success with this technique but it undoubtedly requires considerable expertise on the part of the personnel performing it.

A third group of techniques depends on detecting the release of non-immunoglobulin mediators (the lymphokines) by sensitized (mainly T) lymphocytes when in contact with an antigen to which they have been sensitized. The lymphokine most studied has been that which in animals slows the movement of macrophages [10] —macrophage inhibitory factor (MIF). The technique described by Søborg and Bendixen is an attempt to apply the MIF assay to man and has been widely applied to many different clinical situations (see reference 6 for review). However, the technique remains cumbersome and requires care and expertise on the part of those performing it, the optimal method of antigen presentation remains debatable and categorization of the lymphokines produced and their identity or non-identity with classical macrophage migration inhibitory factor remains to be settled. These problems apart, our own results and those of other groups [11–14] suggest that the leucocyte migration technique is applicable to the study of patients with malignant disease.

The data presented here make the following conclusions possible:

1. Melanoma-derived materials preferentially inhibit the migration of melanoma patients' leucocytes. Similarly prepared materials from other tissues are undoubtedly less active.

2. A minority of control donors have leucocytes which are inhibited by contact with melanoma materials. This may indicate a background of technical artefact, but could also indicate exposure of the reactors to some form of antigenic stimulus identical with or similar to that associated with malignant melanoma.

3. The occurrence of reactions when autologous leucocytes and tumour are combined and similarities in transfusion and pregnancy history in melanoma and control groups are against HL-A disparity being important in the production of the observed reactions.

4. The occurrence of reactions when leucocytes are exposed to homologous tumour indicates that antigens which are at least structurally similar are shared by different melanomas.

5. Reactions were less frequently detectable as disease advanced. The results indicate that intact tumour cells are the form of antigen least suited to this type of study.

6. Surgery, radiotherapy and chemotherapy induce depression of tumour-directed cellular immunity of variable duration and degree.

7. Loss of reactivity in patients shortly after primary surgery ($<$ 2 years) predicts the occurrence of clinically detectable metastases in some patients.

8. Reactions are relatively infrequent in patients who are tumour-free for prolonged periods ($>$ 2 years) after surgery. O'Toole and her colleagues [20] have recorded a similar situation in patients with bladder cancer.

9. The administration of BCG to patients alters many specific and non-specific tests of immunological functions including tumour-mediated leucocyte migration inhibition. Unfortunately, in the small group of patients studied, to date, these changes do not correlate well with clinical status and in our view, such patients are best monitored for clinical effects and apparent complications of therapy by clinical examination.

The continued use of the migration assay depends largely upon two factors. We urgently require a detailed understanding of the mechanisms involved and there should be progress towards simplification of the manipulations involved, the eventual aim being a technique which could be applied easily and reliably to large numbers of patients and which could be performed by technicians. The technique described by Clausen [21] goes some way towards simplifying the procedures but still requires considerable manipulative skill in performance. Another area of interest is in the use of indirect lymphokine assays, in which the supernatants of reacted leucocytes and antigens are assayed for activity against indicator cells.

Two techniques which ostensibly apply the same strategy as leucocyte migration are the macrophage electrophoretic mobility test [22] and the leucocyte adherence inhibition test [23]. Both tests demand considerable skill of those who perform them but have produced interesting results. However, they are undoubtedly too complex for routine use in their present form, but after simplification, may become more widely used, when their relativity to existing tests will become clearer.

ACKNOWLEDGEMENTS

These studies were performed with the aid of funds from the Peel Medical Research Trust, London, the Swedish Cancer Society, the Secretary of State for Scotland and the McMillan Research Funds of the University of Glasgow. We acknowledge the generous co-operation of those clinical colleagues who permitted us to study their patients.

REFERENCES

1. M. Søborg and G. Bendixen, Human lymphocyte migration as a parameter of hypersensitivity. *Acta med. Scand.* **181**, 247 (1967).
2. A.J. Cochran, U.W. Jehn and B.P. Gothoskar, Cell mediated immunity to malignant melanoma. *Pigment Cell* **1**, 360 (1973).
3. A.J. Cochran, W.G.S. Spilg, R.M. Mackie and C.E. Thomas, Post-operative depression of tumour directed cell mediated immunity in patients with malignant disease. *Br. Med. J.* **2**, 67 (1972).

4. C.E. Ross, A.J. Cochran, D.E. Hoyle, R.M. Grant and R.M. Mackie, Formalin-fixed tumour cells
    in the leucocyte migration test. *Lancet*, **ii**. 1087 (1973).
5. U.W. Jehn, L. Nathanson, R.S. Schwarz and M. Skinner, *In vitro* lymphocyte stimulation by a
    soluble antigen from malignant melanoma. *New Engl. J. Med.* **283**, 329 (1970).
6. A.J. Cochran, R.M. Mackie, C.E. Thomas, R.M. Grant, D.E. Cameron-Mowat and W.G.S. Spilg,
    Cellular immunity to breast carcinoma and malignant melanoma. *Br. J. Cancer*, **28** (Suppl. 1), 77
    (1973).
7. R.M. Mackie, W.G.S. Spilg, C.E. Thomas, D.E. Cameron-Mowat, R.M. Grant and A.J. Cochran,
    A comparison of tumour-directed cell-mediated immunity and tumour histology in melanoma
    patients. *Rev. de l'Inst. Pasteur de Lyon*, **6**, 281 (1973).
8. A.J. Cochran, C.E. Thomas, W.G.S. Spilg, R.M. Grant, D.E. Cameron-Mowat, R.M. Mackie and
    G. Lindop, Tumour-directed cellular immunity in malignant melanoma and its modification by
    surgical treatment. *Yale J. Biol. Med.* **46**, 650 (1973).
9. C.E. Ross, A.J. Cochran, D.E. Hoyle, R.M. Grant and R.M. Mackie, Formalinised tumour cells in
    the leucocyte migration inhibition test. *Clin. Exp. Immunol.* **22**, 126 (1975).
10. M. George and J.H. Vaughan, *In vitro* cell migration as a model for delayed hypersensitivity.
    Proc. Soc. Exp. Biol. Med. **111**, 514 (1962).
11. V. Andersen, O. Bjerrum, G. Bendixen, T. Schiødt and I. Dissing, Effect of autologous mammary
    tumour extracts on human leukocyte migration *in vitro*. *Int. J. Cancer*, **5**, 357 (1970).
12. A. Segall, O. Weiler, J. Genin, J. Lacour and F. Lacour, *In vitro* study of cellular immunity
    against autochthonous human cancer. *Int. J. Cancer*, **9**, 417 (1972).
13. J.M. Anderson, F. Kelly, S.E. Wood, K.E. Rodger and R.I. Freshney, Evaluation of leucocyte
    functions six years after tumour autograft in human mammary cancer. *Br. J. Cancer*, **28** (Suppl.
    1), 83 (1973).
14. J.L. McCoy, L.F. Jerome, J.H. Dean, G.B. Cannon, T.C. Alford, T. Doering and R.B. Herberman,
    Inhibitions of leukocyte migration by tumor associated antigens in soluble extracts of human
    breast carcinoma. *J. Nat. Cancer Inst.* **53**, 11 (1974).
15. J.-C. Cerottini and K.T. Brunner, Cell mediated cytotoxicity, allograft rejection and tumour
    immunity. *Adv. Immunol.* **18**, 67 (1974).
16. M. Takasugi and E. Klein, The methodology of microassay for cell mediated immunity. *In vitro
    Methods in Cell-mediated Immunity*, edited by B.R. Bloom and P.R. Glade. Academic Press
    Inc., N.Y., 1971.
17. K.E. Hellström and I. Hellström, Lymphocyte mediated cytotoxicity and blocking serum activity
    to tumor antigens. *Adv. Immunol.* **18**, 209 (1974).
18. J. Stjernswärd, L.E. Almgård, S. Franzén, T. von Schreeb and L.B. Wadström, Tumour-distinctive
    immunological reactions and patients with renal carcinomas. *Clin. Exp. Immunol.* **6**, 965 (1970).
19. E.M. Hersh, J.U. Gutterman, G.M. Mavligit, C.H. Granatek, R.C. Reed, U. Ambus and C. McBride,
    Approaches to the study of tumour antigens and tumor immunity in malignant melanoma.
    Behring Inst. Mitt. **56**, 139 (1975).
20. C. O'Toole, P. Perlmann, B. Unsgaard, L.E. Almgård, B. Johansson, G. Moberger and
    F. Edsymyr, Cellular immunity to human urinary bladder carcinoma. II. Effect of surgery and
    preoperative irradiation. *Int. J. Cancer*, **10**, 92 (1972).
21. J.E. Clausen, Tuberculin-induced migration inhibition of human peripheral leucocytes in agarose
    medium. *Act. Allergol.* pp. 56–80 (1971).
22. E.J. Field and E.A. Caspary, Lymphocyte sensitisation. An *in vitro* test for cancer? *Lancet*, **2**,
    1337 (1970).
23. W.J. Halliday, J.W. Halliday, C.B. Campbell, A.E. Maluish and L.W. Powell, Specific immuno-
    diagnosis of hepatocellular carcinoma by leucocyte adherence inhibition. *Brit. Med. J.* **2**, 349
    (1974).

DETECTION OF CELL-MEDIATED IMMUNITY AGAINST TUMOR-ASSOCIATED ANTIGENS OF HUMAN BREAST CARCINOMA BY MIGRATION INHIBITION AND LYMPHOCYTE-STIMULATION ASSAYS

J.L. McCOY*, J.H. DEAN*, G.B. CANNON*, B.A. MAURER*, R.K. OLDHAM[†]
and R.B. HERBERMAN[†]

ABSTRACT

Direct and indirect migration inhibition assays using allogeneic 3 M KCl tumor extracts were employed to detect cell-mediated immunity (CMI) to tumor-associated antigens (TAA) of human breast carcinoma. Results suggest that breast carcinomas possess common TAA and that many tumor-bearing patients have CMI against these TAA. Further testing with lymphocyte stimulation assays using 3 M KCl extracts of breast carcinoma indicated that allogeneic extracts may induce a primary proliferative response to normal alloantigens rather than to TAA. The problems with interpreting the specificity of the allogeneic reactions were overcome by the use of autologous patient material in the lymphocyte stimulation assay. The autologous tests demonstrated that this assay was also useful in the detection of CMI against TAA of breast carcinoma.

INTRODUCTION

Cell-mediated immunity (CMI) to tumor-associated antigens (TAA) has been described in patients with human breast carcinoma employing assays of delayed skin cutaneous reactions [1–3] as well as *in vitro* lymphocyte microcytotoxicity [4, 5], lymphocyte stimulation (LS) [6–9] and direct leukocyte migration inhibition (LMI) [10–17] assays. Most of these studies have indicated that carcinomas of the breast may possess common TAA.

In studies employing the direct LMI assay and LS tests, TAA in several forms have been used. For example, early work with LMI employed crude particulate saline extracts of breast carcinoma cells [10–13]. Others have exposed the patient's leukocytes to cryostat

* Department of Immunology, Litton Bionetics, Inc., 5516 Nicholson Lane, Kensington, Maryland 20795, U.S.A.
† Laboratory of Immunodiagnosis, National Cancer Institute, Bethesda, Maryland, 20014 U.S.A.
Supported by Contracts NO1-CB-23227 and NO1-CP-43333 from the National Institutes of Health, Bethesda, Maryland 20014, U.S.A.

sections of breast carcinoma tissue [14] or to formalin-inactivated breast tumor cells in LMI assays [17]. Intact tumor cells blocked with mitomycin C have also been successfully employed in LS assays with autologous lymphocytes [18].

More recently, crude soluble 3 M KCl [19] extracts of breast carcinomas have been successfully employed in LMI [15] and LS assays [8, 9]. Whereas, LMI assays do not appear to be complicated by problems associated with histocompatibility antigens in allogeneic 3 M KCl extracts, the LS test seems to measure proliferative responses to normal alloantigens as well as to TAAs in the 3 M KCl extracts [9]. This problem appears to be resolved when autologous combinations are used in LS.

The purpose of the present study was to perform direct LMI assays and LS tests with the peripheral bloods of patients with breast carcinoma to identify TAA in 3 M KCl crude soluble extracts, hypotonic saline membrane extracts or on intact cells of fresh breast carcinoma tissue. Generally allogeneic combinations were run in the LMI assay while both allogeneic and autologous reactions were employed in the LS test. Most of our early work with LMI was performed using the direct test where migration inhibition is measured without knowing whether a lymphokine has been generated. We therefore also employed indirect migration inhibition assays using human polymorphonuclear indicator cells and assayed for the generation of leukocyte inhibitory factor (LIF) as described by Rocklin [20].

MATERIALS AND METHODS

Bloods

Whole blood and tissues from female patients with confirmed breast carcinoma or benign breast disease and from females and males with other cancer were obtained from George Washington University and the Medical University of South Carolina and the Clinical Center of the National Institutes of Health.

Patients were tested at various times before or after surgery and in all stages of disease; i.e. local tumor (Stage 1), extension into the regional lymph nodes (Stage 2) and metastatic disease (Stage 3).

Tumors

Fresh tumor and other tissue extracts were prepared by the crude 3 M KCl extraction procedure as previously described [9, 15, 25] or by crude hypotonic saline extraction of membranes as earlier reported [21]. Single tumor cell suspensions were also cryopreserved by controlled rate freezing to be later used as stimulator cells in autologous mixed leukocyte tumor cell cultures (MLTC).

Some experiments were performed with 3 M KCl extracts of tissue culture cell lines derived from breast carcinomas including MCF-7 [22] and MDA-MB-231 [23]. These cell lines grew as epithelial cells in monolayers and were maintained on RPMI 1640 media supplemented with 20% fetal bovine serum and glutamine.

Direct LMI assay

Direct LMI assays were performed as previously described [15]. Briefly, peripheral blood leukocytes were collected after 1 × g Plasmagel sedimentation. Washed leukocytes were incubated for 1 hr at 37°C with and without appropriate concentrations (ranging from 25 μg to 750 μg) of the various 3 M KCl extracts and then drawn into 25-μl (micro) capillary pipettes (replicates of 4). Cells were then pelleted, capillaries were cut, placed into chambers containing McCoy's 5A media, 10% fetal calf serum and Gentamicin and incubated at 37°C for 18 to 24 hr. The areas of migration were determined by planimetry. The migration index (MI) was calculated by the formula:

$$MI = \frac{\text{Mean migration of replicates with antigen}}{\text{Mean migration of replicates without antigen}}$$

Values of $\leqslant 0.85$ were arbitrarily considered positive. The cut-off value is based on the normal donor observations and is selected so that approximately 10% of the normal donor MI values fall below this cut-off value (i.e. the cut-off is the lower tenth percentile of the normal donor observations).

Indirect LMI assay

Indirect migration inhibition assays to determine if LIF was being generated were performed as described by Rocklin [20]. Briefly, Ficoll Hypaque separated peripheral blood lymphocytes were incubated for 2 hr with or without 3 M KCl extract of MCF-7 (concentration of 15–50 μg per 4×10^6 lymphocytes). Lymphocytes were resuspended in RPMI 1640 media containing 0.5% fetal calf serum, penicillin and streptomycin and incubated at 37°C for 48 hr to generate LIF. Undiluted supernatants were evaluated for the generation of the mediator by tests with human polymorphonuclear (PMN) cells which were obtained from a normal donor and prepared by Plasmagel separation of leukocytes to remove a large percentage of red blood cells followed by Ficoll Hypaque separation of the leukocytes into mononuclear cells and PMNs. Capillary tubes were filled with the PMNs, placed in chambers to which supernatants were added, and incubated for 18 to 24 hr at 37°C. Areas of migration were determined by planimetry. Reactions were considered positive if MI values were $\leqslant 0.85$ as described above.

Micro-culture LS assay

LS assays were performed in replicates of four as earlier described [19]. Ficoll Hypaque separated peripheral blood lymphocytes (4×10^5/well) were placed in 200-μl cultures in Falcon Microtest II plates. RPMI 1640 media supplemented with Hepes buffer (25 mM), 10% human AB serum, glutamine (1%) and Gentamicin (50 μmg/ml) with or without antigen (0.01–10 μg/well) or intact tumor cells in the mixed lymphocyte tumor cell culture (MLTC). Cryopreserved tumor cells blocked with 50 μg/ml mitomycin C were added to lymphocyte cultures at varying ratios (5 to 20 lymphocytes/tumor cell). Cultures were incubated in a humidified 5% CO_2 atmosphere at 37°C and pulsed with 1 μCi of ^3H thymidine 8 hr prior to harvest. Cells were harvested 7 days after culture and the amount of incorporated label was determined by scintillation spectroscopy. A stimulation index (SI) was calculated as the mean counts per minute (CPM) of experimental cultures relative to CPM of control lymphocyte cultures containing no tissue extract. The stimulation index for MLTC was expressed as the CPM of MLTC cultures minus the CPM of mitomycin C blocked tumor cells alone relative to CPM of control lymphocyte cultures containing no tumor cells. Data were considered positive when CPM of experimental cultures were significantly different from control cultures at $p < 0.01$.

RESULTS

The direct LMI assay was performed with leukocytes from normal controls and patients with breast carcinoma, benign breast disease and cancer of other sites (Fig. 1). Antigens were soluble 3 M KCl extracts of breast carcinomas, benign lesions and non-breast cancer tissue. Most tests were allogeneic, i.e. one patient's leukocytes were usually tested against another patient's tumor. A total of 44/78 tests with leukocytes

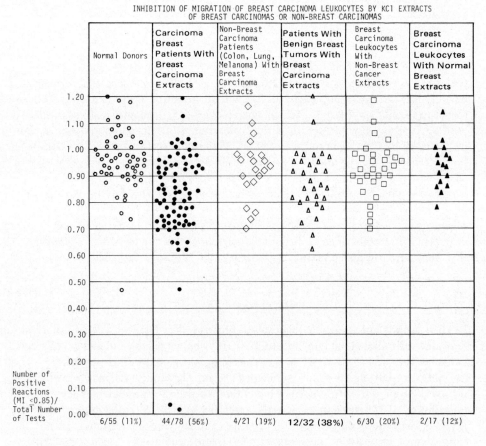

Fig. 1. Results of direct LMI assays with leukocytes from normal donors and breast cancer patients and with 3 M KCl extracts of fresh surgically removed breast carcinomas, benign breast tissues, non-breast cancers and normal breast tissue.

from patients with confirmed breast carcinoma had an MI ≤ 0.85, whereas only 6/55 tests with leukocytes from normal donors and 4/21 with leukocytes from patients with cancer of other sites had MI values ≤ 0.85. Only 6/30 breast carcinoma leukocytes reacted with non-breast cancer extracts and only 2/17 reacted with extracts of normal breast tissue. Of interest was the finding that 12/32 patients with benign breast disease gave positive reactions with extracts of breast carcinoma. This observation is being pursued and includes studying both benign and breast carcinoma patient reactivity with 3 M KCl extracts of benign breast tumors.

There were several instances in which a patient's leukocytes were inhibited by one breast carcinoma extract, but not by another breast carcinoma extract that was active with cells from other breast carcinoma patients suggesting that multiple common breast cancer antigens may be involved in this reactivity.

Table 1 shows the correlation of LMI reactivity of breast carcinoma patients with stage of disease and time after surgical removal of tumor. In evaluating the data in relation to surgery, the lowest incidence of reactivity was observed with the 0 to 10 day post-operative period where 4/13 patients were positive. The levels of reactivity during the pre-operative period and as late as 6 months or more after surgery were quite similar. Patients at all stages of disease reacted with approximately the same frequency.

Different degrees of direct LMI reactivity were seen with various tumor extracts. For example, Table 2 presents the results obtained with three different breast carcinoma extracts. As shown, the extract 3112 elicited more positive reactivity in breast carcinoma patients than extract 3286. Both extracts gave more positive reactions than did the extract 2937.

It was of interest to determine whether 3 M KCl extracts of cell lines derived from breast carcinomas possess TAAs which could be detected by LMI tests. The finding of antigenic cell lines would allow preparation of large, standard 3 M KCl extracts for future testing. Table 3 summarizes direct LMI results with extracts of two cell lines, MCF-7 and MDA-MB-231. Extracts of both cell lines elicited positive reactivity with leukocytes from breast carcinoma patients, while normal donors had low levels or no reactivity. Specificity with the MCF-7 extract was evidenced by the low reactivity of non-breast cancer patients with this extract.

Table 1. *Direct Leukocyte Migration Inhibition Reactivities of Breast Carcinoma Patients as a Function of Stage of Disease and Time after Surgical Removal of Tumor[a]*

Stage of disease	Pre-op.	0–10 days post-op.	11–30 days post-op.	1–6 months post-op.	>6 months post-op.	Totals
1	7/12	4/9	–	–	–	11/21 (52%)
2	4/7	–	–	–	2/2	6/9 (67%)
3	1/4	0/4	–	7/9	16/24	24/41 (59%)
Long-term survivors with no evident disease	–	–	–	–	3/7	3/7 (43%)
Totals	12/23 (52%)	4/13 (30%)		7/9 (78%)	21/33 (63%)	

[a] A positive LMI reaction was defined as MI of ≤ 0.85.

Table 2. *Direct Leukocyte Migration Inhibition Reactions with*
Selected KCl Extracts of Breast Carcinoma

3112		3286		2937	
Normal donors	Breast carcinoma patients	Normal donors	Breast carcinoma patients	Normal donors	Breast carcinoma patients
1.12[a]	0.79	0.91	0.70	1.11	0.89
1.01	0.82	0.98	0.77	0.85	0.98
0.96	0.70	1.04	0.93	0.97	1.02
1.12	0.95	0.96	0.87	1.00	0.87
0.91	0.91	1.17	1.10	1.23	0.70
1.05	0.62	1.02	0.99		0.66
0.91	1.09	0.97	0.75		0.95
					1.15
					1.13
					0.94
					0.93
Total positive Total tested	5/8 (63%)	0/7	3/8 (38%)	1/5 (20%)	2/11 (18%)

[a] Migration index. A reaction is considered positive if the MI is ≤ 0.85.

Table 3. *LMI Reactivity of Breast Carcinoma Patients against KCl Extracts*
of Tissue Cultured Cell Lines Derived from Breast Carcinomas

Leukocyte donors	% positive reactions[a] total no. patients tested	
	MCF-7 cell line	MDA-MB-231 cell line
Breast carcinoma patients	28/37 (78%)	5/11 (45%)
Non-breast cancer patients[b]	4/19 (21%)	N.D.
Normal donors	3/27 (11%)	0/8

[a] Reaction was considered positive if MI ≤ 0.85. Sixteen of the twenty-five positive values had an MI ≤ 0.80.
[b] Included lung carcinoma, melanoma and Ewings sarcoma patients.

The direct LMI assay does not permit analysis of the mechanism of the reaction. We therefore performed indirect assays using human polymorphonuclear indicator cells and assayed for LIF production in supernatants from patients' lymphocytes incubated with 3 M KCl extracts (Table 4). Whereas 6/10 breast carcinoma patients reacted with 3 M KCl extracts of MCF-7 only 1/8 normal donors gave a positive result. There were no positive reactions with a 3 M KCl extract of a lung carcinoma (7661), an extract that has been shown in our laboratory to inhibit the leukocyte migration of lung carcinoma patients in direct LMI assays. These results indicate that significant levels of LIF are probably being produced which can inhibit the migration of polymorphonuclear cells following the interaction of breast carcinoma TAA with lymphocytes from breast carcinoma patients.

Data from fifteen separate lymphocyte stimulation assays employing allogeneic

Table 4. *Reactivity of Peripheral Blood Lymphocytes from Breast Carcinoma Patients to a 3 M KCl Extract of MCF-7 Cell Line as Assayed by Indirect Migration Inhibition Assay*

| Lymphocytes from | 3 M KCl extract | |
	MCF-7	7661 lung carcinoma
Breast carcinoma patients	6/10 (60%)[a]	0/4
Normal donors	1/8 (16%)	0/2

[a] Values were considered positive if MI $\leqslant$ 0.85. (Individual migration indices of breast carcinoma patients with MCF-7 extract were 0.79, 0.78, 0.73, 0.37, 0.56 and 0.54.) The one positive reactive normal had an MI of 0.82.

Table 5. *Lymphocyte Stimulation by Allogeneic Extracts of Breast and Non-breast Tumors and Normal Breast Tissue*

| Type of 3 M KCl | Breast carcinoma patient lymphocytes | | Normal donor lymphocytes | |
	Responders/Tested (%)	Mean SI[a]	Responders/Tested (%)	Mean SI
Allogeneic normal breast tissue	1/7 (14)	3.7	2/10 (20)	3.5
Allogeneic non-breast tumor tissue	2/14 (14)	4.2	7/18 (39)	7.7
Autologous normal leukocyte extracts	N.D.	–	0/8 (0)	–
Allogeneic breast carcinoma tissue	4/26 (15)	5.7	12/30 (40)	9.1

[a] Mean counts per minute (CPM) of ^{3}H-T&R incorporation in lymphocyte microcultures (200 μl) were obtained. Stimulation index (SI) is the ratio of CPM in the experimental lymphocyte cultures containing the appropriate 3 M KCl extracts/CPM of controls. SI values were considered positive if the value was $\geqslant$ 3.

lymphocyte—tumor combinations are summarized in Table 5. Lymphocytes from twenty-six patients and thirty normal individuals were cultured in the presence of several different 3 M KCl extracts of allogeneic breast carcinoma, normal breast tissue or non-breast tumor tissue. Stimulation ratios of ^{3}H-TdR incorporation $\geqslant$ 3 were observed in 4/26 of the breast carcinoma patients studied, while a total of 12/30 normal donors demonstrated positive reaction to the allogeneic breast carcinoma material. Similar degrees of patient and normal donor lymphocyte reactivity were also seen with allogeneic extracts of normal breast tissue or non-breast tumor tissue, but not with autologous leukocyte extracts. Overall, normal donors responded better to the allogeneic extracts than did the breast carcinoma patients. Thus it appears that the LS assay using allogeneic breast extracts cannot be reliably used to measure specific reactivity of breast cancer patients against TAA.

We therefore studied whether the LS assay could measure CMI reactivity against TAA when a completely autologous system was employed. Preliminary testing with autologous 3 M KCl extracts and breast carcinoma patient leukocytes did not yield appreciable reactivity. We subsequently employed intact tumor cells or crude hypotonic saline membrane extracts of breast carcinoma tissue as stimulants in the tests. The results of LS

Table 6. *Lymphocyte Stimulation by Autologous Intact Cells or Autologous Extracts of Breast Carcinoma Tissue*

Form of tumor tissue	Positive tests Total	Mean stimulation index of responders (± SD)[1]	Mean CPM (± SD) of responders
Intact Tumor Cells[2]			
4 × 10⁵ lymphocytes/well	3/5 (60%)	4.8	6,316 (± 1,059)
2 × 10⁵ lymphocytes/well	1/5 (20%)	3.0	2,404 (± 1,393)
Total:	4/10 (40%)	4.3 (1.4)	5,343 (± 1,143)
Hypotonic Saline Membrane Extract[3]			
4 × 10⁵ lymphocytes/well	4/9 (44%)	8.1	11,687 (± 1,245)
2 × 10⁵ lymphocytes/well	1/13 (8%)	10.0	4,372 (± 1,972)
Total:	5/22 (22%)	8.5 (2.8)	10,225 (± 1,397)

[1] Stimulation indices (SI) were considered positive if value ⩾ 3.
[2] Tumor cells were treated with 50 μg/ml of mitomycin C for 30 minutes prior to addition to lymphocytes. A ratio of 10–20 lymphocytes/tumor cell was employed.
[3] Crude membrane extracts of fresh breast carcinoma tissues were prepared by extraction with decreasing concentrations of saline as earlier described [19].

testing using completely autologous material are presented in Table 6. A total of nine positive reactions were obtained with thirty-two patients in these autologous tests when using either intact tumor cells or the membrane material as the stimulant. More significantly, 7/14 positive reactions were obtained with the 4 × 10⁵ lymphocytes/well concentration with these two stimulators. Thus, the LS assay appears capable of detecting CMI against TAA of human breast carcinomas only if autologous testing is performed. It should also be pointed out that in parallel testing, autologous normal breast tissue failed to elicit positive reactivity in zero of five patients tested and in three cases where positive reactivity was obtained with autologous carcinoma tissue material.

DISCUSSION

Earlier studies [6–17] and those reported here have demonstrated the usefulness of migration inhibition assays and lymphocyte stimulation tests with human peripheral blood leukocytes or lymphocytes in the detection of TAA of breast carcinoma. The current results with the direct and indirect LMI assays suggest that different breast carcinomas possess common TAA and that the TAA elicit a CMI response in the tumor-bearing female. Interpretation of data obtained with LS tests was more restricted since only autologous combinations of lymphocytes and stimulator materials yielded specific CMI responses. The data with the LS assay, however, clearly demonstrated that this test could also detect reactivity against breast carcinoma TAA, when autologous tests were done, but no evaluation of antigenic cross-reactivity between different breast carcinomas could be made. Normal breast tissue failed to elicit positive autologous LS reactivity which further supports tumor specific reactivity.

Further analysis of the direct LMI results showed that some patients at all stages of disease including those with widespread metastases had CMI reactivity to TAA. Similarly, patients before surgery and those tested at various times after surgery responded well in LMI. One exception was noted with patients immediately after surgery (0 to 10 days) where a somewhat decreased level of reactivity was observed. Cochran et al. [12] earlier reported that leukocytes from a series of breast carcinoma patients before surgery were significantly inhibited by particulate saline extracts of breast carcinoma tissue, whereas during the immediate post-operative period (0 to 5 days) there was a drop in reactivity. Possibly the drop in reactivity is not related to a specific decrease in patient immunity against TAA, but rather to a general depression in immunological reactivity due to surgical trauma, hormonal factors or other physiological factors.

The reactions in LMI of breast carcinoma patients with the KCl extracts of breast carcinoma appear to be directed against breast carcinoma-associated antigens. The observed inhibition did not appear to be due to toxicity of the tumor extracts since at the concentrations of extracts used in the assays, migration of leukocytes from controls was usually not affected. The observed pattern of results is also not consistent with reactivity against histocompatibility antigens in the extracts even though allogeneic combinations were usually employed. In addition, nine of the normal donors were multiparous females and none of them reacted with the breast carcinoma extracts. Also, our total experience with cancer patients' reactivity against 3 M KCl extracts of normal tissues including liver, colon, lung and breast has been that only 2/76 (3%) had positive LMI reactions (seventeen were breast carcinoma patients tested with normal breast extracts). We did, however, observe 12/32 positive reactions when benign breast disease patients were tested with extracts of breast carcinoma. We do not yet know the specificity of this reactivity. More extensive studies are in progress employing extracts of both breast carcinoma and benign breast disease.

Our studies with the indirect LMI tests using human polymorphonuclear indicator cells strongly support the idea that the LMI assays are measuring reactivities of lymphocytes with TAA, with consequent production of a lymphokine, LIF.

Earlier LMI studies of human breast carcinoma have usually employed particulate antigens [10–13] or cryostat sections of tumors [14]. The 3 M KCl extracts, though still crude, were satisfactory as antigens in the LMI tests, but were somewhat less effective for LS assays. Others have demonstrated the usefulness of this extraction method in yielding soluble HL-A antigens [19] and TAA of animal tumors [24] as well as human solid tumors [8].

Variations in the antigenicity of the 3 M KCl breast carcinoma extracts that we observed could have significantly affected the overall incidence of reactivity. Factors influencing the antigenicity of a given extract may be related to variations in the proportion of breast carcinoma cells versus normal cells in the tumor mass used for extraction, the presence of some type of inhibitors in the tumor, the stage of the tumor used for extraction or a variety of other factors. Black et al. [14] have reported that in situ tumors gave the highest reactivity with breast carcinoma patients. Recently we have evaluated our LMI results [25] on the basis of the stage of the tumor used for our 3 M KCl extraction and have found that local primary tumors with or without node involvement (Stages 1 and 2) appear to be slightly more reactive in tests with breast carcinoma patients than are breast tumors metastatic to the liver or pleural effusions. Due to the limited quantity of extract that is obtained when extracting small primary breast carcinomas we are hopeful that tissue cultured cells derived from breast carcinomas can be used as a source of standard antigen preparations for LMI assay. Finally, our LMI data presented in this study indicate that some cell lines may be excellent sources of specific breast carcinoma TAA.

REFERENCES

1. L.E. Hughes and B. Lytton, Antigenic properties of human tumours: delayed cutaneous hyper-sensitivity reactions. *Br. Med. J.* **209**, 212 (1964).
2. T.N. Stewart, The presence of delayed hypersensitivity reactions in patients toward cellular extracts of their malignant tumors. *Cancer,* **23**, 1368 (1969).
3. C. Alford, A.C. Hollinshead and R.B. Herberman, Delayed cutaneous hypersensitivity reactions to extracts of malignant and normal human breast cells. *Ann. Surg.* **178**, 20 (1973).
4. I. Hellström, K.E. Hellström, H.O. Sjögren and G.A. Warner, Demonstration of cell-mediated immunity to human neoplasms of various histological types. *Int. J. Cancer,* **7**, 1 (1971).
5. G. Fossati, S. Canavari, G. Della Porta, G.P. Balzarini and Y. Veronesi, Cellular immunity to human breast carcinoma. *Int. J. Cancer,* **10**, 391 (1972).
6. P. Fisher, E. Golub, H. Holyner and E. Kunze-Muhl, Comparative effects of tumor extracts on lymphocyte transformation in peripheral blood cultures of healthy persons and patients with breast cancer. *Krevsforsch.* **72**, 155 (1969).
7. H. Savel, Effect of autologous tumor extracts on cultured human peripheral blood lymphocytes. *Cancer,* **24**, 56 (1969).
8. G.M. Mavligit, J.U. Gutterman, C.M. McBride and E.M. Hersh, Cell-mediated immunity to human solid tumors: *In vitro* detection by lymphocyte blastogenic response to cell-associated and solubilized tumor antigens. *Nat. Cancer Inst. Monogr.* **37**, 167 (1973).
9. J.H. Dean, J.S. Silva, J.L. McCoy, C.M. Leonard, M. Middleton, G.B. Cannon and R.B. Herberman, Lymphocyte blastogenesis induced by 3 M KCl extracts of allogenic breast carcinoma and lymphoid cells. *J. Nat. Cancer Inst.* **54**, 1295 (1975).
10. V. Andersen, O. Bjerrum, G. Bendixen, T. Schiødt, and I. Dissing, Effect of autologous mammary tumor extracts on human leukocyte migration *in vitro. Int. J. Cancer,* **5**, 357 (1970).
11. W.H. Wolberg, Inhibition of migration of human autogenous and allogeneic leukocytes by extracts for patient's cancers. *Cancer Res.* **31**, 798 (1971).
12. A.J. Cochran, W.G. Spilg, R.M. Mackie and C.E. Thomas, Postoperative depression of tumor directed cell-mediated immunity in patients with malignant disease. *Br. Med. J.* **2**, 67 (1972).
13. A. Segall, O. Wiler, J. Genin, J. Lacour, and F. Lacour, *In vitro* study of cellular immunity against autochthonous human cancer. *Int. J. Cancer,* **9**, 417 (1972).
14. M.M. Black, H.P. Leis,Jr., B. Shore and R.E. Zachrau, Cellular hypersensitivity to breast cancer —Assessment by a leukocyte migration procedure. *Cancer,* **33**, 952 (1974).
15. J.L. McCoy, L.F. Jerome, J.H. Dean, G.B. Cannon, T.C. Alford, T. Doering and R.B. Herberman, Inhibition of leukocyte migration by tumor-associated antigens in soluble extracts of human breast carcinoma. *J. Nat. Cancer Inst.* **53**, 11 (1974).
16. W.H. Wolberg, Inhibition of leukocyte migration by human tumors. *Arch. Surg.* **109**, 211 (1974).
17. C.E. Ross, A.J. Cochran, D.H. Hoyle, R.M. Grant and R.M. Mackie, Formalin-fixed tumour cells in the leukocyte migration test. *Lancet,* **1**, 1087 (1973).
18. F. Vánky, J. Stjernswärd, G. Klein and U. Nilsonne, Serum-mediated inhibition of lymphocyte stimulation by autochthonous human tumors. *J. Nat. Cancer Inst.* **47**, 95 (1971).
19. R.A. Reisfield, M.A. Pellegrino, and B.D. Kahan, Salt extraction of soluble HL-A antigens. *Science,* **172**, 1134 (1971).
20. R. Rocklin, Products of activated lymphocytes: Leukocyte inhibitory factor (LIF) distinct from migration inhibitory factor (MIF). *J. Immunol.* **112**, 1461 (1974).
21. M.E. Oren and R.B. Herberman, Delayed cutaneous hypersensitivity reactions to membrane extracts of human tumors. *Clin. Exp. Immunol.* **9**, 45 (1971).
22. H.D. Soule, J. Vazquez, A. Long, S. Albert and M. Brennan, A human cell line from a pleural effusion derived from a breast carcinoma. *J. Nat. Cancer Inst.* **51**, 1409 (1973).
23. R. Cailleau, R. Young, M. Olive and W.J. Reeves, Breast tumor cells lines from pleural effusion. *J. Nat. Cancer Inst.* **53**, 661 (1974).
24. M. Meltzer, E. Leonard, H. Rapp and T. Borsos, Tumor-specific antigen solubilized by hypertonic potassium chloride. *J. Nat. Cancer Inst.* **47**, 703 (1971).
25. G.B. Cannon, J.L. McCoy, R.B. Oldham, R.J. Connor, and R.B. Herberman, Variations in reactivity of 3 M KCl extracts of human breast carcinoma and melanoma using leukocyte migration inhibition assays. *J. Nat. Cancer Inst.* (submitted, 1975).

TUMOR ANTIGENS

THE USE OF CEA (CARCINOEMBRYONIC ANTIGEN) AND OTHER CARCINOFOETAL ANTIGENS IN HUMAN CANCER

S. VON KLEIST[*]

Institut de Recherches Scientifiques sur le Cancer, 94000 Villejuif, France

ABSTRACT

Among the numerous carcinofoetal antigens, which have been described in literature, only three have been sufficiently investigated in different laboratories so as to allow clinical application. They are: the CEA, AFP and α-2H-Fe. If these substances, which all circulate in patients' sera, can be considered as markers for malignancy, their respective assays are valid only in a very well-defined, limited field and under certain conditions:

The tests must be performed repeatedly for the same patient.

Their main clinical importance lies in the postoperative surveillance and therapy monitoring of the patient, especially for the early detection of residual or recurrent disease, therapy resistance or relapse, rather than in early diagnosis of cancer.

The tests as they are performed in practice must still be considered as supplementary indices and not as priming clinical data.

INTRODUCTION

Before going into the subject I shall just briefly define what is meant by the term "carcinoembryonic (or carcinofoetal) antigens": when in 1965 Gold and Freedman published their first paper on a cancer specific antigen present in human tumors of the gastrointestinal tract and other organs from the entodermally derived digestive tissue, they coined the expression carcinoembryonic antigen or CEA for this particular substance, because their antigen was also present in foetal gut, liver and pancreas up to the 6th month of gestation [1].

Although it is known now that this original definition is not correct because CEA is present throughout prenatal life and even after birth, this denomination has been adopted universally to designate antigens present in malignant and foetal tissues and/or serum, apparently absent from normal adult organs, as shown principally by the use of heteroantisera. That this definition is somewhat schematic will be seen later on. At the present time there are at least six carcinofoetal antigens known in human malignancies, all of which are not rigorously cancer specific. Four of these antigens are found in

---

[*] Chargée de Recherches à l'Institut National de la Santé et de la Recherche Médicale.

primary carcinomas of organs of the digestive tract, i.e. (1) the alpha-foeto-protein
(AFP), first described by Tatarinov in man as being specific for malignant hepatomas
[2]; (2) the CEA of Gold, independently found also by us [3, 4]; (3) the foeto-
sulphoglyco-protein (or FSA) described by Häkkinen to be present in cancerous gastric
juice [5], and finally (4) the alpha-2-hepatic ferroglobulin (α-2H) which has been
isolated by Buffe *et al.* initially from foetal liver [6].

The two remaining antigens we shall only mention for the sake of completeness—
because their clinical significance has not yet been demonstrated by other laboratories—
are the

carcinofoetal glial antigen (CFGA), which has been described by Trouillas in malignant gliomas [7], and the

Gamma-a foetal antigen (γFA) found by Edynak in a large variety of human neoplasia, and for which quite recently he described a radioimmunoassay [8].

Among all these carcinofoetal antigens only three have been physico-chemically
sufficiently characterized and reproduced as to allow clinical trial and application. They
are the CEA, AFP and α2H Fe and they will be discussed in more detail.

1. THE CARCINOEMBRYONIC ANTIGEN (CEA)

(a) Characterization

The best-known antigen as far as clinical investigations are concerned is the CEA. It
has the following physico-chemical characteristics:

It is soluble in perchloric acid (PCA).

It is a highly antigenic glycoprotein with a carbohydrate moiety of about 45%,
which contains galactose, mannose, fucose, N-acetyl glucosamine and sialic acid.
The peptide moiety of the molecule is rich in glutamic and aspartic acid and their
bases and the twenty-three aminoacids of the N-terminal end have been determined
by Terry [9].

CEA has a sedimentation constant of about 7.2 S, its molecular weight is generally
considered to be about 180,000 D [9].

It is easily demonstrable by immunoelectrophoresis or double diffusion reactions in
PCA extracts of intestinal tumors, where it shows up as one of the principal antigens
migrating towards the cathode (Fig. 1). The high sugar content of the molecule makes
it subject to cross reactions with other glycoproteins (for instance, blood group
substances), which might interfere with the specific CEA reaction. One of these cross-
reacting antigens, the NCA (non-specific cross-reacting antigen), is demonstrated on the
same slide together with the third main antigen of colon tumors, which has an α
mobility. Both these substances will be discussed later.

CEA is widely distributed and has been evidenced by the use of sensitive methods in a
great variety of tissues and fluids (Table 1).

By immunofluorescence microscopy the CEA can be demonstrated abundantly on
the luminal surface of the tumor glands specially of well-differentiated epitheliomas of the
glandular type (Fig. 2), whereas in poorly differentiated tumors it becomes less abundant
and anaplastic tumors can be even negative [10, 11].

The fact that it needs a well-differentiated carcinoma or metastasis in order to get a
clear-cut result impairs greatly the use of this technique for the identification of

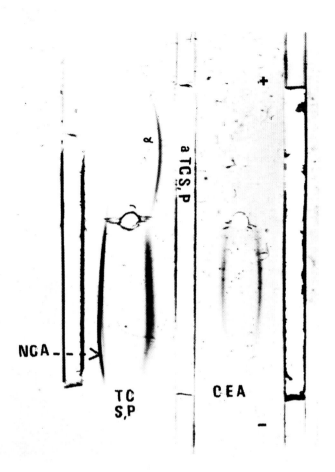

Fig. 1. Immunoelectrophoresis of a PCA extract of colonic tumors (TCS, P) and purified CEA. Left: an anti-CEA revealing also the NCA.

undifferentiated metastases of unknown origin. Furthermore, CEA has been shown by our group to be present in non-cancerous mucosa more than 10 cm off the primary tumor and in well-differentiated polyps and even in hemorrhoids [10, 12]. These findings bring about the crucial question of the cancer specificity of CEA, which has raised so much emotion. In normal, that is noninflammatory, adult colonic mucosa we have not found appreciable amounts of CEA with the methods we employed [13]. Equal findings have been reported for instance by Todd *et al.* [14], Denk [11], Orjasacter *et al.* [15] and Gold [1]. On the other hand, there are the absorption experiments of Martin and Martin which showed the presence of CEA in minute quantities in normal colonic mucosa extracts, thus demonstrating that the cancer specificity of CEA is based on quantitative rather than qualitative differences [16].

Table 1. *Presence of "CEA" in Malignant and Non-malignant Tissues and Body Fluids*

TISSUES		FLUIDS / SECRETIONS
MALIGNANT	NON-MALIGNANT	
Site :		Plasma
		Saliva
Colon	Inflammatory, normal colonic mucosa, polyps, hemorrhoids	Faeces, mucus (meconium)
Stomach	Gastric mucosa with intestinal metaplasia	Gastric juice
Lung	Normal	Malignant pleural effusion
Breast	Lactating	Colostrum
Liver	Normal, cirrhotic	Ascites
Pancreas		
Gall bladder		Bile
Kidney		Urine
Ovary		Prostatic and seminal ; cervical and vaginal secretions
		Amniotic fluid

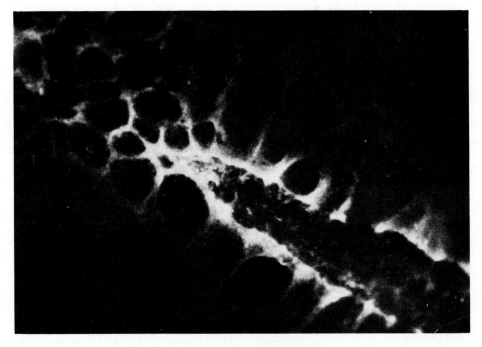

Fig. 2. Immunofluorescence pattern of a frozen section of a colonic tumor incubated with an anti-CEA antiserum (indirect method, × 400).

All results reported until now were exclusively obtained with heteroimmunsera. The question is, can one demonstrate the CEA also with autologous sera, in other words, is the CEA autoantigenic? The answer we give to that question is no! Here we are in controversy with Gold, who described repeatedly circulating antibodies directed against CEA in colonic cancer patients' sera [17]. No one else yet has reproduced his findings [18].

We have worked also on this problem but were not able to demonstrate anti-CEA anti-bodies. The antibodies we found, in patients' sera, were all directed against other tumor proteins as, for instance, the α-protein, which I mentioned before [19].

Apparently CEA does not stimulate cell mediated immunity either, because when Hollinshead *et al.* injected patients intradermally with soluble fractions of autologous colon tumor cell membranes they observed positive delayed-type hypersensitivity skin reactions. They did not see anything alike with purified CEA [20]. Likewise, Lejtenyi of Gold's group did not receive any evidence for a cell mediated immune response in her test system either, which consisted of patients' lymphocytes blastic transformation upon *in vitro* exposure to CEA [21].

One might argue that CEA *in vitro* contains a protein constituent which permits the stimulation of cell mediated immunity and that the acid extraction alters the molecule in such a way that it will no longer stimulate delayed type immunity.

This brings about the problem of possible differences between the extracted and the native antigen, which circulates in patients' sera in nanogram quantities and is hence only measurable by the radioimmunoassay (RIA). Technical details of the different methods employed will not be discussed, because the overall results obtained with various techniques (% of positivity, etc.) are the same.

(b) The RIA of CEA

Ever since the first publication of Thomson [22] from Gold's equipe reporting a unique specificity for only digestive tract cancer of the measurement of serum CEA levels, the clinical (and scientific) interest in this antigen has become world wide. However, all following reports of reproducing laboratories differ from the initial promising one, in that the exclusive specificity of the CEA test has been found neither for digestive cancer nor for other malignancies. All groups confirmed a specially high percentage of CEA positive sera from carcinomas of the digestive tract (Table 2), but they also found an overall positivity of about 50% in tumors of the genito-urinary system, the lung, breast, in neuroblastomas and myelomas. Furthermore, positive CEA values were also found in 30–40% of benign diseases of the gastrointestinal tract and other non-malignant disorders, preferentially alcoholic cirrhosis and pancreatitis [23]. However, in absolute healthy control sera CEA was undetectable. Following the different techniques employed the upper limit for normal varies, but is usually taken at 2.5 ng/ml.

Although it had been proved then that the CEA test had no diagnostic specificity for neoplasia, further investigations evidenced that the RIA kept its clinical interest mainly in two well-defined, limited fields:

1. One is the evaluation of the cancer extension which implicates (long-term) prognosis. It has been shown that elevated CEA levels were seen only in one-third of colonic tumors strictly localized to the intestinal wall, in about half of locally infiltrative carcinomas, but in 80–90% of those with distant metastases [23]. Figure 3 taken from a collaborative Swiss study published by Mach *et al.* illustrates this [24]. The conclusion is that low CEA blood values exclude not a carcinoma but (at most) a widespread one.

Table 3 [25] shows that, indeed, preoperative CEA measurements may be a sensitive indicator for the presence of hepatic metastases. In a series of twenty-two colonic tumor patients all with hepatic metastases verified after laparotomy, nine had no evidence

Table 2. *CEA Serum Levels in Patients with*
Tumors and Other Conditions
(> 25 ng/ml)

DISORDER	No. TESTED	% POS.
INTESTINAL CARCINOMAS	390	81
OTHER CARCINOMAS	512	51
BENIGN DISEASES OF THE GASTROINTESTINAL TRACT	143	39
OTHER NON MALIGNANT DISORDERS	472	32
"NORMAL CONTROLS"	503	1.6
Total	2 020	

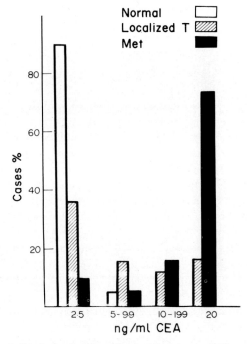

Fig. 3. CEA serum levels as a function of colon cancer spread. (From Mach *et al.* [24].)

(neither clinical nor biochemical) for metastases, seven (or 78%) had elevated (> 15 ng/ml) CEA levels, and three even very high values (> 100 ng/ml). From the thirteen patients with either clinical and/or biochemical abnormalities, only four had both, yet the CEA was augmented in all of them.

Table 3. *CEA Measurement and Presence of Hepatic Metastases*

PREOPERATIVE STATUS	No TOTAL	SERUM CEA LEVELS	
		>15 NG/ML	>100 NG/ML
No preoperative Evidence for hepatic Metastases	9	7	3
Clinical & Biochemical Evidence for hepatic Metastases	13	13	8
Total	22	20	11

CLINICAL DATA FROM : BOOTH. S.N., ET AL., BRIT. MED. J., 664 (1974), 183.

As far as prognosis is concerned, it has been claimed by some investigators, such as Booth *et al.* [25] and Chu *et al.* [26], that elevated preoperative CEA levels mean in most cases poor prognosis. In fact Booth reviewed after 2 years a series of twenty patients, eleven of whom (or 55%) encountered recurrent disease or death. Nine out of eleven of the patients had had preoperatively elevated CEA values (for this author > 15 ng/ml). From the remaining nine patients who were tumor free at that time, four, i.e. 44%, had had elevated CEA levels [25]. These results are in accordance with those of Chu, who observed recurrent disease in five out of six patients with elevated CEA values, elevated meaning here > 7.5 ng/ml. Note that all–sixteen patients–with normal CEA levels stayed tumor free during the same lapse of time.

2. The other most valuable aspect of CEA measurement is that of clinical surveillance of patients for the (postoperative) early detection of residual or recurrent disease and the monitoring of radio- and chemotherapy. It is now generally admitted [27] that above normal CEA blood values, which do not return to normal, usually within a week or so after curative surgery, are an indicative sign of incomplete surgery or hidden metastases (Fig. 4, from Holyoke *et al.* [28]). If the absolute condition of repeated serum tests is respected, then even a slight but constant rise is a reliable precocious signal of recurrency, which might precede the clinical detection by more than a month. Holyoke also showed that chemotherapy can be monitored by CEA evaluations: the therapeutical success as reflected by a clinical remission coincided with a decrease in the CEA serum level which increased again when the patient relapsed.

There is one last aspect, we have not yet mentioned, that of differential diagnosis: is the CEA test of any value in early detection of malignant transformation, for instance in chronic disorders, known to have similar (if not identical) symptomatology with early stage cancer? Studied examples are ulcerative colitis and Crohn's disease, which Booth *et al.* reviewed [29] (Table 4). In their survey of 272 patients they observed only in 9% of rectocolitis and in 22% of long-standing Crohn's disease an elevated CEA serum level. In two ulcerative colitis patients who developed carcinoma, the CEA value was normal. So it is concluded that CEA estimations in chronic intestinal as in other inflammatory or benign disorders are of no assistance in the distinction of malignant degeneration. However, it has been demonstrated, too, that benign lesions seldom give rise to high CEA values so that they would always strongly suggest neoplasia. This, nevertheless, still leaves incipient cancers undetectable.

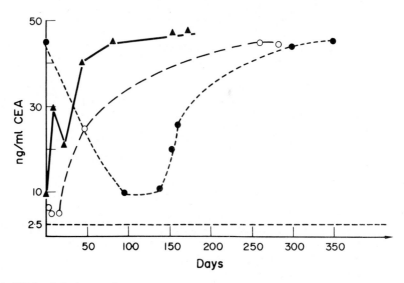

Fig. 4. CEA levels in three patients with residual disease (after partial resection). In no case did CEA fall below normal, in one case there was a partial remission. (From Holyoke *et al.* [28].)

Table 4. *Serum CEA Levels in Inflammatory Bowel Disorders*

DIAGNOSIS	DURATION YEARS	No. TOTAL	CEA ELEVATION		
			> 15 NG/ML	TRANSIENT	PERSISTENT
ULCERATIVE PROCTOCOLITIS	0 - 5	37	2	0	1
	5 - 10	18	1	1	0
– RECTAL & LEFT COLONIC DISEASE	> 10	27	3	1	2
– TOTAL OR EXTENSIVE ULCERATIVE COLITIS	0 - 5	22	4	4	0
	0 - 10	19	2	0	2
	> 10	10	0	0	0
CROHN'S DISEASE	0 - 5	51	8	5	2
	5 - 10	27	4	1	2
	> 10	61	19	4	12

CLINICAL DATA FROM : BOOTH, S.N, ET AL. SCAND. J. GASTROENT., 9,(1974), 651.

3. In conclusion one can say that the RIA of CEA, provided it is repeatedly employed and by experienced hands, already has its clinical importance for
the postoperative surveillance, and
therapy monitoring of the patient, specially for the early detection of residual or recurrent resistance or relapse.
The CEA test cannot be used (yet), because of lack of specificity for diagnostic or screening purposes, except perhaps, as has been pointed out recently by Freedman [30], in very selected high-risk groups such as asbestos workers or uranium miners.
Also one should bear in mind that the whole evaluation of the CEA test is based on

observations made in patients with already established diagnoses; the final word about its clinical interest will be probably delivered only after more "blind" series have been run.

Nevertheless, we shall finish this first section with an optimistic outlook: Plow and Edgington [31, 32] have a paper in press, in which they describe the purification of a species of CEA molecules, which no longer, in the RIA, give rise to so-called false positive reactions, or render them exceptional (as known in heavy smokers, hepatic cirrhoses, etc.). Let us hope that the CEA-S brings back some of the tumor specificity to this antigen, which was its glory 10 years ago.

Table 5. *Antigens Related to CEA*

Abbreviation	Full Name	Reference
FSA	Feto-Sulphoglycoprotein	Hakkinen, J.T., Immunochemistry 9, (1972) 115
NGP	Normal Glycoprotein	Mach, J.P., Pusztaszeri, G., Immunochemistry 9 (1972) 1031
NCA	Non specific Crossreacting Antigen	von Kleist, S. et al. P.N.A.S. (USA), 69 (1972) 2492
CCA III	Colon Carcinoma Antigen III	Newman, E.S. et al. Fed. Proc., 31 (1972) 639
CEX	Associated Protein	Darcy, D.A. et al. Brit. J. Cancer, 28 (1973) 147
BCGP	Breast Cancer Glycoprotein	Tseng-Tong Kuo et al. Int. J. Cancer, 12 (1973) 532
NCA-2	Non specific Crossreacting Antigen - 2	Burtin, P. et al. J. Immunology (1973), 111, 1926

Before discussing AFP, we shall briefly mention that there are several substances known in literature (Table 5, [3]) that cross react with CEA, not all of them having been tested for their possible interference in the RIA of CEA. The best known of these antigens is the NCA (non-specific cross-reacting antigen, [3]), which has been described by Mach [35], Darcy and us under different names, but which are identical. For the NCA it is approximately certain that it does not interfere in the RIA of CEA, though this might not be true for other techniques as, for instance, immunofluorescence [36]. There seems to be little clinical interest in this antigen, which circulates in much greater quantities in normal serum than CEA (Table 6) and which apparently decreases (rather than increases) in some malignancies [37].

II. THE ALPHA-FOETO-PROTEIN (AFP)

In contrast to CEA, the AFP has its animal counterparts in all mammalian species. It was Abelev [38] who described it in sera of hepatoma-bearing mice and named it α foetoglobulin because of its electrophoretic mobility and presence in foetal serum;

Table 6. *NCA in Patients' Sera*

DIAGNOSIS	No.	NG/ML				AGE
		NCA	MEAN	CEA	MEAN	
N.DONORS	50	32 - 510	132	2 - 25	5	22 - 56
BENIGN DISEASES	57	32 - 1000	179	2 - 60	18	15 - 87
CARCINOMAS	84	25 - 1000	157	2 - 125	34	? - 32
	191					

Tatarinov [2] was the first to see it in man, and to claim its specificity for this kind of malignancy. AFP, which is a protein of a M.W. of about 70,000 D and a sedimentation constant of 4.5 S [39] , is the first demonstrable principal embryonic serum protein. It appears in adult serum under various physiological and pathological conditions, specially in primary liver cancer.

Its hepatic synthesis seems to be in relation with the degree of histological differentiation: well-differentiated and highly anaplastic hepatomas do not produce AFP, or very little. Hence it would appear that serum titers are in a certain correlation with the degree of dedifferentiation of malignant hepatomas [40] .

AFP serum concentrations vary considerably, dropping from some mg/ml at about the 11th week of gestation to some μg/ml in newborn sera. In sera of pregnant women and normals, ng/ml quantities are seen, while in hepatoma sera as much AFP can be found as in foetal sera [41, 42] . It follows that the lower limit of sensitivity of the chosen method of detection is of great importance in the AFP test. At the beginning only the simple Ouchterlony double diffusion test has been employed with monospecific heteroimmunsera and a foetal serum as positive control for the demonstration of AFP in hepatoma sera: results varying from 30 to 80% of positivity were obtained in different countries throughout the world for this particular malignancy.

Significantly higher percentages of positivity were obtained in children as compared with adults [43] . In benign liver diseases (including hemochromatosis, hepatitis, etc.) less than 0.5% "false" positive results were obtained in more than 70,000 sera tested with the Ouchterlony method, hence this test was considered specific for hepatic carcinoma. Things have changed slightly since more sensitive methods such as passive hemagglutination or RIA have been used: AFP has been detected also in normal sera and increased levels were found in 13–20% of non-malignant hepatic disorders, especially in acute hepatitis in the regenerative phase, but not only was this augmentation often transitory, but also were the values under those observed in hepatomas [41, 44] . As pointed out by Seppäla and Ruoslahti [45] , in pregnant women, in whom AFP serum levels rise with the progressing gestation, AFP may reach pathological values in case of fetal distress and death.

AFP has also been found in 1% (Ouchterlony) or 14% (RIA) of secondary hepatic cancer (primarily in case of gastric metastases), and in active teratomas and ovarian tumors with a very high incidence of serum positivity again in children (Table 7, [46]); other embryonic tumors, such as neuro- or nephroblastomas, for instance, have been found negative.

Table 7. *AFP in Tumor-bearing Adults and Children*

Positive Cases	Age (Years)		Negative Cases	Age (Years)
Diagnoses	0 - 15 pos./total	22 - 75 pos./total	Diagnoses	0 - 15 pos./total
Hepatoma	21/23*	36/47	Nephroblastoma	0/43
Malignant Teratoma	15/27°	4/27	Sympathoma	0/42
			Osteosarcoma	0/19
Total Positivity	81 %	54 %	Lymphoma	0/17
			Embryonic Sarcoma	0/17
			Brain Tumor	0/ 7
			Miscellaneous	0/ 5
			Total	150

° 11/12 of negative sera came from children either cured or in complete remission.

* Histologically confirmed.

Data from :

Mawas, C. et al, Rev. Europ. Etudes Clin. et Biol., 16 (1971), 430.

Table 8. *Alpha Foetoprotein in the Sera of Tumor-bearing Children*

	Nr. of Cases	Immunodiffusion	
		Simple	Radioautography
Hepatoma	41	38	39
Active Teratoma	29	27	27
In remission	28	0	0
Other Tumors	369	0	3

Clinical Data from : Buffe, D., Gann, 14 (1973), 129.

As has been shown by Buffe [43] (Table 8), it is not necessary in children to use particularly sensitive methods because the AFP serum level in this group of patients is sufficiently elevated as to give positive results with the Ouchterlony test. So it appears that specially in this last group of neoplasia (i.e. paediatric tumors) the AFP test is an uncomplicated and specific test, provided—again—that the same serum is tried repeatedly. The introduction of highly sensitive techniques allows (as for the CEA) early detection of malignancy, often before clinical manifestation [46], and surveillance, both post-operatively and prospective in such high-risk groups as, for instance, postnecrotic cirrhosis or hemochromatosis, where the incidence of hepatoma has been described to be >20% [48, 49]. Here, also, it is commonly agreed, that even a slight but steady rise in the antigen level indicates neoplasia.

A word of caution is necessary, however, as far as AFP augmentation in infants is concerned: as has been demonstrated by Buffe and Rimbaut [50] and Belanger [51] this antigen is increased also in a congenital metabolic disease, the tyrosinaemia. One will have to rule out this illness first before thinking of a tumor.

III. THE ALPHA-2H-FERROGLOBULINE (α-2H-Fe)

The last antigen that will be discussed is the α-2H-Fe, first described and isolated from foetal liver by Buffe *et al.* [6]. (The "H" stands for hepatic.)

It is a glycoprotein rich in iron, which accounts for 10–25% of its molecular mass. Although giving an immunological reaction of identity with ferritin, it seems to be a distinct though closely parental substance for the following two reasons:

α-2H-Fe is practically insoluble in media (i.e. distilled water or PBS) where ferritin is soluble,

it has a carbohydrate moiety, while ferritin has not.

The composition of this complex molecule varies with its tissular origin (as shown by Rimbaut [52]): closest to ferritin is α-2H-Fe present in normal, most different than found in foetal or tumorous tissues, where it is distributed in an ubiquitous fashion. α-2H-Fe also circulates in sufficiently great quantities as to be demonstrable by gel precipitation methods.

The evolution of the α-2H-Fe studies was approximately that of the two preceding antigens: first thought absent from normal adult organs, α-2H-Fe has been found to be present in very small quantities when more sensitive techniques were used. As far as its presence in patients' sera is concerned, more than 4000 sera have been tested now by the mentioned group and other authors [53, 54]—the following results have been obtained (Table 9, [52]): α-2H-Fe is found in 50% of tumor-bearing adults and in 80% of tumorous children, against 20% in adults suffering from non-malignant diseases. Only 9% of healthy or benignly diseased children showed positive α-2H-Fe serum tests. Clinical trials run in paediatrics by Buffe *et al.* [55] clearly demonstrated the great medical interest of this antigen in the follow-up of either chemotherapeutically or surgically treated children with resectable neoplasia. α-2H-Fe disappears after efficient treatment and reappears and increases in case of metastases or recurrency, and this even before AFP does so, as comparative studies of the two antigens have shown.

So summing up, we can say that there are actually three antigenic markers for malignancy: the CEA, AFP and α-2H-Fe. Their respective tests bear a definite clinical interest if some basic rules are respected:

1. The tests should not be considered decisive but rather supplementary to classical medical methodology.
2. It should be remembered that their main application range lies in the follow-up of treated patients.
3. All tests should be performed repeatedly (over a certain period of time) before conclusions are drawn.

Finally, combining one of the tests with another can only improve the informative value of each individual test: this would also help to demonstrate that immunological methods, if widely and critically employed, are helpful tools in the clinic of today.

Table 9. *Positivity of Alpha-2H-Ferroglobulin in Sera of Children and Adults*

ADULTS	No. of cases	Positive	% of pos.
with Tumors	496	254	51
without Tumors	413	83	20
Total	909		

CHILDREN (2m–16 years)	No. of cases	Positive	% of pos.
with Tumors	452	362	80
Healthy or Benign	177	16	9
Total	629		

Clinical Data from : Rimbaut, C., Bull. Cancer, 60 (1973), 411.

REFERENCES

1. Ph. Gold and S. Freedman, Demonstration of tumor-specific antigens in human colonic carcinomata by immunological tolerance and absorption techniques. *J. Exp. Med.* 121, 439 (1965).
2. Yu. S. Tatarinov and A.C. Afanasyeva, The detection of similar antigenic determinants in embryospecific α-globulin of man and certain animals (in Russian). *Bull. Exp. Biol. Med.* 59, 65 (1965).
3. Ph. Gold and S.O. Freedman, Specific carcinoembryonic antigens of the human digestive system. *J. Exp. Med.* 122, 467 (1965).
4. S. von Kleist and P. Burtin, Mise en évidence dans les tumeurs coliques humaines d'antigènes non présents dans la muqueuse colique de l'adulte normal. *C.R. Acad. Sci. Paris,* 263, 1543 (1966).
5. J.P. Häkkinen, L.K. Korhonen and L. Saxen, The time for appearance and distribution of sulphoglycoprotein antigens in the human foetal alimentary canal. *Int. J. Cancer,* 3, 582 (1968).
6. D. Buffe, C. Rimbaut and P. Burtin, Présence d'une protéine d'origine tissulaire l'α2H-globuline dans le sérum des enfants porteurs de tumeur. *Int. J. Cancer,* 3, 850 (1968).
7. P. Trouillas, Carcino-foetal antigen in glial tumours. *Lancet,* 2, 552 (1971).
8. E.M. Edynak, M.P. Lardis and L.M. Pizzaia, Radioimmunoassay for gamma-a-fetal protein in serum of patients with cancer and non malignant diseases. *Surg. Forum,* 25, 126 (1974).
9. W.D. Terry, P.A. Hendart, J.E. Coligan and C.W. Todd, Structural studies of the major glycoprotein in preparations with carcinoembryonic antigen activity. *J. Exp. Med.* 136, 200 (1972).
10. S. von Kleist and P. Burtin, Localisation cellulaire d'un antigène embryonnaire de tumeurs coliques humaines. *Int. J. Cancer,* 4, 874 (1969).
11. H. Denk, G. Tappeiner, R. Eckestorfer and J.H. Holzner, Carcinoembryonic antigen (CEA) in gastrointestinal and extra-gastrointestinal tumors and its relationship to tumor-cell differentiation. *Int. J. Cancer,* 10, 262 (1972).
12. P. Burtin, E. Martin, M.C. Sabine and S. von Kleist, Immunological study of polyps of the colon. *J. Nat. Cancer Inst.* 48, 25 (1972).
13. S. von Kleist, Etude d'un antigène spécifique de tumeurs coliques humaines d'origine embryonnaire. *Biol. Med.* LX, 237 (1971).
14. C.W. Todd, M.L. Egan, J.T. Lautenschleger and J.E. Coligan, Dosage, isolement et caractérisation de l'antigène carcinoembryonnaire. *Ann. Inst. Pasteur,* 122, 841 (1972).
15. H. Orjasaeter, G. Fredriksen and I. Liavac, Studies on carcinoembryonic and related antigens in malignant tumors of colon-rectum. *Acta Path. Microbiol. Scand.*, Section B, 80, 599 (1972).

16. F. Martin and M.S. Martin, Demonstration of antigens related to colonic cancer in the human digestive system. *Int. J. Cancer,* **6**, 352 (1970).
17. J.M. Gold, S.O. Freedman and Ph. Gold, Human anti-CEA antibodies detected by radio-immunoelectrophoresis. *Nature (New Biol.)* **239**, 60 (1972).
18. P. Logerfo, F.P. Herter and S.J. Bennett, Absence of circulating antibodies to carcino-embryonic antigen in patients with gastrointestinal malignancies. *Int. J. Cancer,* **9**, 344 (1972).
19. E. Collatz, S. von Kleist and P. Burtin, Further investigations of circulating antibodies in colon cancer patients on the auto-antigenicity of the carcinoembryonic antigen. *Int. J. Cancer,* **8**, 298 (1971).
20. A.C. Hollinshead, C.G. Macwright, T.C. Alford, D.H. Glew, Ph. Gold and R.B. Herberman, Separation of skin reactive intestinal cancer antigen from the carcinoembryonic antigen of gold. *Science,* **177**, 887 (1972).
21. M.C. Lejtenyi, S.O. Freedman and Ph. Gold, Response of lymphocytes from patients with gastrointestinal cancer to the carcinoembryonic antigen of the human digestive system. *Cancer,* **28**, 115 (1971).
22. D.M.P. Thomson, J. Krupey, S.O. Freedman and Ph. Gold, The radioimmunoassay of circulating carcinoembryonic antigen of the human digestive system. *P.N.A.S.* (USA), **64**, 161 (1969).
23. N. Zamcheck, T.L. Moore, P. Dhar, H.Z. Kupchik and J.J. Sorokin, Carcinoembryonic antigen in benign and malignant diseases of the digestive tract. *Nat. Cancer Inst. Monogr.* **35**, 433 (1972).
24. J.P. Mach, G. Pusztaszeri, M. Dylsi, F. Kapp, B. Bierensaadehaan, R.M. Loosli, P. Grob and H. Isliker, Radioimmunoassay of carcinoembryonic antigen (CEA) in patients with carcinoma. Conclusion from preliminary results of a collaborative study in Switzerland. *Schweiz. Med. Wschr.* **103**, 365 (1973).
25. S.N. Booth, G.C. Jamieson, J.P. King, J. Leonard, G.D. Oates, P.W. Dykes, Carcinoembryonic antigen in management of colorectal carcinoma. *Br. Med. J.* **4**, 183 (1974).
26. T.M. Chu, E.D. Holyoke, G.P. Murphy, Carcinoembryonic antigen. Current clinical status. *N.Y. State J. Med.* **74**, 1388 (1974).
27. M.A. Neville and D.J.R. Laurence, Report of the workshop on the carcinoembryonic antigen (CEA): the present position and proposals for future investigation. *Int. J. Cancer* **14**, 1 (1974).
28. D. Holyoke, G. Reynoso and T.M. Chu, Carcinoembryonic antigen (CEA) in patients with carcinoma of the digestive tract. *Ann. Surg.* **176**, 559 (1972).
29. S.N. Booth, J.P. King, J.C. Leonard and P.W. Dykes, The significance of elevation of serum carcinoembryonic antigen (CEA) levels in inflammatory diseases of the intestine. *Scand. J. Gastroenterol.* **9**, 651 (1974).
30. S.O. Freedman, *Carcinoembryonic Antigen: Clinical Aspects. XI Int. Cancer Congr.,* p. 172, Conf., Symp., Workshops. Florence 1974.
31. E.F. Plow and T.S. Edgington, Isolation and characterization of a homogeneous isomeric species of carcinoembryonic antigen: CEA-S. *Int. J. Cancer,* **15**, 748 (1975).
32. T.S. Edgington, R.W. Astarita and E.F. Plow, Association of an isomeric species of carcinoembryonic antigen (CEA-S) with neoplasia of the gastrointestinal tract. *New Engl. J. Med.* **293**, 103 (1975).
33. S. von Kleist, Substances related to CEA. *Ann. d'Immunol.* **124**, 589 (1973).
34. S. von Kleist, G. Chavanel and P. Burtin, Identification of a normal antigen that cross-reacts with the carcinoembryonic antigen. *P.N.A.S.* (USA) **69**, 2492 (1972).
35. J.P. Mach and G. Pusztaszeri, Carcinoembryonic antigen (CEA)—demonstration of a partial identity between CEA and a normal glycoprotein. *Immunochemistry,* **9**, 1031 (1972).
36. J.T. Tomita, J.W. Saffort and A.A. Hirata, Antibody response to different determinants on carcinoembryonic antigen (CEA). *Immunology* **26**, 291 (1974).
37. S. von Kleist, S. Troupel and P. Burtin, Dosage radioimmunologique comparatif de l'antigène carcinoembryonnaire (CEA) et d'un antigène immunologiquement apparenté (NCA). *Ann. Immunol. (Inst. Pasteur)* **126C**, 100 (1975).
38. G.I. Abelev, S.D. Perova, N.I. Kramkova, Z.A. Postnikova and I.S. Irlin, Production of embryonal serum alpha-globulin by the transplantable mouse hepatomas. *Transplantation,* **I**, 174 (1963).
39. H. Hirai, S. Nishi, H. Watabe and Y. Tsukada, Some chemical, experimental and clinical investigations of alpha-foetoprotein. *Gann Monogr. Cancer Res.* **14**, 19 (1973).

40. T. Shikata and K. Sakakitara, Relationship between alpha-foetoprotein and histological patterns of hepatoma and localization of alpha-foetoprotein in hepatoma cells using the peroxidase antibody technique. *Gann Monogr. Cancer Res.* **14,** 269 (1973).

41. J. Uriel and B. de Nechaud, La recherche d'alpha-foetoprotéine en Pathologie humaine. Etat actuel de la question. *Ann. Inst. Pasteur,* **122,** 829 (1972).

42. R.F. Masseyeff, Factors influencing alpha-foetoprotein biosynthesis in patients with primary liver cancer and other diseases. *Gann Monogr. Cancer Res.* **14,** 3 (1973).

43. D. Buffe, Foetoproteins and children's tumors. *Gann Monogr. Cancer Res.* **14,** 117 (1973).

44. F.G. Lehmann, Tumor antigens. *Dtsch. Med. Wochenschr.* **99,** 410 (1974).

45. M. Seppäla and E. Ruoslahti, Alpha-foetoprotein in normal and pregnancy. *Lancet,* **1,** 375 (1972).

46. C. Mawas, B. Buffe, O. Schweisguth and P. Burtin, Alpha-foetoprotein and children's cancer. *Rev. Europ. Etud. Clin. Biol.* **16,** 430 (1971).

47. Y. Endo, K. Kanai, S. Iino and T. Oda, Clinical significance of alpha-foetoprotein with special reference to primary cancer of the liver. *Gann Monogr. Cancer Res.* **14,** 67 (1973).

48. J.A.P. Chayvialle, C. Touillon, C. Crozier and R. Lambert, Radioimmunoassay of alpha-foetoprotein in human serum. Clinical value in patients with liver diseases. *Ann. J. Dig. Dis.* **19,** 1102 (1974).

49. D.T. Purtilo and L.S. Gottlieb, Cirrhosis and hepatomas occurring at Boston City Hospital (1917–1968). *Cancer,* **32,** 458 (1973).

50. D. Buffe and C. Rimbaut, L'alpha-foetoprotéine dans les atteintes hépatiques et les maladies métaboliques de l'enfant. *Biomed.* **19,** 172 (1973).

51. L. Belanger, M. Belanger and J. Larochelle, Une cirrhose infantile associée à néoproduction d'alpha-foetoprotéine. Perspectives nouvelles dans la tyrosinémie héréditaire. *Nouv. Presse Med.* **1,** 1503 (1972).

52. C. Rimbaut, L'alpha 2 H globuline, glycoprotéine reactionnelle sérique d'origine hépatiques, ses rapports avec les affections malignes. *Bull. Cancer,* **60,** 411 (1973).

53. J.P. Martin, R. Charlionnet and C. Ropartz, Alpha 2 H sérique au cours des hémopathies malignes et cirrhoses. Valeurs évolutive. *Presse Med.* **79,** 2313 (1971).

54. T. Wada, T. Anzai, A. Yachi, A. Takahashi and S. Sakamoto, Incidences of three different foetal proteins in sera of patients with primary hepatoma. In: *Protides of Biological Fluids,* edited by H. Peters, Vol. 18, p. 221. Bruges, 1971.

55. D. Buffe, C. Rimbaut, J. Lemerle, O. Schweisguth and P. Burtin, Présence d'une ferroprotéine d'origine tissulaire, l'alpha 2H globuline dans le sérum des enfants porteurs de tumeur. *Int. J. Cancer,* **5,** 85 (1970).

HL-A IN CANCER

HL-A AND CANCER

A. GOVAERTS

Free University of Brussels, Department of Immunology,
Hôpital St Pierre, Rue Haute, 322, 1000 Bruxelles

ABSTRACT

Association between HL-A antigens and diseases was extensively investigated in the last decade. It is supported by genetic considerations and was clearly established in several diseases, malignant or not. Besides ankylosing spondylitis in which HL-A 27 is strongly prevalent, many autoimmune diseases (or suspected to be so), immunodeficient and metabolic diseases, were systematically studied with encouraging results. In the malignant group, acute lymphoblastic leukemia, chronic lymphoid and myeloid leukemias, Hodgkin's disease, Burkitt's disease and different solid tumors were carefully investigated. The observed associations are discussed according to the most likely hypotheses.

INTRODUCTION

The association between blood antigens and diseases seems to have been one of the most persistent dreams of many immunohematologists in the last half century. May I recall briefly the countless papers devoted to the suspected associations between the ABO system and gastro-duodenal ulcer, gastric and colic cancer, pernicious anemia, diabetes mellitus, rheumatic fever, hypertension and several other somatic or psychiatric diseases. Most of these correlations were due to statistical bias; some of them looked convincing and were accepted as true during years. None is nowadays considered reliable except, of course, the hemolytic anemia of the newborn. In 1956, Wiener [1] wrote: "I am surprised to see how much space is being wasted in the *Lancet* and *British Medical Journal* on articles dealing with blood-groups distribution in various diseases. The hardest things to explain are those which are untrue."

The association between the HL-A system and diseases, malignant or not, was investigated on a rather extensive scale. The reasons for such studies were, in fact, more solid than for erythrocytes: the H_2 system in mice is known to be involved in the development of cancer to oncogenic viruses and, furthermore, geographical association between HL-A genes and the Ir locus on chromosome 6 is now rather well established. On this chromosome, three structural genes (at 1st, 2nd and 3rd loci), each existing in several allelic forms, control the expression of HL-A antigens. Each locus is highly polymorphic and the total number of different antigenic specificities which can be detected on human leucocytes is thus close to 90. Next to the HL-A area, the MLR complex manages the capacity of lymphocytes to be stimulated in allogenic cultures, and the Ir dominant genes are

107

108   CLINICAL TUMOR IMMUNOLOGY

involved in the regulation of specific responses to a variety of defined antigens. Several
of these genes are not completely independent on each other and this dependence is
called linkage disequilibrium. This means that some antigens depending on next loci are
present together more often than expected by random. For instance, the gene frequencies
of HL-A 1 and HL-A 8 are, respectively, 0.12 and 0.07. Their expected frequency on the
same haplotype, assuming random segregation, would be 0.84%; observed is 5.46%.

HL-A AND NON-MALIGNANT DISEASES

The most striking association was shown to be between ankylosing spondylitis and
HL-A 27. In the last 2 years, hundreds of cases of this rheumatoid disease were pheno-
typed and shown to be HL-A 27 with a frequency higher than 80%, and in several series
close to 100%; the mean frequency in a Caucasian population being around 7%. If,
undoubtedly, bearing that HL-A 27 is not sufficient to induce the disease, there is a
strong linkage disequilibrium between both genes. Up to now, no interaction could be
demonstrated with the LD loci or the Ir genes. This prevalence of HL-A 27 is also evident,
although less striking, in Reiter's disease, psoriatic arthritis, juvenile rheumatoid arthritis,
ulcerative colitis and uveitis. However, all of these illnesses are certainly polygenic and
probably environmentally dependent.

Autoimmune diseases were systematically investigated: myasthenia gravis, active
chronic hepatitis, insulin-dependent diabetes mellitus, coeliac disease, Addison's disease,
thyreotoxicosis; all these diseases show an association with the same antigen of the
second locus, HL-A 8. This strange observation will be briefly discussed later on. In the
neurological group, the gene governing susceptibility to multiple sclerosis seems, according to several authors, to be closely associated to HL-A 3 and 7, and LD 7a genes; it could
well be next to the latter [2]. Other diseases, like leprosy, rheumatic fever and heart
disease, polycystic kidneys, psoriasis and aplastic anemia, were also suspected of a genetic
linkage with the HL-A system but the reported cases were somewhat conflicting.

The fast increasing number of reports on the association between HL-A antigens and
disease led Svejgaard [3] to open an international registration of all collected data. This
register will include negative as well as positive results and will thus give an accurate
information for each disease.

Recently Terasaki and Mickey [4] claimed that haplotype frequency should be
considered in place of antigen frequency. They computed the frequency of 150 different
haplotypes in more than 10,000 patients enduring more than seventy different diseases
and compared them to the haplotypes distribution in a similar number of healthy persons.
They noticed that the HL-A 1-8 haplotype which is the most common in the Caucasian
race was absent in ankylosing spondylitis and rheumatoid arthritis, but also in acute
lymphocytic leukemia and in colon and prostate cancers. In psoriasis, the linkage 1-17
is 9 times more frequent than 1-8, and in amyotrophic lateral sclerosis the incidence of
1-22 is 95/1000 instead of 2/1000 in controls. The haplotype 2-12 appears to be 100-fold
decreased in multiple sclerosis, systemic lupus erythematosus and kidney cancer. In
ankylosing spondylitis and Reiter's syndrome, HL-A 27 is markedly increased in association with HL-A 2 but not with HL-A 1. Furthermore, the HL-A 3-27 haplotype is much
more frequent in Reiter's syndrome than in ankylosing spondylitis. From this study,
Terasaki and Mickey conclude that disease susceptibility genes are linked to specific
haplotypes more than to individual genes.

HL-A AND CANCER

The first investigation on correlations between HL-A and cancer was published in 1967 by Kourilsky *et al.* [5] on acute leukemias: 102 cases of acute lymphoblastic leukemia and fourteen cases of acute myeloid leukemia were analyzed; all of them were in remission in order to avoid errors due to typing of leucoblasts. The authors concluded to a normal distribution of the ten HL-A antigens which could be identified at that time. However, several other series published somewhat later presented different results: increase of HL-A 2, decrease of HL-A 9, and conflicting data for other antigens. In 1973 Rogentine *et al.* [6] claimed that HL-A 2 was much more frequent in patients surviving acute lymphoblastic leukemia more than 5 years (84%) than in the normal population (44%). Because of the strong cross-reaction between HL-A 2 and HL-A 28, and to some extent HL-A 9, the authors analyzed their pooled material for the three suspected antigens; they found that at least one of them was present in 94% of the long survival cases. According to Lawler, Klouda *et al.* [7], however, HL-A 2 and 28 are not more frequent in survivors than in normal controls but HL-A 9 patients have the longest median survival time.

These series are thus suggestive that the increased frequency of the suspected antigen is associated not with increased susceptibility but with increased resistance to acute leukemia. This correlation would be due to a linkage disequilibrium between the concerned HL-A genes and an anti-leukemia immune response gene, probably located in the Ir complex. Unfortunately for this hypothesis, several more recent studies did not confirm such a correlation: Dausset *et al.* [8], for instance, typing for twelve antigens at the first locus and sixteen at the second, did not find any difference between forty acute lymphoblastic leukemias and the normal population. As stated before, Terasaki described a significant reduction of the HL-A 1-8 haplotype frequency.

Similar studies were devoted to chronic lymphoid and myeloid leukemias. Inconsistent deviations to normal were observed: some reduction of HL-A 12 frequency in myeloid leukemia and variable results in lymphoid leukemia. In the latter, a technical pitfall is likely: antibodies cytotoxic for B cells only have been described in mice and men [9]; such antibodies present in HL-A antisera may give additional positive reactions. Delmas-Marsalet *et al.* [10] studying the HL-A genotypes in a family with four leukemic haplo-identical siblings suggested a linkage between HL-A and susceptibility to the disease. Hors and Dausset [11] also found an unexpected number of haplo-identity among siblings sharing the same malignant disease. Altogether, collected data suggest a weak association which is far from being established.

Due to several suggestive publications, Hodgkin's disease was strongly suspected to be HL-A linked. An unusual effort was made to confirm or disprove this hypothesis: during the Fifth Histocompatibility Workshop in 1972, eleven teams studied 300 cases of the disease with the same antisera. The pathological diagnosis was established on very strict criteria and the different groups were working in double blind. These extensive investigations concluded in favor of the absence of any correlation between HL-A and the disease, with the possible exception of W5 or T4.

Burkitt's disease was also studied by several authors, on a pool of 106 patients [12]. No significant difference could be observed with a normal negroid population.

In other groups of solid tumors, results are rather clearcut. A total of nearly 600 patients with breast cancer were typed in different laboratories [13]; the combined analysis did not show any association with HL-A antigens. Malignant melanoma was investigated in 350 patients [13] without any correlation between single HL-A antigens and the disease. However, the W30-HL-A 12 haplotype appears much more frequently than in normal subjects. Lymphomas display a usual high incidence of the HL-A 9-5 haplotype whereas kidney cancers have seldom the haplotype 2-12 and stomach cancer the haplotype 3-7. Last of all, haplotype 1-8 is much less common than expected in colic, prostate and tongue cancers.

DISCUSSION

Several general reviews have discussed the possible mechanisms which could explain associations between HL-A determinants and diseases. Let us briefly consider the most likely hypotheses. Immune response or Ir genes are now well documented in several animal species including man. They are located on chromosome 6, next to the major histocompatibility complex, and they regulate the T cell dependent antibody response. A linkage disequilibrium between some Ir and HL-A genes would then easily explain the observed associations; moreover, the Ir complex is known to be closer to the second locus than to the first, and it is a fact that most of the described associations between HL-A and disease involve antigens, like HL-A 8, depending on the second locus. The concerned Ir gene might, of course, confer an increased resistance as well as an increased sensitivity to the disease. This hypothesis, however, remains unproved. Some experiments do not support it: i.e. attempts of immunizing rhesus negative volunteers with rhesus red blood cells reveal both good responders and non-responders. Among them, no significant difference was observed of the HL-A distribution in each group, ruling out a linkage disequilibrium between HL-A and a specific immune response gene, in this particular case at least.

Another hypothesis relies on the supposed cross-antigenicity between some HL-A determinants and microorganisms. Such cross-tolerance was named molecular mimicry and would make these fortunate microorganisms acceptable by the immune system which would be unable to distinguish them from the self HL-A antigens. This theory would explain the dominant susceptibility to infections but it remains completely conjectural, in spite of Rappaport's observations that allograft immunity can be induced by sensitization with streptococci.

Other tentative explanations have been proposed but they do not elucidate more convincingly the mechanisms of these undeniable but most polymorphic associations between HL-A and disease. Many, and perhaps all, of the associated diseases are polygenically controlled: it is thus unwise to expect one single explanation for the observed associations. In this field cancer is, once more, still more evasive than other diseases.

REFERENCES

1. A.S. Wiener, Blood groups and disease. *Lancet*, **2**, 1308 (1956).
2. L. Degos and J. Dausset, Histocompatibility determinants in multiple sclerosis. *Lancet*, **1**, 307 (1974).
3. A. Svejgaard, C. Jersild, L. Staub-Nielsen and W.F. Bodmer, HL-A antigens and disease. Statistical and genetical considerations. *Tissue Antigens*, 4, 95 (1974).
4. P.I. Terasaki and M.R. Mickey, HL-A haplotypes of 32 diseases. *Transplant. Rev.* **22**, 105 (1975).
5. F.M. Kourilsky, J. Dausset, N. Feingold, J.M. Dupuy and J. Bernard, Etude de la répartition des antigènes leucocytaires chez des malades atteints de leucémie aigüe en rémission. In: *Advances*

in Transplantation, p. 515, Munksgaard, Copenhagen, 1967.

6. G.N. Rogentine, R.J. Trapani, R.A. Yankee and E.S. Henderson, HL-A antigens and acute lymphocytic leukemia: the nature of the HL-A2 association. *Tissue Antigens* **3**, 470 (1973).

7. S.D. Lawler, P.T. Klouda, P.G. Smith, M.M. Till and R.M. Hardisty, Survival and the HL-A system in acute lymphoblastic leukemia. *Br. Med. J.* **1**, 547 (1974).

8. J. Dausset and J. Hors, Some contributions of the HL-A complex to the genetics of human diseases. *Transpl. Rev.* **22**, 44 (1975).

9. L. Legrand and J. Dausset, Immunogenetics of a new lymphocyte system. *5th Int. Congress of the Transplant. Soc.*, Jerusalem, p. 12 (1974).

10. Y. Delmas-Marsalet, J. Hors, J. Colombani and J. Dausset, Study of HL-A genotypes in a case of familial chronic lymphocytic leukemia (CLL). *Tissue Antigens*, **4**, 441 (1974).

11. J. Hors and J. Dausset, Maladies malignes identiques au sein d'une même famille. *Nouv. Presse Médicale*, **3**, 1237 (1974).

12. J.G. Bodmer, W.F. Bodmer, P. Pickbourne, L. Degos, J. Dausset and H.M. Dick, Combined analysis of three studies of patients with Burkitt's lymphoma. *Tissue Antigens*, **5**, 63 (1975).

13. A. Svejgaard, P. Platz, L.P. Ryder, L. Staub-Nielsen and M. Thomsen, HL-A and disease associations–a survey. *Transpl. Rev.* **22**, 3 (1975).

CLASSIFICATION OF LEUKEMIAS
AND LYMPHOMAS

IMMUNOLOGICAL APPROACHES TO THE IDENTIFICATION OF LEUKAEMIC CELLS

M.F. GREAVES, G. BROWN,* D. CAPELLARO, G. JANOSSY and T. REVESZ†

*Imperial Cancer Research Fund, Tumour Immunology Unit,
Zoology Department, University College, London*

ABBREVIATIONS

Cells	FACS	Fluorescence activated cell sorter
	T-cell	Thymus derived lymphocyte
	B-cell	Bursa-equivalent derived lymphocyte
	AUL	Acute undifferentiated leukaemia
	ALL	Acute lymphoblastic leukaemia
	AML	Acute myeloblastic leukaemia
	AMML	Acute myelo-monocytic leukaemia
	CML	Chronic myeloid leukaemia
	CGL	Chronic granulocytic leukaemia
	CLL	Chronic lymphocytic leukaemia

Surface markers:

HuTLA	Human T-lymphocyte antigen
HuBLA	Human B-lymphocyte antigen
HuMA	Human monocyte/macrophage antigen
E rosette	Reaction of lymphocytes with sheep erythrocytes
EAHu	Reaction of lymphocytes (and other cells) with human rhesus positive red cells coated with anti-D-antibody
EAC rosette	Reaction of lymphocytes and other cells with antibody (A) plus complement (C) coated erythrocytes (E)
AggIgG	Heat-aggregated immunoglobulin G
SmIg	Surface membrane immunoglobulin
EBV	Epstein Barr Virus

* Present address: Department of Biochemistry, Oxford University.
† Present address: 2nd Department of Paediatrics, Semmelweis University of Medicine, Budapest, Hungary.

CELL SURFACE PHENOTYPING

Leukaemic cells in man have in the past been identified and classified by morphological and histochemical criteria. Recent advances in immunology now promise to provide an exciting new approach which both supplements older methods and adds a greater degree of discrimination. The principle of the immunological technique can be referred to as *cell surface phenotyping.* I have recently reviewed elsewhere both the philosophy and technology of this approach [1] and I shall therefore restrict my introduction to a few general comments. The central concept is that cells which are morphologically anonymous may advertise their true nature and origin by the existence of certain *cell surface* structures or molecules. The latter can be identified with the aid of selectively binding probes or *markers* which can be labelled (e.g. by fluorescent dyes). By using a combination or "panel" of markers one therefore builds up a picture or phenotype of the cell surface which is used as a guide to identify, distinguish and enumerate cells of interest. These methods have a very broad applicability to both basic biological problems (in heterogeneous cell systems) and to clinical investigation [1].

In the context of human leukaemia two approaches can be taken which differ in some important respects.

Normal or "differentiation" markers on leukaemic cells

Over the past few years methods have become available for identifying different populations and subsets of lymphoid cells (see refs. 2, 3, 4). Human T (thymus derived) and B (Bursa-equivalent derived) lymphocytes can now be adequately distinguished by a variety of cell surface markers and although it is recognized that considerable heterogeneity exists within these two major populations, the general cell surface phenotype of T- and B-cells is fairly clear (Table 1).

Markers for T- and B-cells have now been fairly extensively used for "typing" leukaemic cells and lymphomas [1, 5, 6]. The results are interpreted to suggest that the leukaemia being studied is of T-cell type (or origin), B-cell type or neither. The limitations of this approach, although generally ignored, are fairly obvious and have been discussed at length elsewhere [1]. I would stress, however, that this approach can only be

Table 1. *Cell Surface Phenotype of Human Blood Mononuclear Cells*

Marker	T-axis	B-axis	Monocytes
HuTLA	+	−	−
E rosettes	+	−	−
HuBLA	−	+	−
SmIg	−	+	−
EBV	−	+	−
EAC	±	±	+
AggIgG	±	+	+
EAHu	−	−	+
HuMA	−	−	+

+ − > 98%; − = < 2%; ± = subset reactive.
See refs. 1–4 for full description of these marker systems.

Table 2. *Cell Surface Phenotype of Human Leukaemic Cells*
(Current data from prospective study at University College, London)

Leukaemia		No. of cases[a]	Cell surface phenotype		
			T-like	B-like	non-T non-B-like
Lymphoid	ALL	(68)	15	3[c]	50
	CLL	(32)	1(b)	30	1
Hairy cell	leukaemia	(2)	–	2[d]	–
Myeloid	AML	(37)	–	–	–
	AMML	(21)	–	–	All
	CML	(6)	–	–	
Monocytic		(1)	–	–	1
Undifferentiated		(6)	–	–	6
Erythroid	Erythroleukaemia	(2)	–	–	2
Others	Plasma cell leukaemia	(1)	–	1	–
	IgG myeloma	(2)	–	2	–
	Thymoma	(1)	1	–	–

Phenotype description (cf. Table on "normal" mononuclear cell suspensions)
T-like: E^+, $HuTLA^+$, $HuBLA^-$, $SmIg^-$, $HuMA^-$, $(EAC^\pm, AggIgG^\pm)$
B-like: E^-, $HuTLA^-$, $HuBLA^+$, $SmIg^+$, $HuMA^-$, $(EAC^\pm, AggIgG^\pm)$

References: 1, 20.

[a] All high count (> 30,000 mm³) patients. Mostly prior to treatment although a few relapse cases are included. Fresh cells studied except in AML and AMML where approximately one-third were frozen (liquid N_2) samples.
[b] A prolymphocytic leukaemia.
[c] Burkitt lymphoma-like cases (cf. ref. 7).
[d] Phenotype in these two cases was found to be E^-, $HuTLA^-$, $SmIg^+$, $HuBLA^+$ (ref. 4).

Table 3. *Reactivity of Human Leukaemias with*
Anti-macrophage Serum (HuMA test)

Leukaemias		HuMA positive?
1. AMML	(21)	> 70% cells[a] in 19/21 cases
2. AML	(15)	50% cells[a] in single case 0.5–30% cells[a] in 14 cases
3. A. Monocytic L	(1)	> 90% +
4. ALL T	(4)	Less than 3% cells positive in all cases
non-T	(7)	
5. CLL	(6)	Less than 5% cells positive in all cases

[a] Taken from ref. 1.

reliably applied to samples from patients with very high white cell counts since the markers do not, by definition, distinguish normal cells from leukaemic cells. E rosette tests, for example, would clearly not distinguish a low count T-leukaemia from infectious mononucleosis or probably even a common cold! Another serious limitation is the clear indication that most acute leukaemias are not derived from differentiated T- or B-cells and therefore can not be positively identified with markers for these cells.

Despite these difficulties, cell surface phenotyping for T- and B-cell markers has given very revealing results. In Tables 2 and 3 I have summarized current results from a prospective study at University College. The main conclusions to be drawn from these

Table 4. *Binding of Cholera Toxin to Membrane* G_{M1}:
Leukaemic versus Normal Cells

		Reactivity		
Cells		−	±	++
Normal white cells/lymphoblasts				all
Leukaemic cells:	ALL	17	0	0
	AML	9	3	1
	AMML	1	0	0
	CGL	0	0	15
	CLL	0	0	10
	Pro-L.L.	2	1	3

Legend:
− negative,
± weakly reactive,
++ strong positive
(assessed by FACS).

All blood cells from high count > 50,000 untreated patients.

Data taken from Revesz and Greaves, 1975 [11] and unpublished.

Assay system: purified cholera toxin is added to cells (at 4°C for 15 min) followed by fluorescent antibodies to the toxin.

data are:

1. Chronic lymphocytic leukaemia (CLL) is, with rare exceptions, a B-cell neoplasia. Analysis of cell surface immunoglobulin establishes its probable monoclonality [5].

2. Acute lymphoblastic leukaemia (ALL) is divisible into a major group (~ 75%) which expresses no T- or B-markers, a minor group (~ 25%) which are clearly T-cell-like, and a rare group (~ 1%) which are B-cell-like and classifiable as Non-African Burkitt's lymphomas/leukaemias [7]. It has been suggested that the T-cell ALLs have a poorer prognosis [8, 9] and it will be extremely important to establish this point unequivocally.

Most non-T and T ALLs examined so far have a common lymphocyte antigen on their surface which can be identified by an antiserum raised against thymus cells and absorbed with AML and CGL cells (Brown and Greaves, unpublished). This antigen is shared by ALL, CLL and normal T- and B-cells and is absent in myeloid leukaemia. We take this observation to suggest that non-T, non-B ALLs could be derived from a lymphocyte committed precursor or stem cell.

3. Myelo-monocytic leukaemias (AMML) have a monocyte–macrophage differentiation antigen (HuMA) on their surface [1, 10]. This marker is absent from lymphoid leukaemias but is present on a minority of cells in acute myeloid leukaemia (AML).

4. Acute leukaemias *irrespective of morphological type* can be distinguished from chronic leukaemias irrespective of morphological type by their lack of a common cell surface membrane glycolipid–G_{M1} ganglioside, the receptor for cholera toxin [11] – Table 4. This observation is of particular interest since gangliosides have been implicated in growth control [12]. The lack of G_{M1} in acute leukaemias may be telling us either that this glycolipid has been lost as a primary or secondary consequence of the neoplastic transformation or alternatively, that acute leukaemias are all derived from normal progenitor cells which themselves lack G_{M1}. The latter explanation seems unlikely to be the

Table 5. *Reactivity of Human Leukaemias with Anti-ALL Sera*

Leukaemias		Number tested	Result
ALL, non-T:	untreated	(36)	$33^+/3^-$
	relapse (B)	(3)	$3^+/0^-$
	relapse (CSF)	(1)	$1^+/0^-$
ALL, T-like:	untreated	(10)	$0^+/10^-$
	relapse (B)	(1)	$0^+/1^-$
	relapse (CSF)	(1)	$0^+/1^-$
ALL, B-like:	relapse (B)	(1)	$0^+/1^-$
AUL	untreated	(7)	$6^+/1^-$
AML	untreated	(43)	$1^+/43^-$
AMML	untreated	(8)	$0^+/8^-$

B   = blood.
CSF = cerebro-spinal fluid.

case for the T-cell-like leukaemias since all identifiable cells of the T developmental axis (i.e. thymocytes, T-lymphocytes, T-lymphoblasts) have a strong expression of G_{M1}.

Leukaemia specific or leukaemia "associated" cell surface antigens

An alternative approach to the "typing" of human leukaemia cells is to use antisera which seek to distinguish different leukaemias not only from each other but also from all normal cells. As discussed in detail elsewhere [1] the great potential value of this approach is that leukaemia cells can be identified with a high degree of precision *even when present at relatively low frequencies*. The assumption here is obviously that leukaemia specific antigens exist and that suitable antisera can be raised. This is by no means an easy matter but several different approaches have given encouraging preliminary results [13, 14, 15, 16, reviewed in 1]. We have raised antisera in rabbits by injecting non-T ALL cells coated with antibodies to "normal" lymphocyte antigens (using an anti-tonsil serum) [15, 16]. Why this approach works is not entirely clear although there are several clear precedents [1].

We have routinely assayed reactivity of leukaemic cells with this antiserum using indirect immunofluorescence. The results are evaluated both by standard ultra-violet microscopy (with Plume illumination) and by using the Fluorescence Activated Cell Sorter (FACS-1, Becton Dickinson, Mountain View, California, refs. 17, 18). The latter electronic instrument measures fluorescence intensity of individual cells at a high rate (10^4-10^5/sec) and provides a rapid, sensitive and objective means to evaluate binding of cell surface reactive fluorescent markers [1].

After adsorption with red cells, liver and tonsils, the sera no longer reacted with lymphocytes from any source. However, detailed analysis by FACS showed that they still reacted with a small proportion (1–5%) of cells in normal or non-leukaemic bone marrow and a very high proportion (> 90%) of mononuclear cells in early (10–13 week) foetal liver. These reactive cells were physically separated using FACS and shown to be myelocytes (which reacted weakly) and a subset of intermediate normoblasts which stained very strongly. Extensive cross-absorption studies [16] revealed that the antisera

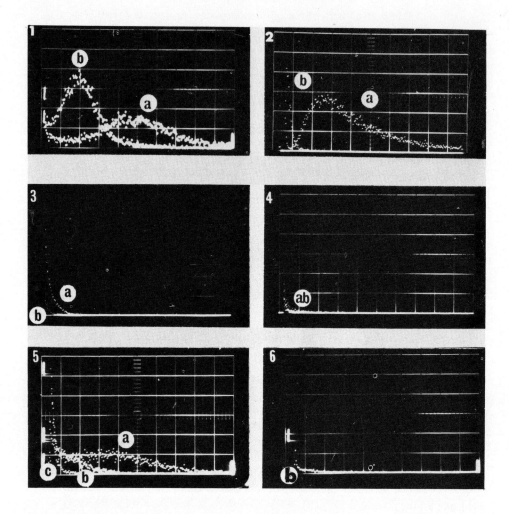

Fig. 1. FACS analysis of leukaemic cells with anti-ALL sera.
    Legend: Vertical: relative number of cells.
                Horizontal: relative fluorescence intensity. 40,000 cells counted per sample.
    1. Blood lymphoblasts from untreated ALL patient. a = anti-ALL absorbed tonsil (i.e. still
       contains anti-normoblast and weak anti-myeloid activity—see text and compare with picture
       4). b = anti-ALL absorbed tonsil + foetal liver (i.e. reactivity with leukaemia specific deter-
       minant only).
    2. Cerebro-spinal fluid lymphoblasts from ALL patient in CNS relapse. a = anti-ALL (as in 1a).
       b = normal rabbit serum (absorbed as with anti-ALL).
    3. AML blood sample from high count (> 100,000 mm³) untreated patient. a = anti-ALL as in
       1a). b = normal rabbit serum.
    4. Lymphoblasts from blood of high count (> 100,000 mm³) untreated patient with T-like ALL.
       a, b, as in 2.
    5. Bone marrow sample from ALL patient in remission showing probable existence of
       leukaemic cells (see refs. 1, 16). a = tonsil absorbed anti-ALL (as in 1a). b = tonsil + bone
       marrow absorbed anti-ALL (cf. 1b)—leukaemia specific determinant only detected. c =
       normal rabbit serum.
    6. Normal bone marrow sample. a, b, c, as in 5.

identified three leukaemia "associated" antigens. One shared by ALL, myelocytes and normoblasts, one shared by ALL and normoblasts, and another which is restricted to ALL. The latter antigen is a glycoprotein and a strong candidate for a leukaemia specific antigen although we cannot at present exclude the possibility that it is a "normal" antigen of an infrequent stem cell [19].

After additional absorption of anti-ALL sera with AML *and* bone marrow or early foetal liver cells they can be used to distinguish non-T ALLs from both T-cell ALLs and other leukaemias (Table 5, Fig. 1). Significantly, six out of seven acute *undifferentiated* leukaemias were also positive. In five of the non-T ALL cases we identified 1 to 5% positive cells in the blood when the haematologist's report had suggested no blasts were present. In *all* cases bone marrow had a very high proportion of reactive cells.

We believe this type of reagent, particularly when combined with the analytical capacity of FACS, may have very considerable practical value. It clearly discriminates between normal cells and different leukaemias and therefore has diagnostic attributes. We believe the level of sensitivity is such that we should be able to detect early or pre-leukaemic conditions and distinguish true from false–positive relapse. Our principal aim is to use this approach to monitor patients throughout treatment and perhaps identify the existence or re-emergence of leukaemic cells prior to overt or haematologically identifiable relapse. Our preliminary studies on children with non-T ALL in remission have been very encouraging in this respect since we appeared to pick up the only two out of a group of fifteen who relapsed [16, 1].

ACKNOWLEDGMENTS

This work was carried out in collaboration with many other colleagues and in particular Dr N. Rapson and Dr A. Hayward (Inst. Child Health), Dr A. Lister (St. Bartholomew's Hospital). The authors are supported by the Imperial Cancer Research Fund (M.F.G., D.C., G.J.), the Medical Research Council (G.B.) and the IARC (T.R.).

REFERENCES

1. M.F. Greaves, *Pro. Haematol.* **IX** (1975).
2. WHO-IARC Technical Workshop Report. *Scand. J. Immunol.* (1974).
3. *Transpl. Rev.*, Ed. G. Moller, Vol. 16, 1973.
4. M.F. Greaves, G. Brown and A. Hayward. In: *Proc. 8th Miles Immunopathology Symp.*, Raven Press, N.Y., 1975.
5. M. Seligmann, J.L. Preud'homme and J.C. Brouet, *Transpl. Rev.* **16**, 85 (1973).
6. R.J. Lukes and R.D. Collins, *Br. J. Cancer*, **31**, Suppl. II, p.1 (1975).
7. G. Flandrin, J.C. Brouet, M.T. Daniel and J.L. Preud'homme, *Blood*, **45**, 183 (1975).
8. L. Borella and L. Sen, *J. Immunol.* **111**, 1275 (1973).
9. D. Catovsky, J.M. Goldman, A. Okos, B. Frisch and D.A.G. Galton, *Brit. Med. J.*, p.643 (1974).
10. M. Baker, J. Falk and M.F. Greaves, *Brit. J. Haematol.* (in press, 1975).
11. T. Revesz and M.F. Greaves. In: *Lymphocyte Receptors*, edited by M. Seligmann, F. Kourilsky and J.L. Preud'homme. North-Holland Publ., Amsterdam, 1975.
12. S. Hakomori, *Biochem. Biophys. Acta*, **417**, 55 (1975).
13. T. Mohanakumar, R.S. Metzgar and D.S. Miller, *J. Nat. Cancer Inst.* **52**, 1435 (1974).
14. M.A. Baker and R.N. Taub, *Nature New Biol.* **241**, 93 (1973).
15. M.F. Greaves, G. Brown, N. Rapson and A. Lister, *Clin. Immunol. Immunopath.* **4**, 67 (1975).
16. G. Brown, D. Capellaro and M.F. Greaves, *J. Nat. Cancer Inst.* (in press, 1975).
17. H.R. Hulett, W.A. Bonner, R.G. Sweet and L.A. Herzenberg, *Clin. Chem.* **19**, 831 (1973).
18. W.A. Bonner, H.R. Hulett, R.G. Sweet and L.A. Herzenberg, *Rev. Scient. Instr.* **43**, 404 (1972).
19. G. Brown and M.F. Greaves, *Nature*, **258**, 454 (1975).
20. G. Brown, M.F. Greaves, N. Rapson, A. Lister and M. Papamichael, *Lancet*, ii, 753 (1974).

LYMPHOCYTE MEMBRANE MARKERS IN B-CELL PROLIFERATIONS AND HUMAN NON-HODGKIN'S LYMPHOMAS

J.C. BROUET, J.L. PREUD'HOMME and M. SELIGMANN

Laboratory of Immunochemistry (INSERM U 108), Research Institute on Blood Diseases, Hôpital Saint-Louis, Paris 10ème, France

ABSTRACT

Lymphocyte membrane markers have provided new approaches and concepts in the study of human lymphoid diseases of B-cell origin. Most lymphoid malignancies featured by a B-cell proliferation appear to be of monoclonal origin, as outlined by the study of membrane-bound immunoglobulins which constitute a clonal marker. The second concept brought forward by the study of these markers is that monoclonal B-cell proliferations vary considerably with respect to the type(s) of proliferating cells and their level within the normal pathway of differentiation of a B-cell clone.

The study of human non-Hodgkin's lymphomas showed in most cases that the proliferating cells were of monoclonal B-cell origin; only rare cases of T-cell lymphomas were found whereas some lymphomas could not be classified in terms of B- or T-cell origin; the latter situation occurred in most cases of so-called histiocytic lymphomas.

INTRODUCTION

The lymphoid cells may be identified by an increasing number of membrane markers. The use of these markers has been rewarding in order to attempt improved classifications of leukemias and lymphomas and to provide new insights into the pathogenesis of several of these diseases. Waldenstrom's macroglobulinemia, Burkitt's lymphoma, most chronic lymphocytic leukemias (CLL) or poorly differentiated lymphomas were shown to be B-cell malignancies. On the other hand, the proliferating cells in the Sezary syndrome, in rare cases of CLL and in about 30% of the patients with common acute lymphoblastic leukemia (ALL) are of T-cell origin.

We do not intend to discuss here all these results in detail (see reviews 1–5) and will focus on two topics: the basic characteristics of B-cell proliferations and recent results obtained in non-Hodgkin's lymphomas.

METHODS AND THEIR CRITICAL EVALUATION

The main membrane markers presently used for the identification of human B- and T-cells are listed in Table 1. A description of the methods used in the present work has

Table 1. *Main Markers of Human B- and T-cells*

Marker	B-lymphocytes	T-lymphocytes	3rd Population[a]	Comments
Easily detectable SmIg	+ (actual cell product)	−	−	Reliable B-cell marker only if its actual synthesis is proved
C receptors (EAC rosettes)	+ (only a sub-population)	−[b]	+	Receptors for C3b, C3d and C4
Fc receptor EA rosettes	+ or −	−[b]	+	Results with B-cells depending upon nature of erythrocytes and of sensitizing IgG antibody
Aggregated IgG binding	+	−[b]	±	Number of positive B-cells close to that obtained with SmIg
EBV receptor	+	−	−	
Specific anti-B antisera	+	−	?	
E rosettes	−	+	−	A modified technique identifies only a subset of T-cells. Expressed on some non-lymphoid cells
Helix pomatia hemagglutinin	−	+	?	
Specific anti-T	−	+	?	As for anti-B sera specificity often only relative. Many sera usable by cytotoxicity only

[a] A term coined by Fröland and Natvig for unidentified lymphocyte-like cells possibly involved in antibody-dependent cytotoxicity (K-cells). However, the relationship of these cells with the monocytic series is still open to question.

[b] Some T-cells (mostly "activated" T-cells) are positive for these markers.

previously been reported [6–7]. We will therefore limit ourselves to the discussion of some methodological problems.

It is well established that those lymphocytes producing surface immunoglobulins (Ig) detectable by rather insensitive methods such as direct immunofluorescence are B-cells. The use of monospecific antisera to the various Ig chains is of utmost importance to establish a possible clonal origin of the leukemic cells. However, the mere finding of Ig determinants at the surface of a cell does not prove its B-cell origin since exogenous Ig molecules may be bound to the cell surface. For instance, immune complexes may be attached to the Fc or complement receptors of B-, K- and some T-cells. Antibodies to lymphocyte surface antigens, such as autoantibodies to T-cells or antibodies directed to neo-antigens in some malignant diseases, can be revealed by methods used to detect surface Ig. It is therefore important to prove the synthesis of surface Ig by the cells, for instance by trypsinization followed by short-term *in vitro* culture [7].

The problem of the identification of monocytic cells is often difficult in cell suspensions. These cells bear receptors for complement components and for IgG. They bind serum IgG and are usually labeled by antisera to γ-, κ- and λ-chains in direct immunofluorescence tests; they may also bind rabbit IgG used as reagents. They may be identified by their phagocytic properties and enzymic activity (i.e. the cytochemical detection of endogeneous peroxidase [8]).

Finally, a classification of cells in terms of B or T origin may not be valid when extrapolated to neoplastic cells. Leukemic cells may express some membrane antigens only at certain stages of the cell cycle or experience surface changes which could prevent their identification. For instance, the receptor for C3b is frequently lacking on B-lymphocytes in CLL. Furthermore, the results obtained with anti-T or anti-B antisera must be carefully evaluated, in particular when using antisera obtained by immunization with fetal thymocytes or leukemic B-cells which may contain antibodies to non-B, non-T tumor associated antigens.

In view of these possible pitfalls in the identification of B- or T-lymphocytes, one must emphasize the need to use several membrane markers in order to reach a correct interpretation of the nature of the cells.

CHARACTERISTICS OF B-CELL PROLIFERATION

Two major concepts have emerged from the study of these B-cell proliferative diseases; most of if not all these disorders are of clonal origin and different patterns with respect to the cell type and maturation process of the neoplastic clone may be observed and vary from one disease to another.

The study of surface Ig with reagents specific for the various Ig heavy and light chains led to the concept of monoclonal B-cell proliferation. Indeed in common B CLL, the surface Ig present on all leukemic lymphocytes are restricted to a single light chain type and heavy chain class (Table 2). In CLL with IgG-bearing lymphocytes the surface IgG belong to a single subclass and show allelic exclusion [2]. The monoclonal nature of CLL is not disproved by the finding in 17% of the cases of what we called a mixed staining pattern, characterized by the simultaneous presence of μ-, γ-, κ-, and λ-chain determinants on freshly drawn cells. In all these cases, in vitro experiments showed that the cells synthesize indeed only a monoclonal surface IgM. The meaning of this false polyclonal appearance is not univocal [6]. In some cases the monoclonal surface IgM had a rheumatoid factor activity and bound normal native IgG leading to an apparently polyclonal pattern on freshly drawn cells [7]. In other patients, the mixed staining was due to the attachment of immune complexes to the surface of the lymphocytes or to the binding of antibodies directed to cell surface determinants.

Further evidence of the monoclonal origin of the disease came from the few instances where a precise antibody activity of the surface Ig was demonstrated. Several cases with an anti-Ig [7] or anti-blood group I antibody activity of the surface Ig [6–8] and a single case with anti-Forsman antigen antibody activity [9] were observed. In these cases the surface Ig of the proliferating cells share the same antibody activity and thus presumably identical variable regions of heavy and light chains. The last clue to the monoclonal nature of CLL came from the demonstration that surface Ig from all lymphocytes share similar idiotypic determinants [10–12].

Table 2. *Lymphocyte SmIg in 153 CLL Patients*

Serum monoclonal Ig	Total number	μ κ	μ λ	γ κ	γ λ	α κ	α λ	Biclonal	Mixed staining	Not detectable
None	119	45	18	12	7	0	1	1	17[a]	18[d]
IgM	13	7	3						3[a]	
IgG	19	1[b]	1[b]	8[c]	4			4	1	
IgA	2							2		
Total	153	75		31		1		7	21	18

[a] IgM synthesized *in vitro* in the seven cases studied.

[b] SmIgM synthesized *in vitro*, IgG being found on freshly drawn cells.

[c] IgG proved to be an actual cell product in six cases.

[d] T-cell origin demonstrated in eleven cases (including two patients with Ig attached to but *not* synthesized by the cells).

With the exception of multiple myeloma, the majority of B-cell proliferative diseases are featured by a surface IgM. IgG-producing clones are rarely involved and a single IgA CLL was observed in our series (Table 2). Thus the distribution of heavy and light chains among CLL patients roughly reflects the distribution of surface Ig on normal blood lymphocytes [6]. Most IgM-bearing normal and leukemic lymphocytes also synthesize surface IgD. This important exception to the rule that leukemic lymphocytes bear a single light and heavy chain does not invalidate the concept of monoclonality since surface IgD and IgM share the same light chain, the same eventual antibody activity and identical idiotypes [11–14].

These studies also revealed that B neoplastic clones may experience a normal maturation process or that their development may be "frozen" at a given stage of their differentiation pathway. Waldenström's macroglobulinemia offers the example of a clone with a normal maturation process. A large predominance of monoclonal IgM-bearing lymphoid cells is found in the bone marrow and blood of such patients. The density of fluorescent spots, their size and brightness vary greatly from cell to cell. Intracytoplasmic staining for monoclonal IgM is restricted to plasma cells and to a limited number of lymphocytes. By contrast in CLL, the fluorescence pattern is homogeneous from one cell to the other in individual patients. The staining of the positive lymphocytes is usually very faint. In some cases the surface Ig are undetectable by direct immunofluorescence although the study of other cell markers demonstrates the B origin of the cells. We interpret these findings as an evidence for a block at an early stage of the maturation process of the B-cell clone. The persistence of some degree of maturation of the proliferating B clone appears likely in most cases of CLL with a serum monoclonal Ig. In this situation the serum monoclonal Ig is usually identical to that found on the leukemic B-cells and both Ig share common idiotypic determinants [10–12]. These cases may be considered as intermediate between the common CLL with a complete block in the maturation process and Waldenström's macroglobulinemia with persistent maturation of the proliferating clone into secreting plasma cells.

The study of surface IgD in these diseases provides additional information with respect to the maturation process of the proliferating B-cell clone. In Waldenström's macroglobulinemia the majority of the cells bear μ and δ determinants, but the density of IgD seems to decrease on IgM-secreting cells [14]. In CLL, variable amounts of IgD and IgM are found on leukemic lymphocytes, with an homogenous pattern in individual patients. The ratio of density of μ- and δ-chains varies from one patient to another and may characterize the level of maturation reached by the leukemic clones "frozen" in their differentiation. It is noteworthy that some blastic proliferations such as "poorly differentiated" lymphomas may be misnamed with regard to their stage of differentiation since they possess a high density of surface Ig and in fact correspond probably to transformed B-lymphocytes.

These two concepts of monoclonal B-cell proliferations and variable maturation blocks are most useful to interpret some unusual lymphoid diseases. Biclonal proliferations, with two clones featured by different surface Ig, are not exceptional (Table 3). In

Table 3. *Summarized Data in Five Patients with Biclonal Lymphoid Proliferation*

Case	Diagnosis	Lymphocyte SmIg markers	Intracytoplasmic staining	Serum monoclonal Ig
1	CLL	$\gamma\lambda + \mu\kappa$	Negative	None
2	CLL	$\mu\lambda + \alpha\kappa$	$\alpha\kappa$ (plasma cells)	IgA κ
3	CLL + myeloma	$\mu\lambda + \alpha\lambda$	$\alpha\lambda$ (plasma cells)	IgA λ
4	CLL	$\mu\lambda + \gamma\lambda + \mu\gamma\lambda$	$\gamma\lambda$ (lymphocytes and plasma cells) $\mu\lambda$ (crystals in lymphocytes)	IgG λ
5	Wald. macr.	$\mu\lambda + \gamma\kappa$	$\mu\lambda + \gamma\kappa$ (plasma cells and some lymphocytes)	IgG κ + IgM λ

these cases the surface Ig of the two clones may be completely different or conversely have similar light chains. This latter situation is probably similar to that known for double paraproteinemias with two serum monoclonal Ig having identical light chains and variable regions but different constant regions of the heavy chains. All the possible situations with respect to cell maturation have been encountered in biclonal proliferations: no one, one or both clones may pursue some maturation into plasma cells resulting either in the absence or in the presence of one or two monoclonal serum Ig.

Acute blastic proliferations such as acute lymphoblastic leukemias or "histiocytic" lymphomas may supervene on CLL or Waldenström's macroglobulinemia. Whereas the cell morphology is totally different in the chronic and the acute phase of the disease, the study of surface Ig clearly shows that the same clone of B-cells is involved at the two different stages of the process and that the blastic cells do not represent the emergence of a new malignant clone (Table 4).

MEMBRANE MARKERS IN HUMAN NON-HODGKIN'S LYMPHOMAS

The study of membrane markers in non-Hodgkin's lymphomas was performed with the hope of improving the current classification which is merely based upon morphological criteria. The results show that, although most lymphomas are of B-cell origin, there is a striking heterogeneity within morphologically homogeneous lymphomas. In

Table 4. *"Blast Cell" Proliferations Supervening on Chronic B-lymphocyte Proliferations*

Chronic disease		Basic proliferation	
Diagnosis	Lymphocyte SmIg	Diagnosis	Blast cell SmIg
CLL	μκ	ALL	μκ
CLL	μκ [a]	ALL	μκ [a]
CLL	ND	ALL	μλ
CLL	ND	Mixed lymphocytic "histiocytic" lymphoma	γλ
WM	μκ	Poorly differentiated "histiocytic" lymphoma	μκ
CLL	ND	Id	μκ

[a] Same antibody activity of the S.Ig synthesized by both the lymphocytes and the lymphoblasts.

addition, some proliferations such as "histiocytic" lymphomas are ill defined by the present membrane markers.

In the majority of cases of poorly differentiated lymphocytic lymphomas in adults studied by us (Table 5) the proliferating cells were of monoclonal B-cell origin. Except for a single case the blast cells bore monoclonal surface IgM molecules together with IgD. IgM with λ-chains predominated in diffuse lymphocytic lymphomas. A single IgG-bearing proliferation was found (in a diffuse lymphoma). In most cases the fluorescence staining was bright suggesting a high density of surface Ig. The cells appeared to be of T-cell origin in one case whereas they were not identified by the current markers in two other cases. One of these patients was the only child studied in this series.

A monoclonal B-cell proliferation was documented in four cases of mixed "lymphocytic histiocytic" lymphomas. Three of these patients were affected with nodular lymphomas and all cells, whether lymphocytic or so-called histiocytic, bore the same surface Ig demonstrating the appurtenance to the same clone of these two types of cells with a different morphologic appearance.

A striking heterogeneity was apparent in patients with "histiocytic" lymphomas (Table 5). It is noteworthy that in our series those two cases which were of B-cell type occurred in patients previously affected with a B CLL. A single lymphoma was definitely

Table 5. *Membrane Markers in Non-Hodgkin's Lymphomas (Rappaport's classification)*

	No. studied	B-cell origin	T-cell origin	Monocytic origin	No markers
Well differentiated, lymphocytic	2	2			
Poorly differentiated, lymphocytic	19	16	1		2
Mixed lymphocytic-"histiocytic"	6	4			2
Poorly differentiated, "histiocytic"	9	2 [a]	1	?1	5
Undifferentiated, non-Burkitt	2	2			
Undifferentiated, Burkitt's type	8	8			

[a] Lymphoma supervening on CLL or WM.

of T origin whereas in five cases the blast cells were not identified. In two of these five cases, the use of anti-T and anti-B sera did not allow any improvement in the classification of the abnormal cells. However, the absence of B or T markers does, of course, not exclude a possible lymphoid origin for these cells. We have studied the cells from eight patients with an acute leukemic disease characterized by blast cells identical to Burkitt's tumor cells by morphologic criteria. These blast cells belonged to a monoclonal B-cell proliferating on. Although such a leukemic presentation is distinctly unusual in Burkitt's disease [15] these findings suggest a close relation of this particular form of ALL to Burkitt's lymphomas.

Three patients with immunoblastic lymphadenopathies [16] (or angioimmunoblastic lymphomas [17]) were studied. In all these cases the characteristic features were observed, including auto-immune hemolytic anemia and a very high polyclonal hypergammaglobulinemia [18]. This polyclonal Ig pattern was also found at the level of the lymph node cells either by cytoplasmic staining or by surface immunofluorescence (Table 6). Perhaps the most unusual finding was the high percentage (between 30 and 50%) of cells not identified by the surface markers used in this study. One may therefore wonder if these lymphomas represent the first instance of a polyclonal B-cell malignant proliferation in man.

Table 6. *Immunoblastic Lymphadenopathy*

Intracellular Ig						Surface Ig						IgG aggregates	E rosettes
δ	μ	γ	α	κ	λ	δ	μ	γ	α	κ	λ		
ND	1	3	3	4	5	ND	23	20	10	18	23	50%	7%
ND	1	20	3	15	8			ND				ND	50%
0	7	19	3	18	16	1	12	12	2	14	11	25%	29

These results in malignant non-Hodgkin lymphomas extend our previous data [19] and are in general agreement with other reports [20–22]. There is much hope that the study of further cases and a careful follow up of those patients whose malignant cells have been characterized with respect to their surface properties will provide useful information for prognosis and perhaps for an improved therapeutic approach.

ACKNOWLEDGEMENTS

We are grateful to Dr G. Flandrin for his help in cytological study of the patients and to Mrs Labaume and Miss Chevalier for skillful technical assistance. This work was performed with grants from DGRST (74.70607), INSERM (ATP 1.73. 16.17) and CNRS (ERA 239).

REFERENCES

1. J.L. Preud'homme and M. Seligmann, Surface immunoglobulins on human lymphoid cells. In *Progress in Clinical Immunology*, edited by R.S. Schwartz, Vol. 2, p. 121. Grune & Stratton, New York, 1974.

2. S.S. Fröland and J.B. Natvig, Identification of three different human lymphocyte populations by surface markers. *Transpl. Rev.* **16,** 114 (1973).
3. Z. Bentwich and H.G. Kunkel, Specific properties of human B and T lymphocytes and alteration in disease. *Transpl. Rev.* **16,** 29 (1973).
4. E.M. Shevach, E.S. Jaffe and I. Green, Receptors for complement and immunoglobulin on human and animal lymphoid cells. *Transpl. Rev.* **16,** 3 (1973).
5. M. Seligmann, J.L. Preud'homme and J.C. Brouet, B and T cell markers in human proliferative blood diseases and primary immunodeficiencies, with special reference to membrane bound immunoglobulins. *Transpl. Rev.* **16,** 85 (1973).
6. J.L. Preud'homme and M. Seligmann, Surface-bound immunoglobulins as a cell marker in human lymphoproliferative diseases. *Blood,* **40,** 777 (1972).
7. J.L. Preud'homme and M. Seligmann, Anti-human IgG activity on membrane-bound monoclonal immunoglobulin M in lymphoproliferative disorders. *Proc. Nat. Acad. Sci. U.S.* **69,** 2132 (1972).
8. T. Feizi, P. Wernet, H.G. Kunkel and S.D. Douglas, Lymphocytes forming red cell rosettes in the cold in patients with chronic cold agglutinin disease. *Blood,* **42,** 753 (1973).
9. J.C. Brouet and A.M. Prieur, Membrane markers on chronic lymphocytic leukemia cells: a B cell leukemia with rosettes due to anti-sheep erythocytes antibody activity of the membrane bound IgM and a T cell leukemia with surface Ig. *Clin. Immunol. Immunopath.* **2,** 481 (1974).
10. P. Wernet, T. Feizi and H.G. Kunkel, Idiotypic determinants of immunoglobulin M detected on the surface of human lymphocytes by cytotoxic assay. *J. Exp. Med.* **136,** 650 (1972).
11. S.M. Fu, R.J. Winchester, T. Feizi, P.D. Walzer and H.G. Kunkel, Idiotypic specificity of surface immunoglobulin and the maturation of leukemic bone marrow derived lymphocytes. *Proc. Nat. Acad. Sci. U.S.* **71,** 4487 (1974).
12. F. Salsano, S.S. Fröland, J.B. Natvig and T.E. Michaelson, Some idiotype of B lymphocyte membrane IgD and IgM: formal evidence for monoclonality of chronic lymphocytic leukemia cells. *Scand. J. Immunol.* **3,** 841 (1974).
13. J.L. Preud'homme, J.C. Brouet, J.P. Clauvel and M. Seligmann, Surface IgD in immunoproliferative disorders. *Scand. J. Immunol.* **3,** 853 (1974).
14. B. Pernis, J.C. Brouet and M. Seligmann, IgD and IgM on the membrane of lymphoid cells in macroglobulinemia. Evidence for identity of membrane IgD and IgM antibody activity in a case with anti-IgC receptors. *Europ. J. Immunol.* **4,** 776 (1974).
15. G. Flandrin, J.C. Brouet, M.T. Daniel and J.L. Preud'homme, Acute leukemia with Burkitt's tumor cells. A study of six cases with special reference to lymphocyte surface markers. *Blood,* **45,** 183 (1975).
16. R.J. Lukes and B.H. Tindle, Immunoblastic lymphadenopathy: a hyperimmune entity resembling Hodgkin's disease. *New Engl. J. Med.* **292,** 1 (1975).
17. G. Frizzera, E.M. Moran and H. Rappaport, Angio-immunoblastic lymphadenopathy with dysproteinemia. *Lancet,* **1,** 1070 (1974).
18. G. Flandrin, M.T. Daniel and G. El Yafi, Sarcomatoses ganglionnaires diffuses à différenciation plasmocytaire avec anémie hémolytique auto-immune. In *Actualités hématologiques,* edited by J. Bernard, p. 25. Masson, Paris, 1972.
19. J.C. Brouet, S. Labaume and M. Seligmann, Evaluation of T and B lymphocyte membrane markers in human non-Hodgkin lymphomas. *Br. J. Cancer,* **31,** suppl. II, 121 (1975).
20. A.C. Aisenberg and J.C. Long, Lymphocyte surface characteristics in malignant lymphomas. *Am. J. Med.* **58,** 300 (1975).
21. J.H. Leech, A.D. Glick, J.A. Waldron, J.M. Flexner, R.G. Horn and R.D. Collins, Malignant lymphomas of follicular center origin in man. I. Immunologic studies. *J. Nat. Cancer Inst.* **54,** 11 (1975).
22. E.S. Jaffe, E.M. Shevach, E.H. Sussman, M. Frank, I. Green and C.W. Beraud, Membrane receptor sites for the identification of lymphoreticular cells in benign and malignant conditions. *Br. J. Cancer,* **31,** suppl. II, 107 (1975).

CLASSIFICATION OF LEUKEMIAS AND HEMATOSARCOMAS BASED ON CELL MEMBRANE MARKERS AND SCANNING ELECTRON MICROSCOPY

D. BELPOMME*, D. DANTCHEV*, R. JOSEPH*†, A. SANTORO*‡,
F. FEUILHADE DE CHAUVIN*, N. LELARGE*, D. GRANDJON*, D. PONTVERT*
and G. MATHE*

ABSTRACT

New methods helpful in the classification of leukemias and hematosarcomas have recently become available. Among the most valuable procedures have been those detecting cell membrane markers and the ultrastructural analysis permitted by convention and scanning electron microscopy (SEM). The results of these studies, taken together with a meticulous morphologic examination on Giemsa smears, allow a more subtle classification on these neoplasias.

Among the most interesting points one can list:

(a) The observation that in typical acute lymphoid leukemia (ALL), T-markers may be found in the prolymphocytic, microlymphoblastic and macrolymphoblastic varieties, but not in the prolymphoblastic one.

(b) T or B immunoblastic acute lymphoid leukaemias are a fifth type of ALL.

(c) Chronic lymphoid leukemia (CLL) is usually a monoclonal cell disease. Cases with atypical cell membrane phenotypes are, however, sometimes observed as well as CLL with T-cell markers.

(d) Hairy cell leukemias (HCL) may be an heterogeneous disease in terms of B-cell membrane markers; SEM allow a clear distinction between CLL, chronic monocytoid leukemia (CMoL) and HCL.

(e) Leukemic lymphosarcomas (LLS) are classified as B in a majority of cases. Cell membrane typing may eventually permit differential diagnosis between early LLS and primary ALL.

(f) The lymphosarcomas (LS) which can be histologically nodular (composed of B cells) or diffuse (composed of cells presenting B, T or no detectable markers) can be cytologically prolymphocytic or lymphoblastic (lymphoblastoid) if they are nodular; prolymphocytic, lymphoblastic, or immunoblastic if they are diffuse.

(g) The diagnosis of reticulosarcoma (RS) which was in the past abusively carried out (because of confusion with immunoblastic lymphosarcoma) is based on the presence of many reticulin fibers at histological examination; there are no detectable T or B membrane markers.

(h) Reed Sternberg cell, which has been considered as an abnormal lymphocyte, may in fact be of histiocytic or B lymphocytic origin.

---

* Institut de Cancérologie et d'Immunogénétique, 14–16 av. Paul Vaillant Couturier, 94800 Villejuif, France.

† Temple University School of Medicine, Philadelphia, Pa., U.S.A.

‡ Institute of Medical Pathology, University of Messine, Italy.

INTRODUCTION

The identification several years ago of membrane markers on the mononuclear cell population of both animals [1] and humans [2, 8] has permitted differentiation of this population into T (thymo-dependent) and B (thymo-independent) lymphocytes and monocytes.

More recently, scanning electron microscopy (SEM) has provided an additional means of distinguishing the various mononuclear compartments in normal individuals [9, 10] .

It is the purpose of this paper to review the methods routinely available for the characterization of human mononuclear cells and to report our findings in the application of these techniques to the study of lympho-monocytoid disorders. Data reported here concern a personal investigation of 150 cases of malignant hematological disorders.

METHODOLOGICAL CONSIDERATIONS

Table 1 summarizes the various membrane markers and the test currently used to differentiate normal T- and B-lymphocytes and monocytes.

Although these tests are widely accepted we stress that problems are still encountered in their practice: they are summarized in Table 2. We would like to emphasize two particular difficulties:

1. The wide variations in published data regarding the mean percentage value of E rosettes with sheep red blood cells in normal human tissues [11] : this is due to the use of various technical conditions; from Fig. 1 one can note that at least four variable parameters are involved in this test.
2. The frequent confusion between "surface" immunoglobulins (sIg) and membrane immunoglobulins (mIg). Only the latter are specific of B-lymphocytes, since sIg may be antibodies coating the membrane of various cells or serum immunoglobulins (Ig) adhering to Fc receptors of monocytes or activated T-lymphocytes. As reported by Seligmann et al. [7] , to demonstrate the presence of mIg on lymphocytes, it is necessary to prove that these Ig are synthetized by trypsinized or in vitro incubated cells.

Other technical difficulties have to be considered when applying these techniques in the classification of hematological disorders:

1. There is a loss of cells during purification of mononuclear elements and thus possibly a cell selection.
2. Presence of both normal and neoplastic cells in tumor tissues requires systematic cytological control to verify which cells possess the markers.

Finally data on cell surface appearance on SEM have to be correlated with other markers: first because several intermediate forms cannot be recognized as either typical T- or B-cells and second because some E-rosette-forming cells (T-lymphocytes) can have a villous appearance similar to normal B-cells [9, 12] . These general considerations stress the need to use a battery of tests rather than any single one when using these tests in an attempt to categorize hematological neoplasias.

Table 1. *Cell Membrane Markers, for T and B Normal Lymphocytes and Monocytes in Humans*

Marker	Test	T	B	Monocyte
SRBC receptors	E rosette	+	0	0
MRBC receptors	E rosette	0	+	0
Fc ag IgG receptors	EA rosettes	0	+	+
Fc Ig receptors	Immunofluorescence with anti-Ig	0	+	+
Fc'Ig receptors	Immunofluorescence with heat-aggregated Ig	0	+	0 (?)
Activated C_3' (d or b) receptor	EAC rosette	0	+	+
mIg	Membrane immuno-fluorescence	0	+	0
Specific T or B hetero antigen(s)	Cytotoxicity or immunofluorescence	+, 0	0, +	0,0
EBV receptors	Rosettes	0	+	0

SRBC: sheep red blood cells.   MRBC: murine red blood cells.   E: spontaneous rosettes with red blood cells (RBC).   EA: rosettes with RBC coated with anti-RBC Ig.   EAC: rosettes with RBC coated with anti-RBC IgM in the presence of C_3'.   Fc ag IgG: Fc receptors for antigen IgG antibody complexes.   Fc Ig: Fc receptors for free immunoglobulins (Ig).   Fc'Ig: Fc receptors for heat aggregated Ig. C_3': activated C_3 complement receptors: two subvarieties C_3'b and C_3'd (see text).   mIg: membrane Ig.

Table 2. *Criticisms of the Test Procedures for Detecting Membrane Markers*[*]

E rosette tests	Variability of the test (differing results according to experimental conditions).
EA rosette tests	EA receptors may be detected on some educated T-lymphocytes, on some B-, K-cells (?) as well as on monocytes.
EAC rosette tests	No good control distinguishing the EA receptors from the EAC.
Membrane immunofluorescence	Difficult to obtain specific antisera. mIg have to be distinguished from sIg. Ig monoclonicity is required for neoplastic B-lymphoid cells.
Specific anti-T or B heterosera	Difficult to obtain specific hetero antisera. Immunofluorescence test is not useful. Cytotoxicity test does not allow correlation with morphological studies.
EBV membrane receptors	Difficulty due to the use of an EBV + permanent cell line.

[*] For abbreviations see Table 1.

RESULTS

1. Normal mononuclear cells

The membrane phenotypes of the different normal mononuclear cells are based on the previously discussed methods reported in Table 3.

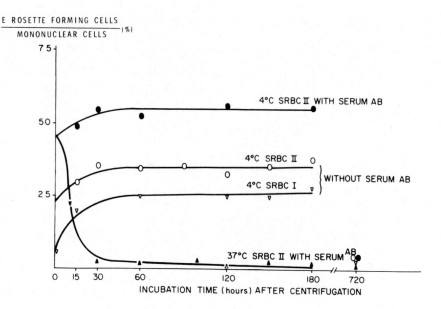

Fig. 1. Variable parameters involved in the E rosette test procedure. Experimental data concern the peripheral blood of six normal adult subjects. Note that the temperature, the quality of SRBC (preparations I and II), the incubation time and the eventual addition of human AB serum (which has been heat decomplemented and absorbed with SRBC) have to be considered.

Table 3. *Immunological Membrane Phenotypes of T- and B-lymphocytes and Monocytes in Humans*

T-cell	= mIg (–), Fc AgIg* (–), Fc (–), C_3 (–), E (+), Em (–), T ag (+), B ag (–)
B-cell	= mIg (+), Fc AgIg (+), Fc (+), C_3 b (+), C_3 d† (+), E (–), Em (+), T ag (–), B ag (+)
"Monocyte"	= mIg (–), Fc agIg (+), Fc (–), C_3 b (+), C_3 d† (+), E (–), Em (?), T ag (–), B ag (–)

* Positive on educated T-cells (?); possible characteristic of K-cells (?).
† Involved in the immune adherence phenomenon.

mIg   Membrane immunoglobulins
Fc AgIg Fc receptors for antigen Ig antibody complexes
Fc   Fc receptors for free immunoglobulins
C_3 Activated C′, complement receptors; two subvarieties C_3 b and C_3 d   (see text)
E   Spontaneous rosette formation with sheep red blood cells
Em   Spontaneous rosette formation with murine red blood cells
T ag   Specific T heteroantigen(s)
B ag   Specific B heteroantigen(s)

2. Primary acute lymphoid leukemias

2.1. Typical acute lymphoid leukemias (ALL)

In typical ALL, we found that in 25% of cases, leukemic cells possess T-membrane properties, while in the remaining 75% of cases, no cell membrane markers could be detected with the technique used (Table 4) [8, 13, 14]. It is noteworthy that in our study, four of the seven cases with T-cell marker were of the prolymphocytic variety, two of the macrolymphoblastic and one of the microlymphoblastic, according to the

Table 4. *Cell Membrane Markers in Classical Acute Lymphoid Leukemias (30 cases studied)*

Cases	Observations	Interpretation
25%*	mIg (−), Fc AgIg (−), Fc (−), C_3 (−), E (+)	T
75%	mIg (−), Fc AgIg (−), Fc (−), C_3 (−), E (−)	No marker[†]

* Four out of the six T-cell cases were of the prolymphocytic variety, while all prolymphoblastic ALL were included in the group with no detectable markers.
† In three cases cells were smooth surfaced at scanning microscopy.

cytological classification used [15, 16]. Five of these patients were children and two young adults. None had mediastinal lymph node enlarged. No particular clinical features were evidenced to differentiate these cases from those who had no detectable cell membrane markers except that all T-cell cases were characterized by a poor prognosis [17].

In three cases lacking membrane markers, SEM revealed that cells were smooth surfaced, while surprisingly it showed that in two cases with T-markers cell surface could in fact possess a degree of villosity [9, 14].

2.2. Primary immunoblastic ALL

In addition to typical ALL we have described an unusual form of this disorder which has been called "immunoblastic" ALL [18]. We showed that this fifth variety of ALL has characteristic cytological and clinical features distinguishing it from the four previously described varieties of typical ALL [15]. We observed that cells possess a deeply basophilic vacuolated cytoplasm, and a relatively immature nucleus with one visible nucleolus in some. Electron microscopy confirmed that there were numerous ribosomes in the cytoplasm. A striking feature was the observation of the absence of ergastoplasm, which led us to distinguish these cells from proplasmocytes. Investigation with membrane markers in four cases so far studied showed that one case was B, one was T, while the two others had no detectable membrane markers (Table 5).

Table 5. *Cell Membrane Markers in Primary "Immunoblastic" Acute Lymphoid Leukemias*

Cases studied	Observations	Interpretation
2	mIg (−), Fc (−), C_3' (−), E (−)	No marker
1	mIg (+), Fc (+), C_3' (+), E (−)	B
1	mIg (−), Fc (+)*, C_3' (−), E (+)	T

* Presence of Fc receptors on normal educated lymphocytes has been demonstrated in animals.

3. Primary acute myeloid leukemias (AML) and acute monoblastic leukemias (AMoL)

In all twelve cases of AML studied, whatever the cell variety (i.e. promyeloblastic, myeloblastic, myelomonoblastic), no cell membrane markers, i.e. Fc receptors for immune complexes and activated complement receptors, could be detected with the technique used.

In seven out of these cases surface immunoglobulins were detected on fresh cells, but after *in vitro* incubation there was no detectable membrane immunofluorescence, suggesting that cells were in fact not able to synthetize mIg [12, 17]. In one case of AMoL there were no detectable cell membrane markers, while in another case, activated complement receptors could be evidenced in 40% of leukemic cells [17].

4. Chronic lymphoid leukemias (CLL)

It is now well established that CLL is usually a B-cell neoplasia because of the consistent evidence that a majority of lymphocytes can synthetize monoclonal membrane immunoglobulins [4, 7, 8, 12, 14] and bear B-cell receptors [6, 8].

Our results dealing with thirty-eight cases did not lead us, however, to always settle this rule. From Table 6 it is concluded that:
1. All cases of CLL cannot be definitely typed as B. Details of cases in which there were no mIg + cells have been previously reported [14].
2. All B-cell cases of CLL cannot be proved to be monoclonal because there is in some of them a mixed immunofluorescence pattern, even after *in vitro* incubation procedures.
3. In addition we observed that all B-lymphocytes do not possess other B-markers such as Fc receptors for immune complexes and activated complement receptors [12, 14].
4. Finally, a striking observation is that in patients investigated for both membrane IgM and IgD, it can be proved that cells synthetizing monoclonal IgM can in addition synthetize IgD of the same light chain.

Table 6. *Heterogeneity of B-lymphoid Cells in Chronic Lymphoid Leukemia* (CLL)*

I.	34/38 cases: B CLL because of prevalence of mIg (+) cells
II.	30/34 cases monoclonal: IgM: 24 μk: 15; μ: 9 IgG: 5 γk: 2; $\gamma\lambda$: 3 IgA: 1 αk Mixed pattern: 4
III.	All mIg (+) cells of the 34 B-cell cases do not possess other receptors mIg (+), Fc ag Ig (+), C_3 (+), Em (+) 85% 30% 40% 51%
IV.	Monoclonal Ig D with the same light chain are detected on 15 to 80% of monoclonal IgM (+) cells (8 cases studied)

* For abbreviations see Table 3.

5. Hairy cell leukemias (HCL)

Another difficulty in cell typing is presented by HCL. We know that this unusual chronic leukemia has in the past been considered to be monocytic [20–22].

In our study, we showed that in two cases there was a monoclonal population of B-neoplastic cells suggesting a B-lymphocytic nature of the disease.

In two other cases, although the presence of Fc receptors for antigen–antibodies complexes and activated complement receptors were detected on hairy cells, we could not in fact prove after *in vitro* procedures that these cells were able to synthetize membrane immunoglobulins and thus the disease could not be definitely typed as B (Table 7). SEM of these two cases showed a cell surface appearance which does not evoke the typical feature usually found to be associated with CLL of the B type (see for comparison Figs. 2 and 3).

Table 7. *Cell Membrane Markers in Hairy Cell Leukemias*

Cases studied	Membrane phenotype	Interpretation
2	mIg (+), Fc agIg (+)*, C_3 (+)*, E (−), Em (+)*	B[†]
2	mIg (−), Fc agIg (+)*, C_3 (+)*, E (−), Em (?)	?

* On 20 to 50% of cells.
[†] 80-90% of cells; monoclonal $\mu\lambda$: 1 case; γk: 1 case.

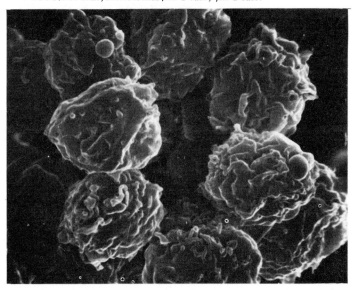

Fig. 2. Scanning electron microscopy appearance of a case of hairy cell leukemia (HCL) without detectable membrane immunoglobulins (× 6000): note that these cells cannot be confused with those from CLL.

6. Leukemic lymphosarcomas (LLS)

Investigation of membrane markers in fifteen cases of LLS revealed that eight cases were of the B type while five had no detectable membrane markers. Only two cases were typed as T.

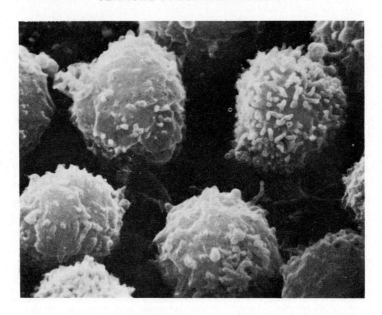

Fig. 3. Scanning electron microscopy appearance of a case of chronic lymphoid leukemia (CLL) (× 6000). Note the relative heterogeneity of the monoclonal B-cell population.

We have recently proposed a cytological classification of LLS based on predominant cells, and showed that this classification had prognostic value [23]. We distinguish the immunoblastic, lymphoblastic (or lymphoblastoid) and prolymphocytic types. As presented in Table 8 our preliminary results still do not permit us to define a correlation between the cytological types and the membrane markers pattern.

Table 8. *Membrane Markers in Leukemic Lymphosarcomas (15 patients)*

Cytological type	Number of cases	Histology of the first localization			Suspected nature of the leukemic cells		
		Diffuse	Nodular	ND	T	B*	NDMN
Immunoblastic	2	1			1		
				1			1
Lymphoblastic (lymphoblastoid)	4	1				1	
			2			2	
				1			1
Prolymphocytic	9	5			1	3	1
			2			1	1
				2		1	1
Total	15	7	4	4	2	8	5

* All cases which have been typed for mIg were monoclonal IgM.
ND: Not determined.   NDMM: No detectable membrane markers.

7. Chronic monocytoid leukemia

In one case studied, activated complement receptors could only be detected on pathological cells. Investigation with SEM of this case showed a particular cell surface appearance which led us to distinguish the cells from those of either CLL or HCL (Fig. 4).

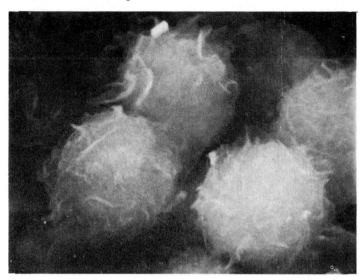

Fig. 4. Scanning electron microscopy appearance of a case of chronic monocytoid leukemia (CMoL) (× 6000). Note that these cells with crested surface cannot be confused with those from either CLL or HCL.

8. Non-leukemic non-Hodgkin's lymphomas

Investigation of membrane markers in spleen and lymph node tissues of fourteen cases of non-leukemic lymphosarcomas showed that a majority of cases were B or had no detectable membrane markers, while only two cases could be definitely typed as T.

Table 9. *Cell Membrane Markers in Lymph Nodes of Six Patients with Non-leukemic Lymphosarcomas*

Patients	Sex/Age	Histology	Cytology	Membrane markers (total cell population)				Interpretation (pathologic cells)
				E(+)	Fc(+)	C_3(+)	mIg(+)	
A	F 51	Diffuse	Immunoblastic	44*	27	28	30	B (?)
B	M 15	Diffuse	Lymphoblastic	80†	40	20	12	T
D	M 69	Nodular	Prolymphocytic	42*	9	5	4	NDMM
A	M 52	Nodular	Prolymphocytic	10*	4	0	90	B (γk)
M	M 45	Nodular	Prolymphocytic	40*	17	33	47	B (μk)
B	M 51	Diffuse	Prolymphocytic	20*	46	38	85	B (μk)

* Rosette-forming cells were differentiated lymphoid cells.
† Rosette-forming cells were exclusively lymphoblastoid cells.
NDMM: No detectable membrane markers.

Table 9 summarizes the results obtained in lymph nodes of six patients with non-leukemic lymphosarcomas (LS). Two out of three nodular LS were typed as B, while the other had no detectable membrane markers. In the three diffuse LS, one immunoblastic and one prolymphocytic cases were typed as B, while the lymphoblastic one was typed as T.

In two reticulosarcomas distinguished from lymphosarcomas by the presence of intercellular reticulin fibers there were no detectable membrane markers.

8.1. Hodgkin's disease

It has been believed that Reed Sternberg cells may be modified T-lymphocytes but more recently we suggested, as did others, that these neoplastic cells might in fact be of B-cell or histiocytic nature [16, 24, 25]. We showed that Reed Sternberg cells do not form spontaneous rosettes with sheep blood cells. Furthermore, we detected Fc receptors for antigen–antibodies complexes and activated complement receptors on some presumed Reed Sternberg cells.

We were, however, unable in our experimental conditions to prove membrane immunoglobulin synthesis by these cells as reported by others [25]. In addition the heterogeneous surface appearance of presumed Reed Sternberg cells on SEM may suggest an histiocytic rather than a B-lymphocytic nature of these cells (Fig. 5). The significance of this finding remains, however, questionable in the light of possible cell-surface modification induced by the neoplastic process [12, 26, 27].

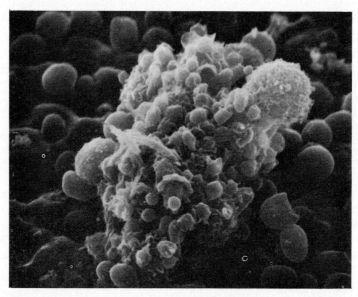

Fig. 5. Scanning electron microscopy appearance of a presumed Reed Sternberg cell (× 3000). Note that lymphocytes (T-lymphocytes?) are attached to the cell, suggesting that these lymphocytes interact with the Reed Sternberg cell.

DISCUSSION

From the data reported here as well as from other studies, it is evident that investigation of cell membrane markers is useful in the study of hematological neoplasia.

In primary typical ALL 25% of cases can be distinguished by the presence of T-membrane markers. Since this original observation [8, 28, 29], several investigators have reported comparable data [30–32], while still others, using hetero-antisera in addition to rosette test procedures, found higher percentages of cases with cells bearing T characteristics [34]; these interesting results require, however, confirmation since specificity of anti-T-heterosera generally remains questionable. In our study, in contrast to other findings [32, 34], there were no typical primary ALL with B-cell membrane markers. We have postulated that this discrepancy may result from a confusion between primary ALL and early leukemic lymphosarcomas [12, 17, 23].

In this study the observed prevalence of B-cell cases in leukemic lymphosarcomas is in fact a striking difference between these cases and those of primary ALL and thus may eventually permit differential diagnosis of the two diseases. In primary immuno-blastic ALL we found, however, that one case was typed as B and another as T, suggesting that the pathological cells may derive from either T or B lymphoid cells, as normal immunoblasts do. In two cases, however, there were no detectable membrane markers.

In all cases of AML studied we found similar negative results, whatever the cytological variety of the disease. A striking observation was the detection of a positive membrane immunofluorescence on fresh myeloid leukemic cells, suggesting the presence of anti-bodies coating the membrane.

In chronic lymphoid leukemia, we confirmed that the great majority of cases could be definitely typed as B and that most of them consisted of a monoclonal cell proliferation. In addition, we confirmed as reported by others [35, 36] that monoclonal membrane IgD could be synthetized by B-lymphocytes in association with monoclonal membrane IgM, and that both mIg are composed of the same light chain. Our data suggest, however, that there are cases with atypical membrane phenotypes [12, 14]. In one case, for example, cells have been typed as T [37] suggesting, as reported by others [38, 39], that CLL may be an heterogeneous disease. We should, however, be very careful in classifying such diseases as true T CLL since this group has to be clearly distinguished from early prolymphocytic leukemic lymphosarcomas of the T-type [23, 37] and from other T-prolymphocytic leukemias [40].

In hairy cell leukemia, we confirm other reports [41], suggesting that the disease can be typed as B-monoclonal. In two cases, however, we were unable to prove that hairy cells were definitely B-lymphocytes [42]. So these data do not allow us to exclude that hairy cells may be, in some cases, derived from other cells such as monocytes or K-cells.

In lymphosarcomas, our preliminary investigation confirmed other studies showing that nodular LS is usually associated with B markers [43, 44], while diffuse LS may be typed as B, T or has no detectable markers [45, 49].

Finally, in Hodgkin's disease, it is interesting to note that membrane typing of Reed Sternberg cells does not favor the T-cell hypothesis [50]. Although it suggests more an histiocytic rather than a B-lymphocytic nature, our data cannot definitely exclude that a Reed Sternberg cell is a modified B-lymphocyte [14, 16, 26, 27, 51].

From the data reported here, it is evident that it is through extended use of this type of investigation that progress can be made towards improved classification of neoplastic hematological disorders. Perhaps the greatest value of such studies will ultimately be in the increased understanding of the physiopathology of these diseases.

REFERENCES

1. M.C. Raff, Two distinct populations of peripheral lymphocytes in mice distinguishable by immunofluorescence. *Immunology*, **19**, 637 (1970).
2. H. Hainz, Human monocytes: distinct receptor sites for the third component of complement and for immunoglobulin G. *Science*, **1662**, 1281 (1968).
3. S. Froland and J.B. Natvig, Surface-bound immunoglobulin as a marker of B lymphocytes in man. *Nature (New Biol.)* **234**, 251 (1971).
4. J.D. Wilson and G.J.V. Nossal, Identification of human T and B lymphocytes in normal peripheral blood and in chronic lymphocytic leukemia. *Lancet*, **2**, 788 (1971).
5. J. Wybran, M.C. Carr and H.H. Fudenberg, The human rosette forming cells as a marker of a population of thymus derived cells. *J. Clin. Invest.* **51**, 2537 (1972).
6. G.D. Ross, E.M. Rubellino, M.J. Polley and H.M. Grey, Combined studies of complement receptor and surface immunoglobulin bearing cells and sheep erythrocyte rosette forming cells in normal and leukemic human lymphocytes. *J. Clin. Invest.* **52**, 377 (1973).
7. M. Seligmann, J.L. Preud'homme and J.C. Brouet, B and T cell markers in human proliferative blood diseases and primary immuno-deficiencies, with special reference to membrane bound immunoglobulins. *Transpl. Rev.* **16**, 85 (1973).
8. D. Belpomme, D. Dantchev, E. du Rusquec, D. Grandjon, R. Huchet, P. Pouillart, L. Schwarzenberg, J.L. Amiel and G. Mathé, T and B lymphocyte markers on the neoplastic cells of 20 patients with acute and 10 patients with chronic lymphoid leukemia. *Biomedicine*, **20**, 109 (1974).
9. D. Dantchev, D. Belpomme and G. Mathé, Usefulness of scanning electron microscopy in classification of human neoplastic hematological disorders. *Biomedicine* (in press, 1976).
10. A. Polliack, N. Lampen, B.D. Clarkson, E. de Harven, Z. Bentwich, F.P. Siegal and H.G. Kunkel, Identification of human B and T lymphocytes by scanning electron microscopy. *J. Exp. Med.* **138**, 607 (1973).
11. D. Belpomme, D. Pontvert and G. Mathé, Une nouvelle méthode d'exploration des lymphocytes et monocytes par leurs marqueurs de membrane: son intérêt en pathologie. p. 25 in: *Rencontre Biologique*, 1975, Expansion Scientifique, ed.
12. D. Belpomme, D. Dantchev, R. Joseph, A. Santoro, F. Feuilhade de Chauvin, D. Grandjon and G. Mathé, Cell membrane markers of T and B lymphocytes and monocytes in leukemias and hematosarcomas. VI International Symposium, Copenhagen, May 13–16, 1975, in: *Biological Characterisation of Human Tumors*, Excerpta Medica, Amsterdam, ICS 375, p. 298, 1976.
13. D. Belpomme, D. Dantchev, E. du Rusquec, D. Grandjon, R. Huchet, F. Pinon, P. Pouillart, L. Schwarzenberg, J.L. Amiel and G. Mathé, La nature T ou B des cellules néoplastiques des leucémies lymphoides. *Bull. Cancer*, **61**, 387 (1974).
14. D. Belpomme, D. Dantchev, R. Joseph, R. Huchet, D. Grandjon, A. Santoro and G. Mathé, Further studies of acute and chronic leukemias: T and B cell membrane markers and scanning electron microscopy. 3rd C.I.S.M.E.L. Symposium, San Giovanni Rotondo, Italy, 12–14 September 1974, in: *Current Studies on Standardization Problems in Clinical Pathology, Haematology and Radiotherapy in Hodgkin's Disease*, Excerpta Medica, Amsterdam, ICS 348, p. 143, 1975.
15. G. Mathé, P. Pouillart, M. Sterescu, J.L. Amiel, L. Schwarzenberg, M. Schneider, M. Hayat, F. de Vassal and C. Jasmin, Subdivision of classical varieties of acute leukemia. Correlation with prognosis and cure expectancy. *Europ. J. Clin. Biol. Res.* **16**, 554 (1971).
16. G. Mathé and D. Belpomme, T and B lymphocytic nature of leukemias and lymphosarcomas: a new but still uncertain parameter for their classification. *Biomedicine*, **20**, 81 (1974).
17. D. Belpomme, D. Dantchev, R. Joseph, H.G. Botto, R. Huchet, and G. Mathé, Cell membrane markers in hematologic neoplasia in man. I. Acute leukemia. (In press, 1976).
18. G. Mathé, D. Belpomme, D. Dantchev, P. Pouillart, C. Jasmin, J.L. Misset, M. Musset, J.L. Amiel, J.R. Schlumberger, L. Schwarzenberg, M. Hayat, F. de Vassal and M. Lafleur, Immunoblastic acute lymphoid leukemia. *Biomedicine*, **20**, 333 (1974).
19. J.L. Preud'homme and M. Seligmann, Surface bound immunoglobulins as a cell marker in human proliferative diseases. *Blood*, **40**, 777 (1972).

20. B.A. Bouroncle, B.K. Wiseman and C.A. Doan, Leukemic reticuloendotheliosis. *Blood*, 13, 609 (1958).
21. Y. Rabinowitz and R. Schrek, Monocytic cells of normal blood, Schilling and Naegli leukemia and leukemic reticulo-endotheliosis in slide chambers. *Blood* 20, 453 (1962).
22. G. Flandrin, M.T. Daniel, M. Fourcade and N. Chelloul, Leucémie à tricholencocyte (hairy cell leukemia). Etude clinique et cytologique de 55 observations. 13, 609 (1973).
23. G. Mathé, D. Belpomme, D. Dantchev, P. Pouillart, J.R. Schlumberger and M. Lafleur, Leukemic lymphosarcomas: respective prognosis of the three types: prolymphocytic, lymphoblastic (or lymphoblastoid) and immunoblastic. *Blood Cells*, 1, 25 (1975).
24. H. Rappaport, Tumor of the hematopoietic system. *A.F.I.P. Washington D.E.* 111 F, 8,48 (1966).
25. J. Leech, Immunoglobulin positive Reed Sternberg cells in Hodgkin's disease. *Lancet*, 1, 265 (1973).
26. D. Belpomme, H. Rappaport and G. Mathé, Histopathologie et histogénèse de la maladie de Hodgkin. *Rev. Prat.* 24, 3911 (1974).
27. D. Belpomme, R. Joseph, L. Navares, R. Gerard-Marchant, R. Huchet, I. Botto, D. Grandjon and G. Mathé. Increased percentage of T lymphocytes associated with Reed Sternberg cells in the spleen of Hodgkin's disease bearing patients. *New Engl. J. Med.* 291, 1417 (1974).
28. L. Borella and L.T. Sen, Cell surface markers on lymphoblasts from acute lymphocytic leukemia. *J. Immunol.* 111, 1257 (1973).
29. J.H. Kersey, A. Sabad, K. Gajl-Peczalska, H.M. Hallgren, E.J. Yunis and M. Nesbit, Acute lymphoblastic leukemic cells with T (thymus-derived) lymphocyte markers. *Science*, 182, 1355 (1973).
30. D. Catovsky, J.M. Goldman, A. Okos, B. Frisch and D.A.G. Galton, T lymphoblastic leukemia: a distinct variant of acute leukemia. *Brit. Med. J.* 2, 643 (1974).
31. A.H. Chin, J.H. Saiki, J.M. Trujillo and R.C. Williams, Peripheral blood T and B lymphocytes in patients with lymphoma and acute leukemia. *Clin. Immunol. Immunopath.* 1, 499 (1973).
32. J.C. Brouet, T.R. Toben, A. Chevalier and M. Seligmann, T and B membrane markers on blast cells in 69 patients with acute lymphoblastic leukemia. *Ann. Immunol. (Inst. Past.)*, 125C, 691 (1974).
33. J.H. Kersey, M.E. Nesbit, H.R. Luckasen, H.M. Hallgren, A. Sabad, E.J. Yunis and K.J. Gajl-Peczalska, Acute lymphoblastic leukemic and lymphoma cells with thymus derived (T) markers. *Mayo Clinic Proc.* 49, 584 (1974).
34. K. Gajl-Peczalska, C.D. Bloomfield, M.E. Nesbit and J.H. Kersey, B cell markers on lymphoblasts in acute lymphoblastic leukemia. *Clin. Exp. Immunol.* 17, 561 (1974).
35. R.T. Kubo, H.M. Grey and B. Pirofsky, IgD: a major immunoglobulin on the surface of lymphocytes from patients with chronic lymphatic leukemia. *J. Immunol.* 112, 1952 (1974).
36. J.L. Preud'homme, J.C. Brouet, J.P. Clauvel and M. Seligmann, Surface IgD in immunoproliferative disorders. *Scand. J. Immunol.* 3, 853 (1974).
37. D. Belpomme and D. Dantchev, Cell membrane markers and scanning electron microscopy aspect of lymphoid and monocytoid leukemias and lymphoreticulosarcomas. *Immuno-oncology Week*, Paris (in preparation, 1976).
38. I. Lille, A. Desplaces, L. Meeus and R.T. Saracino, Thymus derived proliferating lymphocytes in chronic lymphocytic leukemia. *Lancet*, 2, 263 (1973).
39. J.C. Brouet and G. Flandrin, Chronic lymphocytic leukemia of T cell origin. An immunological and clinical evaluation in eleven patients (in preparation, 1976).
40. D. Catovsky, J.M. Goldman, A. Okos, B. Frisch and D.A.G. Galton, T lymphoblastic leukemia: a distinct variant of acute leukemia. *Brit. Med. J.* 2, 643 (1974).
41. D. Catovsky, J.E. Petit, J. Galetto, A. Okos and D.A.G. Galton, The B lymphocyte nature of the hairy cell of leukemic reticuloendotheliosis. *Brit. J. Haematol.* 26, 29 (1974).
42. D. Belpomme, R. Joseph, D. Dantchev and G. Mathé, Further investigations of hairy cell leukemia: T and B cell membrane markers and scanning electron microscopy (in preparation 1976).
43. E.S. Jaffe, E.M. Shevach, M.M. Frank, C.W. Beraud and I. Green, Nodular lymphoma: evidence for origin from fillicular B lymphocytes. *New Engl. J. Med.* 290, 813 (1974).
44. A.C. Aisenberg and J.C. Long, Lymphocyte surface characteristics in malignant lymphomas. *Am. J. Med.* 58, 300 (1975).
45. G. Mathé and H. Rappaport, *Histological and Cytological Typing of the Neoplastic Diseases of the Hemapoietic and Lymphoid Tissues*, 1 vol. Organisation Mondiale de la Santé (Edit.), Genève (in press, 1976).
46. R.B. Mann, E.S. Jaffe, R.C. Braylan, J.C. Eggleston, L. Ransom, H. Kaizer and C.W. Beraud, Immunologic and morphologic studies of T cell lymphoma. *Am. J. Med.* 58, 307 (1975).
47. C.R. Peter and M.R. Mackenzie, T or B cell origin of some non Hodgkin's lymphomas. *Lancet*, 2, 686 (1974).

48. G. Mathé, D. Belpomme and D. Dantchev, La révision actuelle de la nomenclature et de la classification des hématosarcomes ou lymphomes non hodgkiniens. *Nouv. Presse Med.* 4, 241 (1975).
49. G. Mathé, D. Belpomme, D. Dantchev and P. Pouillart, Progress in the classification of lymphoid and/or monocytoid leukemias and of lympho and reticulosarcomas (non Hodgkin's lymphomas). *Biomedicine*, 22, 177 (1975).
50. D. Dantchev, D. Belpomme, M. Martin and G. Mathé, Immunological studies of Reed Sternberg cell and lymphocytes in Hodgkin's disease. *XVth Congress of International Society of Hematology, Jerusalem, Sept. 1974.*
51. R. Joseph and D. Belpomme, T and B lymphocytes in spleen in Hodgkin's disease. *Lancet*, 1, 747 (1975).

IMMUNOTHERAPY

PRECLINICAL APPROACHES IN TUMOR IMMUNOCHEMOTHERAPY

ABRAHAM GOLDIN and DAVID P. HOUCHENS

National Cancer Institute, Division of Cancer Treatment,
National Institutes of Health, Bethesda, Maryland 20014, U.S.A.

In any attempt to maximize chemotherapeutic response to antitumor agents it is important to take into account the interrelationships of host, tumor and drug [1–3]. An active drug exerts an inhibitory effect against the tumor and the extent of this effect is generally limited by the toxicity for the host or the origin of resistance. Also, the host itself may react immunologically against the tumor and the question arises as to the approaches that may be employed with the combination of host immunity and chemotherapy for the improvement of treatment of neoplastic disease. Several important reviews may be cited on tumor immunotherapy in which there is also reference to studies in immunochemotherapy [4–6]. In the current review preclinical approaches to the combined modality immunochemotherapy are presented.

In the treatment of leukemia L1210 in mice it is possible to achieve considerable increases in the survival time of the animals as the result of chemotherapy. In general, this treatment is more successful when it is initiated early following leukemic inoculation, at a time when there is a small number of leukemic cells. However, against advanced systemic disease in which treatment is initiated several days prior to the expected time of death of controls, it is still possible to achieve definitive increases in survival time of the leukemic animals. In one study, treatment with folic acid antagonists was initiated on the 7th day following leukemic inoculation of CDF_1 hybrid mice and continued to the 90th day [7]. The median survival time of the controls was approximately 10 days. Treatment with the folic acid antagonist methotrexate yielded a substantial increase in survival time of the animals. Two analogs of folic acid, $3'5'$-dichloromethotrexate (DCM) and $3'$bromo-$5'$chloromethotrexate (BCM), were capable of increasing the survival time of the animals very extensively and a considerable number of the animals lived indefinitely.

The question arose as to whether the surviving mice would be immune to reinoculation of the leukemic cells. To test this, the animals that were alive at 160 days without evidence of disease were reinoculated with leukemic cells. These animals, apparently cured of advanced systemic leukemia L1210 either as the result of treatment with DCM or BCM, were resistant to reinoculation of the disease [8]. In 70% of the survivors resulting from treatment with DCM and 50% of the survivors with BCM, the tumor failed to grow on reinoculation. These results were considered of interest because it is apparently necessary for the disease to be systemic at the time of initiation of treatment [8] in order to obtain an appreciable refractory response. When treatment was initiated shortly after leukemic inoculation and the disease totally eradicated, the animals generally were not refractory to leukemic reinoculation.

Following eradication of the initial advanced leukemia, in instances where the animals were only partially resistant to the reinoculum the tumor grew slowly and achieved a large size at the subcutaneous site of reinoculation prior to death [8]. Also, death occurred considerably later than was observed in a set of control animals. In this study leukemic deaths following reinoculation of the partially resistant animals ranged from 8 to 50 days, whereas controls receiving a primary inoculum died in a narrow range with a median of 10 days. Apparently, in the partially immune animals there is some inhibition of metastasis and the tumor grows locally but progressively, eventually metastasizing and killing the animals. This refractory state could not be attributed to the advanced age of the animals nor to any retention in the host of DCM or BCM, and it did not occur following initial inoculation of blood or spleen cells of normal DBA/2 or CDF_1 animals.

Studies were conducted to determine whether the survivors of systemic leukemia L1210 would be immune to an antifolic resistant subline of leukemia L1210 as well as to the initial sensitive line. It was observed that there was, in fact, a considerable degree of refractoriness to reinoculation not only of the sensitive L1210 leukemia but also of the L1210 M46R, a subline of leukemia L1210 that is resistant to methotrexate and partially cross-resistant to dichloromethotrexate [9]. It may be of interest that there was not as extensive host resistance to the M46R subline as to the parent L1210. The partially resistant subline appeared to grow somewhat more readily, although there was nevertheless considerable residual immune response. On subsequent reinoculation there was also resistance to the growth of a second subline of leukemia L1210 resistant to antifolics (M66-3R). Again, although there was resistance to reinoculation it was not as extensive as that observed with the initial sensitive line of leukemia L1210. In any event, there certainly was a considerable degree of transplantation immunity to the growth of the resistant lines. Whether the more extensive growth of the resistant lines represents some alteration in tumor cell antigenicity cannot be judged from these experiments, although later studies do indicate that for drug-induced resistant lines alteration of tumor cell antigenicity may occur [10–12].

Since advanced leukemic mice successfully treated with DCM or BCM are immune to both sensitive and folic-acid-resistant leukemic cells, it was considered that it might be possible to take advantage of the immune response against the sensitive line, on therapy, to effectively treat an antifolic resistant line of leukemia L1210. In one experiment [13] the sensitive line of leukemia L1210 was inoculated into the flank of the animals and, when the disease was systematic, daily treatment with DCM was initiated. At that time or at subsequent times the resistant line was introduced in the opposite flank of the animal and treatment was continued. The survival time of the animals was determined, as well as the extent of local tumor growth for the sensitive line and the incidence of tumor "takes" and tumor growth for the resistant line. In this experiment the untreated sensitive leukemic L1210 controls had a median survival time of 10 days. On daily treatment of the sensitive line with DCM from the 7th day, the median survival time was greater than 74 days. The untreated controls for the resistant line (M46R) also had a median survival time of 10 days and treatment of the resistant line with DCM approximately doubled the survival time indicating that there was a marked degree of resistance for this tumor as compared with the sensitive line. However, when the L1210 sensitive line was inoculated into the animals and treatment was initiated with DCM on the 7th day and the M46R resistant cells inoculated into the animals on either the 7th, 14th, 21st or 28th day, the resistant line was also sensitive to the therapy and the animals lived for an extended period of time. In addition to the increase in survival time of the animals the resistant M46R tumor either did not grow at the site of inoculation or grew at a reduced rate. It was necessary to continue treatment with DCM in order to elicit the augmented therapeutic response, indicating that the extent of immunity resulting from the effective treatment of the sensitive line had not been very extensive. Thus, the combination of an apparently moderate immune response to the sensitive leukemic cells coupled with continuous therapy with DCM resulted in an extensive increase in the survival time of the animals despite the presence of antifolate resistant leukemic cells.

A similar result was obtained in a second experiment [13]. In this experiment there was an additional group in which both the sensitive line and resistant line were inoculated at the same time that DCM treatment was initiated. In this group no therapeutic advantage was observed. Apparently, then, it is necessary to have advanced systemic disease when the treatment is initiated in order to obtain the augmented response against the resistant cells.

Augmentation of therapeutic response was also obtained when the sensitive line of leukemia L1210 was inoculated intracerebrally (day 0), and treatment with BCM was initiated at a subsequent time (day 7) and a resistant subline also inoculated intracranially or subcutaneously (day 14) [14].

Another manner in which immunity plus chemotherapy was shown to be capable of improving therapeutic response involved partial immunization of the host prior to inoculation of the leukemic cells, followed by therapy with 1,3 bis-2-chlorethyl-1-nitrosourea (BCNU) [15]. In this experiment the animals were immunized with a single treatment of X-irradiated L1210 leukemic cells (25×10^6 cells) 21 days before challenge with viable leukemia L1210. Prior immunization alone did not lead to any increase in the survival time of the animals. The dose of BCNU employed (20 mg/kg) gave a moderate increase in the survival time of the animals. But the combination of pre-immunization plus subsequent treatment with BCNU resulted in an extensive increase in the survival time of the animals.

Adoptive immunochemotherapeutic approaches are receiving current attention. In one type of study the combination of therapy plus the inoculation of syngeneic spleen or bone marrow cells has been employed. The spleen or bone marrow cells may be either normal cells or cells taken from animals that had been preimmunized. This is illustrated in an experiment involving leukemia L1210 in CDF_1 hybrid animals in which treatment with cyclophosphamide followed 6 hr later by inoculation of syngeneic immune spleen cells or immune bone marrow cells resulted in a therapeutic advantage as compared with treatment with cyclophosphamide alone (Table 1) [16]. Marked increases in survival time and an increase in the number of survivors occurred with the combination modality at a dose of cyclophosphamide which was only moderately effective by itself. Also, it may be noted that the inoculation of immune spleen cells without the contribution of prior treatment with cyclophosphamide was essentially ineffective in increasing the survival time of the animals.

Chemotherapy plus adoptive immunotherapy is also being attempted employing treatment with drug followed by inoculation of allogeneic cells. This is illustrated in an

Table 1. *Influence of Transplantation with Isogeneic Cells on the Survival Time of Mice Treated with Cyclophosphamide (Cytoxan)* *

Cytoxan† dose mg/kg	Experiment 1					Experiment 2				
	Drug alone	Spleen cells‡ (3×10^7)		Bone marrow cells‡ (3×10^6)		Drug alone	Spleen cells‡ (3×10^7)		Bone marrow cells‡ (3×10^6)	
		Normal MST§	Immune (days)	Normal MST§	Immune (days)		Normal MST§	Immune (days)	Normal MST§	Immune (days)
0	9	8.5	9	9	8	8	8	8	8	8.5
39	10	10	10	10.5	10	10	10	11	10	11
65	11	11	11.5	12	12	11	12	13	12	12
108	13	14.5	14.5	13.5	25.5	13	13.5	16.5	13.5	14
180	16.5	20	>60(7)	17	>60(7)	16	17	>60(6)	17	19
300	>60(5)	>60(6)	>60(8)	17	>60(7)	26	42(3)	>60(8)	22.5	>60(8)

* CDF₁ mice inoculated intraperitoneally (IP) with 10^5/0.25 ml leukemic L1210 ascites cells on day 0.

† Treatment IP on day 3 only.

‡ Donor CDF₁ mice immunized for 12 weeks (Experiment 1) and for 6 weeks (Experiment 2). Donor cells were transplanted 6hr following treatment with cytoxan.

§ MST median survival time of eight mice per group. Figures in parentheses denote 60-day survivors.

From Vadlamudi *et al.* [16].

experiment with leukemia L1210 in DBA/2 mice in which the animals were treated with cyclophosphamide followed 6 hr later by inoculation of unimmunized DBA/2, BALB/c, or C57BL/B10.A spleen cells. With inoculation of spleen cells, without prior chemo-therapy, there were no increases in survival time [16]. Cyclophosphamide alone increased the survival time to 12 days compared to 8 days in controls. Treatment with cyclophosphamide followed by inoculation of DBA/2 cells or BALB/c cells increased the survival time to 15 and 16 days respectively. When cyclophosphamide therapy was followed by inoculation of allogeneic C57BL cells the survival time was increased to 20 days. Although treatment with cyclophosphamide plus the allogeneic spleen cells did provide a rather substantial increase in survival time, the problem of graft versus host disease would have undoubtedly proved a limiting factor if the treatment had been somewhat more successful.

Studies on chemotherapy plus adoptive immunotherapy have also been conducted in viral tumor systems. An experimental procedure employed by Glynn et al. [17] involving immunochemotherapy of a transplantable Moloney leukemia (LSTRA) originally induced in BALB/c mice is represented schematically in Fig. 1. The tumor is inoculated into BALB/c mice subcutaneously and is treated with drug after it becomes palpable and systemic. LSTRA or MBL-1 tumor cells (both induced by Moloney virus) are X-irradiated and employed to immunize hybrid CDF_1 mice. The semi-syngeneic immune spleen cells from these mice are then inoculated into the BALB/c animals, usually 6 hr following the chemotherapy. In this study [17] treatment of advanced

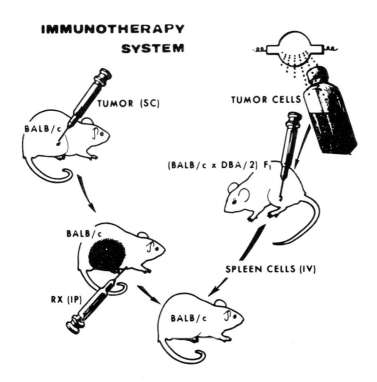

Fig. 1. Schematic representation of procedure used for immunochemotherapeutic treatment of Moloney leukemias. From Glynn et al. [17].

Moloney leukemia (LSTRA) with cyclophosphamide alone gave moderate increases in the survival time of the animals. Treatment with cyclophosphamide followed by inoculation of normal CDF_1 spleen cells provided no further advantage in therapy. However, treatment with cyclophosphamide followed by inoculation of specifically sensitized allogeneic spleen cells yielded marked increases in survival time. In this experimental model the possibility of the animals dying of graft versus host disease was precluded by the employment of immunized spleen cells from the CDF_1 hybrid. At the termination of the experiment (day 90) all of the survivors had detectable levels of DBA/2 donor type gammaglobulin of CDF_1 spleen cells. Most of the animals lived for a 292-day observation period and in a number of them, the DBA/2 allotype persisted, indicating stable chimera formation. The utilization of cyclophosphamide served (a) to exert its own therapeutic effect, and (b) to sufficiently suppress the immune response of the host so that the inoculated allogeneic sensitized lymphocytes resulted in chimera formation.

In another type of experiment involving chemotherapy plus adoptive immunotherapy, BALB/c mice bearing LSTRA Moloney lymphoma were treated with cyclophosphamide and this was followed by administration of spleen cells from BALB/c or DBA/2 mice immunized with murine Moloney sarcoma virus [18]. For the immunization the Moloney sarcoma virus had been inoculated intramuscularly and the tumor permitted to develop and regress. The animals then received one or more additional doses of the Moloney sarcoma virus. In this system, also, treatment with cyclophosphamide followed by inoculation of syngeneic BALB/c spleen cells immunized against the Moloney sarcoma virus resulted in a marked increase in the survival time of the animals [18]. This did not occur when the immunized spleen cells were killed. It also did not occur with the combination of cyclophosphamide plus BALB/c spleen cells immunized against C57BL tissue. In a second experiment employing cyclophosphamide plus adoptive immunotherapy with DBA/2 spleen cells immunized against the Moloney sarcoma virus there was again a marked increase in the survival time of the animals [18].

In an additional type of experiment adoptive immunochemotherapy was attempted against the primary Moloney sarcoma virus-induced tumor [19]. When the Moloney sarcoma virus was introduced into the animals (BALB/c), the tumor developed at the site of inoculation and without treatment the tumors ordinarily regressed. Cyclophosphamide administration, after the tumor developed, was apparently capable of exerting only moderate antitumor effect but also suppressed the immune response so that the tumor grew progressively and all of the animals (9/9) succumbed. Where the cyclophosphamide therapy was followed by injection of unimmunized BALB/c spleen cells, no protection was afforded against the progressive growth of the tumor and 9/9 deaths ensued. On the other hand, when treatment with cyclophosphamide was followed by administration of spleen cells of BALB/c mice hyperimmunized against the Moloney sarcoma virus there was marked regression of the tumor and extension of survival time. Ten out of thirteen animals were alive at the termination of the experiment at 100 days. For the three of the thirteen animals that died of tumor, the tumors grew relatively slowly. Apparently then, with the combination modality, there was a moderate therapeutic effect exerted by the cyclophosphamide, which, followed by injection of the hyperimmune spleen cells, yielded a marked therapeutic response. Alternatively, it is possible that the cyclophosphamide suppressed the immune response to such extent that it permitted the hyperimmune spleen cells to become established and to thereby exert a therapeutic response.

There has been somewhat limited experience with chemotherapy plus serotherapy. In one investigation [20], established primary Moloney sarcoma was treated with cyclophosphamide plus serotherapy with moderate success. Since serotherapy has been demonstrated to be capable of enhancing tumor growth [21] there are evident risks in this type of combined modality.

Immunological aspects of the phenomenon of collateral sensitivity are worthy of consideration. Collateral sensitivity describes a situation in which resistance to a drug leads to increased response to a second chemotherapeutic agent. The phenomenon is illustrated in a study in which a subline of leukemia L1210 resistant to 6-mercaptopurine and also to 8-azaguanine showed increased sensitivity to methotrexate [22, 23]. The phenomenon of collateral sensitivity demonstrated in several laboratories [22–26] may have an immunological contribution [10–12, 25–28]. There is the indication that accompanying the origin of resistance there may occur an alteration of the antigenicity of the tumor cells and that the immunological response of the host is coupled with the chemotherapeutic effect, resulting in a form of immunochemotherapy.

Evidence that treatment with an antitumor agent may indeed alter the antigenicity of tumor cells is provided by studies of Bonmassar *et al.* [11] in which it was observed that treatment of leukemia L1210 with the imidazole carboxamide derivative DIC over a series of generations leads to the alteration of the antigenicity of the tumor cells. The antigenically altered tumor cells fail to grow in the host of origin (CDF_1) unless the animals are treated with DIC (Table 2). Growth apparently occurs on treatment since the tumor cells of the DIC subline are resistant to the drug and the immunosuppressant action of the drug prevents any immunoresponse to altered antigen. When the animals are immunosuppressed by injection of cyclophosphamide prior to inoculation of the tumor the growth of the DIC subline is progressive, indicating further that failure to grow in untreated animals is a result of altered antigenicity of the tumor cells.

That DIC has immunosuppressant action is indicated by the observation that treatment with DIC resulted in inhibition of allograft responses and in a reduction of the

Table 2. *Mortality Data for Normal and Immunosuppressed CDF_1 Mice Given Transplants of L1210 Leukemia and DIC Transformed L1210 (C_1)*

Tumor line	Transplant generation	Recipient animals					
		Non-treated		Treated with DIC 50 mg/kg (days 1–10)		Pretreated with cytoxan 180 mg/kg (day 1)	
		MST*	D/T†	MST	D/T	MST	D/T
L1210	—	8	8/8	—	—	—	—
C_1	0	8	8/8	11	8/8	8	8/8
	2	12	8/8	12	8/8	NT‡	
	4	14	8/8	13	8/8	NT	
	6	28	8/8	14	8/8	NT	
	8	—	0/8	13	8/8	14	8/8

* MST = median survival time.
† D/T = death over total number tested.
‡ NT = not tested.
    From Bonmassar *et al.* [11].

plaque-forming cell capacity of the spleen in CDF_1 male mice that had been immunized with sheep red blood cells [11]. Further studies indicated that the mechanism of DIC action is not specifically related to the induction of drug-resistance since a naturally resistant line of L1210 leukemia became highly immunogenic following treatment with drug [27].

The collateral sensitivity of one of the transformed L1210 DIC sublines (C_1) to BCNU is illustrated in BDF_1 mice, pretreated with cyclophosphamide in order to permit progressive growth of the tumor [11]. Treatment with BCNU at the dose levels employed was moderately effective in increasing the survival time of mice inoculated with the sensitive line but resulted in survival of most of the animals carrying the C_1 line, indicating in the latter instance collateral sensitivity resulting from a combination of an immune response to altered antigenicity plus the therapeutic response to BCNU.

In order to determine whether the contribution of altered antigenicity to collateral sensitivity is a generalized phenomenon a series of sublines of leukemia L1210 resistant to various drugs was examined [12]. In general, when the animals were inoculated with an equivalent number of tumor cells, the untreated controls of the resistant sublines lived moderately longer (1–5 days) than the animals carrying the sensitive line. When cyclophosphamide was administered a day before leukemic inoculation, in a number of instances there was a reduction in the survival time of the animals. With all of the resistant sublines there was increased sensitivity to BCNU as compared with the response of the sensitive line, and in a number of instances the animals lived indefinitely. When the animals were pretreated with cyclophosphamide there was a reversal of the therapeutic augmentation resulting from treatment with BCNU, again indicating that the collateral sensitivity could be reversed by immunosuppression of the host.

That there may be specificity with respect to the altered antigenicity is indicated in a study of Nicolin *et al.* [12] who found evidence of humoral antibodies specific for an altered subline of leukemia L1210. Using [51]Chromium release it was observed that antiserum to an L1210 cytosine arabinoside resistant subline acted against the cytosine arabinoside leukemic cells but not against the sensitive cells. Conversely, antiserum against the sensitive cells did not act against the resistant cells.

Further, employing an *in vitro* assay for cell-mediated immunity it was found that spleen cells of mice immunized against a DIC altered subline of leukemia L1210 (L1210/Ha/DIC) were specifically cytotoxic to the cells of the same leukemia subline, as evaluated by the ^{51}Cr-release technique [29]. They showed little or no cytotoxic activity for a series of other tumor or normal cells from syngeneic or allogeneic donors. The specificity of the cytotoxic reaction was supported further by the inhibition of ^{51}Cr release resulting from addition of unlabeled L1210/Ha/DIC cells to the ^{51}Cr-labeled L1210/Ha/DIC cells.

Additional studies in our laboratory have shown that, despite the specificity of the drug-induced antigenic alteration of tumor cell, mice which have rejected DIC-treated sublines which originated in conventional or athymic mice were relatively resistant to a subsequent inoculum of the parental lines [30]. This observation indicates that the DIC-treated sublines retain at least a portion of the antigenic makeup of parental lymphomas. It has been suggested [30] that if the immunogenic character of human tumors can be altered by drug treatment in athymic mice this might serve as a possible approach to clinical immunotherapy.

In recent years there has been much interest in non-specific stimulation of the immune system by the use of various drugs or biological agents. Such studies have included the

Table 3. *Combined Chemotherapy and Immunostimulation Therapy of LSTRA* in BALB/c Mice*

Group	Treatment BCNU 20 mg/kg (day 7 after LSTRA)	BCG 2–4 × 10⁶ organisms (day after LSTRA)	C. parvum 100 mg (day after LSTRA)	Survivors at day 85 (%)
1	–	–	–	0
2	+	–	–	12
3	–	7	–	0
4	–	–	7	0
5	+	10	–	25
6	+	13	–	25
7	+	16	–	35
8	+	19	–	68
9	+	–	10	76
10	+	–	13	23
11	+	–	16	25
12	+	–	19	32

* 10^4 LSTRA cells given sc.
From Pearson *et al.* [36].

use of Bacillus Calmette-Guérin (BCG) and *Corynebacterium parvum* [31, 32], levamisole and tetramisole [33], pyran copolymer and tilorone [34]. It is apparent from the various studies that the dose, route and time of administration in relation to tumor are of great importance. Other studies have indicated that agents such as BCG may, in fact, be detrimental to the host in some instances [35].

In one study employing BCG or *C. parvum* plus 1,3-bis (2-chloroethyl)-1-nitrosourea against LSTRA, a murine lymphoma, Pearson *et al.* [36] demonstrated that the immunostimulants could be used more effectively with chemotherapy than either treatment alone (Table 3). Their study suggested that the BCG was effective when administered at a later interval in relation to drug administration while *C. parvum* was more effective at a shorter interval. This suggested that BCG may enhance tumor-specific response at a time when there are increasing amounts of tumor antigen during relapse while *C. parvum* may simply be acting by non-specific stimulation of the immune system.

In summary, areas have been outlined in which there have been illustrations of an increased therapeutic response on treatment with a combination of immunotherapy plus chemotherapy. In one instance an immune response to a sensitive line of leukemia L1210 was capable of improving the therapeutic response against a resistant line of leukemia. In another example, moderate preimmunization of the animals against the leukemic line improved therapeutic response to chemotherapy. Adoptive immunologic procedures were capable of improving therapeutic response to a drug for not only leukemia but also a transplantable Moloney leukemia as well as primary Moloney sarcoma-virus-induced sarcoma. Progressive therapy with a drug may result in an alteration of the antigenicity of the tumor cells and these cells may be protected by the origin of drug resistance. The presence of antigenically altered cells may in turn lead to improved therapeutic response to a second drug. There would appear to be some specificity in the origin of this new antigenicity. The ability to alter tumor cell antigenicity in athymic mice suggests that it may be possible to alter antigenicity of human tumors in these mice, and taking advantage of residual common antigen, to employ such tumors in immunotherapeutic investigations. There has been considerable emphasis over many years in chemotherapy and emphasis and interest in immunotherapy. The approaches and studies reviewed here suggest that the two modalities may be combined profitably in the form of immuno-chemotherapy for the improvement of therapeutic response. There has really been only a modest start in this direction employing animal model systems.

REFERENCES

1. E.K. Marshal, Jr., The dosage schedule of chemotherapeutic agents. *Pharmacol. Rev.* **4**, 85 (1952).
2. A. Goldin, J.M. Venditti and N. Mantel, Preclinical screening and evaluation of agents for the chemotherapy of cancer: a review. *Cancer Res.* **21**, 1334 (1961).
3. A. Goldin and R.K. Johnson, Evaluation of actinomycins in experimental systems. *Cancer Chemother. Rep.,* Part 1, **58**, no. 1, 63 (1974).
4. G.A. Currie, Eighty years of immunotherapy: a review of immunological methods used for the treatment of human cancer. *Br. J. Cancer,* **26**, 141 (1972).
5. A Fefer, Tumor immunotherapy. In: *Antineoplastic and Immunosuppressive Agents,* edited by A.C. Sartorelli and D.G. Johns, Part 1, Springer-Verlag, New York, 1974.
6. R.T. Smith, Possibilities and problems of immunologic intervention in cancer. *New Eng. J. Med.* **287**, 439 (1972).
7. A. Goldin, S.R. Humphreys, J.M. Venditti and N. Mantel, Prolongation of the lifespan of mice with advanced leukemia (L1210) by treatment with halogenated derivatives of amethopterin. *J. Nat. Cancer Inst.* **22**, 811 (1959).
8. A. Goldin and S.R. Humphreys, Studies of immunity in mice surviving systemic leukemia L1210. *J. Nat. Cancer Inst.* **24**, 283 (1960).
9. A. Goldin, S.R. Humphreys, G.O. Chapman, M.A. Chirigos and J.M. Venditti, Immunity of mice surviving systemic leukemia (L1210) to antifolic resistant variants of the disease. *Nature,* **185**, 219 (1960).
10. E. Mihich, Modification of tumor regression by immunologic means. *Cancer Res.* **29**, 2345 (1969).
11. E. Bonmassar, A. Bonmassar, S. Vadlamudi and A. Goldin, Immunological alteration of leukemic cells *in vivo* after treatment with an antitumor drug. *Proc. Nat. Acad. Sci.* **66**, 1089 (1970).
12. A. Nicolin, S. Vadlamudi and A. Goldin, Antigenicity of L1210 leukemic sublines induced by drugs. *Cancer Res.* **32**, 653 (1972).
13. A. Goldin, S.R. Humphreys, G.O. Chapman, J.M. Venditti and M.A. Chirigos, Augmentation of therapeutic efficacy of 3'5'-dichloroamethorpterin against an antifolic-resistant variant of leukemia (L1210-M46R) in mice. *Cancer Res.* **20**, 1066 (1960).
14. M.A. Chirigos, L.B. Thomas, S.R. Humphreys, J.P. Glynn and A. Goldin, Therapeutic and immunological response of mice with meningeal leukemia (L1210) to challenge with an antifolic-resistant variant. *Cancer Res.* **24**, 409 (1964).
15. E. Bonmassar, S. Vadlamudi, W. Vieira and A. Goldin, Influence of Tween 80 on the antileukemic activity of 1,3-bis-(2-chloroethyl)-1-nitrosourea (NSC-409962). *Arch. It. Pat. Clin. Tumori,* **12**, 163 (1969).
16. S. Vadlamudi, M. Padarathsingh, E. Bonmassar and A. Goldin, Effect of combination treatment with cyclophosphamide and isogeneic spleen and bone marrow cells in leukemic (L1210) mice. *Int. J. Cancer* **7**, 160 (1971).
17. J.P. Glynn, B.L. Halpern and A. Fefer, An immunochemotherapeutic system for the treatment of a transplanted Moloney virus-induced lymphoma in mice. *Cancer Res.* **29**, 515 (1969).
18. A. Fefer, Adoptive chemoimmunotherapy of a Moloney lymphoma. *Int. J. Cancer,* **8**, 364 (1971).
19. A. Fefer, Immunotherapy and chemotherapy of Moloney sarcoma virus-induced tumors in mice. *Cancer Res.* **29**, 2177 (1969).
20. A. Fefer, Immunotherapy of primary Moloney sarcoma-virus-induced tumors. *Int. J. Cancer,* **5**, 327 (1970).
21. R.W. Baldwin and C.R. Barker, Antigenic composition of transplanted rat hepatomas originally induced by 4-dimethylaminoazobenzene. *Br. J. Cancer,* **21**, 338 (1967).
22. L.W. Law, V. Taormina and B.J. Boyle, Response of acute lymphocytic leukemias to the purine antagonist 6-mercaptopurine. *Ann. N.Y. Acad. Sci.,* **60**, 224 (1954).

23. J.M. Venditti and A. Goldin, Drug synergism in antineoplastic chemotherapy. In: *Advances in Chemotherapy,* **1,** 397, Academic Press Inc., New York, 1964.

24. D.J. Hutchison, Cross-resistance and collateral sensitivity studies in cancer chemotherapy. In: *Advances in Cancer Research,* edited by A. Haddon and S. Weinhouse, **7,** 235 (1963).

25. F.A. Schmid and D.J. Hutchison, Collateral sensitivity of resistant lines of mouse leukemias L1210 and L5178Y. *Proc. Am. Ass. Cancer Res.* **12,** 23 (1971).

26. E. Mihich, Synergism between chemotherapy and immunity in the treatment of experimental tumors. In: *Proc. of the 5th International Congress of Chemotherapy,* edited by K.H. Spitzy and H. Haschek, **3,** 327, Wiener Medizinischen Akademie, Vienna, 1967.

27. E. Bonmassar, A. Bonmassar, S. Vadlamudi and A. Goldin, Antigenic changes of L1210 leukemia in mice treated with 5-(3,3-dimethyl-1-triazeno) imidazole-4-carboxamide. *Cancer Res.* **32,** 1446 (1972).

28. A. Nicolin, S. Vadlamudi and A. Goldin, Increased immunogenicity of murine lymphatic tumors by pyrazole-4-carboxamide, 3 (or 5)-amino (NSC-1402; PCA). *Cancer Chemother. Rep.* **57,** 3 (1973).

29. A. Nicolin, A. Bini, P. Franco and A. Goldin, Cell-mediated response to a mouse leukemic subline antigenically altered following drug treatment *in vivo. Cancer Chemother. Rep.* **58,** 325 (1974).

30. F. Campanile, D.P. Houchens, M. Gaston, A. Goldin and E. Bonmassar, Increased immunogenicity of two lymphoma lines following drug treatment in athymic (nude) mice. *J. Nat. Cancer Inst.* **55,** 207 (1975).

31. R.C. Bast, Jr., B. Zbar, T. Borsos and H.J. Rapp, BCG and cancer, part 1. *New England J. Med.* **290,** 1413 (1974).

32. J.C. Fisher, W.R. Grace and J.A. Mannick, The effect of nonspecific immune stimulation with *Corynebacterium parvum* on patterns of tumor growth. *Cancer* **26,** 1379 (1970).

33. R.K. Johnson, D.P. Houchens, M. Gaston and A. Goldin, Effects of Levamisole (NSC 177023) and Tetramisole (NSC 102063) in experimental tumor systems. *Cancer Chemother. Rep.* **59,** 697 (1975).

34. P.S. Morahan, J.A. Munson, L.G. Baird, A.M. Kaplan and W. Regelson, Antitumor action of pyran copolymer and tilorone against Lewis lung carcinoma and B16 melanoma. *Cancer Res.* **34,** 506 (1974).

35. R.C. Bast, Jr., B. Zbar, T. Borsos and H.J. Rapp, BCG and cancer, part 2. *New Engl. J. Med.* **290,** 1458 (1974).

36. J.W. Pearson, G.R. Pearson, W.T. Gibson, J.C. Chermann and M.A. Chirigos, Combined chemoimmunostimulation therapy against murine leukemia. *Cancer Res.* **32,** 904 (1972).

LEVAMISOLE IN RESECTABLE HUMAN BRONCHOGENIC CARCINOMA

W. AMERY*

ABSTRACT

Levamisole per os appears to diminish the number of post-surgical recurrences and metastatic deaths, in patients operated upon because of primary bronchial cancer. This effect is especially apparent in patients with epidermoid carcinoma and in patients with great tumors. Moreover, levamisole does not seem to influence the incidence of intrathoracic relapses, but its effect on distant metastases is rather marked.

These are the conclusions from a first interim analysis evaluating the data of 111 patients, followed-up for at least 1 year after surgery and treated in a strictly double-blind way with levamisole (50 mg t.i.d. for 3 consecutive days every fortnight, started 3 days before surgery) or placebo.

Suggestions for the design of future trials, studying immunotherapy in connection with surgery, are proposed.

INTRODUCTION

Levamisole (Fig. 1) is a chemotherapeutic agent which has been used as an anthelmintic for several years. In 1971 it was first described to possess immunotropic properties [1] and since that time evidence has been accumulating that levamisole restores host defense mechanisms when these are inefficient, but that it has almost no effect upon a normal immunity (see reviews: 2, 3). Similarly, levamisole does not seem to influence the primary growth or the dissemination of experimental tumors [2], unless such tumors are studied in newborn animals [4], but it prolongs the remission period and even increases the number of long-time survivors if given after cytoreductive chemotherapy [2, 5, 6]. In cancer patients, levamisole has been shown to restore delayed-type skin reactivity

* Chairman of the Study Group for Bronchogenic Carcinoma, whose composition is as follows:
Cooperating centres:
    Utrecht (Prof. J. Swierenga, Dr. H.C. Gooszen and Dr. R.G. Vanderschueren); Leuven (Prof. J. Cosemans, Dr. A. Louwagie and Dr. E. Stevens); Amsterdam (Dr. J. Stam, Dr. R.W. Veldhuizen and Prof. E. Lopes Cardozo)
Consultants:
    G. De Ceuster for *computer*; Dr. L. Desplenter for *tumor immunology*; J. Dony for *statistics*; Prof. A. Drochmans for *radiotherapy and cytostatics*; Dr. P.A.J. Janssen for *pharmacology*; Dr. W. Tanghe for *pathology*
    Co-ordination: E. Denissen.
Address for reprints:
    W. Amery, M.D., Janssen Pharmaceutica, B-2340 Beerse (Belgium)

LEVAMISOLE

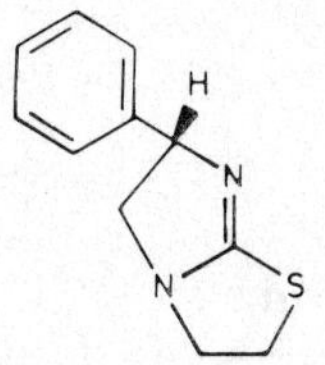

l - 2,3,5,6 - tetrahydro - 6 - phenyl -
imidazo [2,1- b] thiazole HCl

Fig. 1. Structural formula of levamisole.

[7–9] and, in Hodgkin patients, E-rosette formation *in vitro* [10]. The latter effect is probably related to the finding that levamisole restores azathioprine-suppressed T-cell function *in vitro* also [11]. Another interesting observation as regards the mechanism of action of levamisole is that this substance enhances the activity of the mononuclear phagocytic system in CDI and C_3H mice, which have a relatively low carbon clearance rate as compared with some other strains [12].

This paper reports on the data obtained so far in the first 111 patients with resectable lung cancer, who all came into the study at least 1 year before the present evaluation.

PATIENTS

All 111 patients had primary bronchial carcinoma and were considered operable. The vast majority of them were males and their ages ranged from 42 to 77 (median 60) years. Their weights were almost normal (median 74 kg; range 53–121 kg) and so was the erythrocyte sedimentation rate (ESR) in most of them (median: 23 mm after 1 hr; range: 2–115 mm). A histological diagnosis was available for all patients, except two, and it was classified according to the WHO criteria (Kreyberg's classification).

METHODS (Fig. 2)

One tablet containing 50 mg of levamisole or placebo was given three times daily on the last 3 days before surgery, and a similar 3-day course of treatment has been given every second week thereafter. The study is still in progress. The medication is individually coded, strictly double-blind, and separately randomized for each centre into levamisole or placebo.

If surgery revealed that the patient was inoperable or that no malignancy was present, he was excluded from the study.

Both the double-blind treatment and the follow-up are to be continued for at least 2 years, unless relapse is evident. In the latter case, appropriate cytoreductive therapy is given, but as long as no proven recurrence has been found, the use of cytostatics, corticosteroids and radiotherapy is prohibited.

At least 15 days before surgery, the patients were sensitized with 2 mg DNCB and several data concerning the patient and his tumor were recorded. Five days before

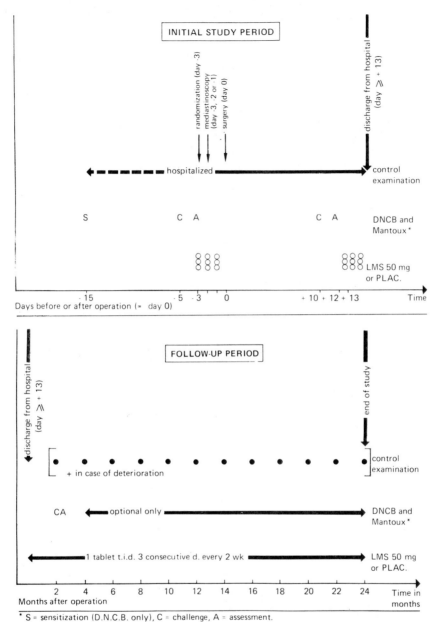

Fig. 2. Design of the study.

surgery a skin test with 25, 50 and 100 μg of DNCB, and an ID reaction with 10 I.U. of PPD was performed, followed by an assessment 48 hr later (i.e. just before the start of the double-blind therapy). Such skin tests were repeated 10 days and 2 months after surgery also.

The surgically removed tumor was fixed with formalin 10% or Bouin fixative and its greatest and smallest diameters were measured. Moreover, the regional extent of the

Table 1. *Definition of Regional Extent Grouping Categories*

CATEGORY 1 a:	lesion limited to the lung, no positive regional lymph nodes are found and there is no pathologic evidence of blood-vessel invasion.
CATEGORY 1 b:	the same as 1 a, but includes blood-vessel invasion as found by the pathologist.
CATEGORY 2:	lesion confined to the lung and hilar or mediastinal lymph nodes. It is thought that all involved tissue is resected.
CATEGORY 3 a:	there is histological evidence of tumor cells at the lines of resection or there is involvement of the thoracic wall (including the parietal pleura).
CATEGORY 3 b:	the surgeon thinks that tumor tissue has remained.

Table 2. *Definition of Total Tumor Extent*

GRADE I:	(1) primary lesion with largest tumor diameter $\leqslant$ 3 cm except for cases with positive resection margin (= Groupings 3 a + 3 b), *and*
	(2) lesion limited to the primary site without blood-vessel invasion (= Grouping 1 a) except for lesions with a largest tumor diameter $\geqslant$ 7 cm.
GRADE II:	other combinations of tumor diameter and grouping.

tumor was assessed by a slightly modified category grouping system, previously described by Slack [13]: its definitions are given in Table 1. Eventually the primary tumor size (i.e. the largest diameter) and the regional extent category were combined into a grading system describing the total tumor burden present, as summarized in Table 2.

After discharge from the hospital, all patients were asked to show up for examination every second month or each time their treating physician should feel an examination to be advisable. In case of relapse, the location was noted and suitable therapy was started as soon as possible.

All data have been stored in an IBM 370/135-computer, and the statistical analysis has been performed by means of the Fisher exact probability test, two-tailed, unless otherwise stated, using a Wang 2200.

RESULTS

The two treatment groups, as studied in the present analysis, were well comparable as to the duration to follow-up, general patient data, skin test reactivity, and tumor

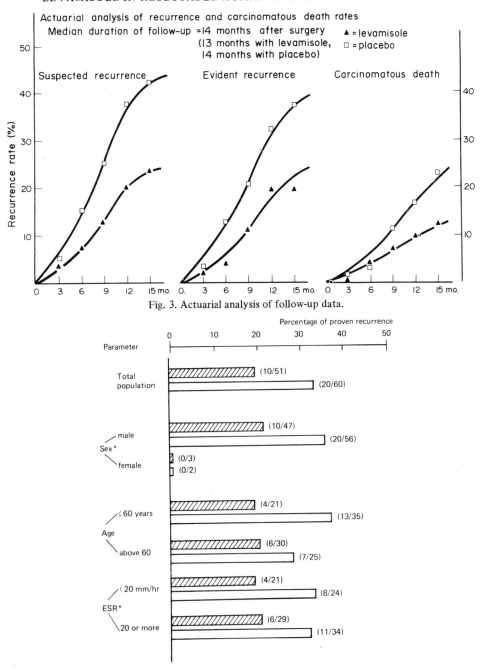

Fig. 3. Actuarial analysis of follow-up data.

Fig. 4. Recurrence rate as related to general patient data.

characteristics (two-tailed probability according to the median test or the chi-square test, n × k table). Fifty-one patients have been receiving levamisole and sixty placebo.

There was no difference between levamisole and placebo as far as side-effects are concerned, as previously reported [14], although there was somewhat more gastric intolerance, nervousness and subfebrility with levamisole.

For the three end-points, i.e. suspected recurrences, proven relapses and carcinomatous deaths, there was a clear but not statistically significant trend in favor of levamisole, and this was the case in the three co-operating centres. The actuarial analysis of the three end-points is shown in Fig. 3. Because of this similarity in the trends, only the number of proven recurrences will be given further on, unless otherwise stated.

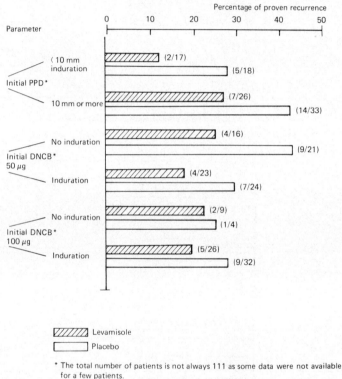

* The total number of patients is not always 111 as some data were not available for a few patients.

Fig. 5. Recurrence rate as related to skin test reactivity.

The difference between levamisole and placebo proved to be related to neither most of the general patient data (Fig. 4) nor to the skin test reactivity (Fig. 5). However, amongst the general tumor data (Fig. 6), the histological diagnosis appeared to be of relevance, since recurrences were less frequent with levamisole in patients with epidermoid carcinoma, but not in those with adenocarcinoma (the number of patients with other histological diagnoses is altogether too small to make a sensible statistical analysis). Although the incidence of proven relapses and that of carcinomatous deaths has not been significantly different so far, a significant difference ($P = 0.035$) was found regarding suspected recurrences in patients with epidermoid carcinoma.

The initial tumor extent (Fig. 7), on the other hand, proved to be of prime importance. Regarding the largest tumor diameters, the statistical analysis revealed that:

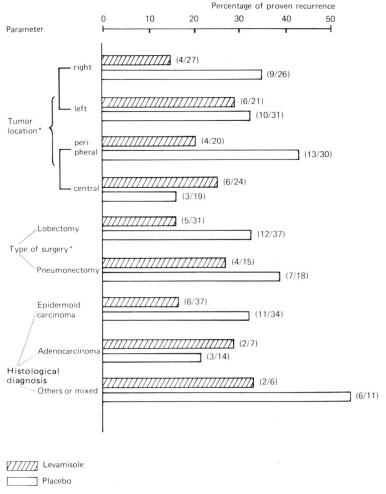

Fig. 6. Recurrence rate as related to general tumor data.

in small tumors (i.e. ≤ 3 cm) levamisole was not different from placebo;

in intermediate tumors (4—6 cm) there were fewer suspected recurrences with levamisole ($P = 0.045$) and a clear but not significant trend was found in favor of levamisole concerning evident recurrences and carcinomatous deaths;

in large tumors (≥ 7 cm) levamisole was better than placebo ($P < 0.05$) for each of the three end-points studied.

Moreover, in contrast to the data in the placebo group where the incidence of recurrences increased with the diameter of the tumor (see Fig. 7), this incidence seemed no longer related to the initial tumor size when levamisole had been given.

The analysis according to the regional grouping categories gives a similar trend: no difference at all between the two groups in the prognostically most favorable category 1a, but a clear difference in the other categories, where there was evidence that the

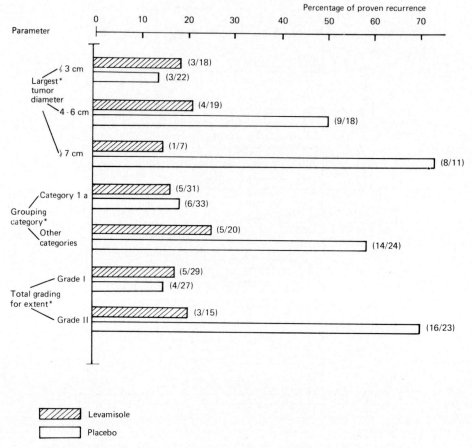

* The total number of patients is not always 111 as some data were not available for a few patients.

Fig. 7. Recurrence rate as related to initial tumor extent.

tumor might have or had spread outside its primary site. This difference was significant for both the suspected and the evident relapses, but not yet for the carcinomatous deaths.

The total extent grading data confirm the above-mentioned findings: no difference in Grade I patients, but a significant ($P < 0.01$ for the two types of recurrences and $P < 0.05$ for the disease mortality) difference in patients with Grade II.

In order to study the possible connection between the histological diagnosis and the initial tumor extent, a cross-table analysis was made (Table 3). This shows that the difference found in epidermoid carcinoma patients can hardly be explained by a difference in tumor extent between these patients and those with another histological diagnosis. Therefore, the initial tumor extent and the histological diagnosis seem to be independent factors as far as the effectiveness of levamisole is concerned.

In patients showing relapse, the disease-free interval was similar in the two groups with a median interval of 8.5 months (range: 3–20 months) with levamisole and of 8 months (range: 1–19 months) with placebo.

Finally, another puzzling phenomenon was apparent (Fig. 8): the influence of

Table 3. *Correlation between Histological Diagnosis and Tumor Extent*[a]

Histological diagnosis	Largest tumor diameter (cm)			
	≤ 3	4–6	≥ 7	Totals
Epidermoid carcinoma	25	25	12	62
Other	14	12	6	32
Totals	39	37	18	

Histological diagnosis	Grouping		
	1a	1b through 3b	Totals
Epidermoid carcinoma	43	28	71
Other	20	16	36
Totals	63	44	

[a] The total gradings for tumor extent are not included as these are a composition of the two parameters described in the table.

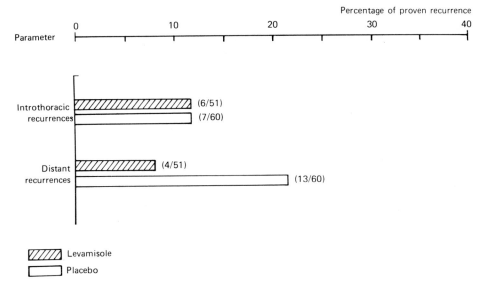

Fig. 8. Site of recurrence in the two treatment groups.

levamisole proved to be quite different according to the site of the recurrences, since no difference at all was found between levamisole and placebo as to the intrathoracic recurrences, but a clear difference, although not yet significant ($P = 0.06$), was noted when the incidence of distant metastases was studied.

COMMENTS

This first interim analysis has revealed some important aspects, which should be taken into consideration when further trials with levamisole or other types of immunotherapy are planned in patients with operable lung cancer (and possibly also other types of cancer).

Apart from the histological diagnosis, which should be documented in every type of study in cancer patients, a great effort should be made to obtain a good description of the tumor burden at the time of operation and to collect accurate data regarding the location of the relapses. Also, since treatment in our study was started before surgery, the timing of immunotherapy could be of major importance.

The significance of the tumor burden, which is present before the start of the therapy, has recently been confirmed [15] since it was found that intermittent treatment with levamisole after successful irradiation of breast cancer decreases the disease mortality in Stage IV patients but not in Stage III (stages according to the TNM definitions [16]).

REFERENCES

1. G. Renoux and M. Renoux, Effet immunostimulant d'un imidothiazole dans l'immunisation des souris contre l'infection par *Brucella abortus. C. R. Acad. Sci. Paris*, **272**, 349 (1971).
2. J. Symoens, The effect of levamisole on host defense mechanisms. A review. Proceedings of a meeting held at the National Institute of Health, Bethesda, Maryland, December 1974.
3. Editorial, Levamisole. *Lancet*, **1**, 151 (1975).
4. L. Thiry, S. Sprecher-Goldberger, L. Tack, M. Jacques and J. Stienon, Comparison of the immunogenicity of hamster cells transformed by adenovirus and herpes simplex virus. *Cancer Res.* (in press, 1975).
5. M.A. Chirigos, J.W. Pearson and J. Pryor, Augmentation of chemotherapeutically induced remission of a murine leukemia by a chemical immunoadjuvant. *Cancer Res.* **33**, 2615 (1973).
6. A. Mantovani and F. Spreafico, Characterization of the immunostimulatory activity of levamisole. *Boll. Ist. Sieroter. Milan* **53**, 302 (1974).
7. D. Tripodi, L. C. Parks and J. Brugmans, Drug-induced restoration of cutaneous delayed hypersensitivity in anergic patients with cancer. *New Eng. J. Med.* **289**, 354 (1973).
8. Y. Hirshaut, C. Pinsky, H. Marquardt and H.F. Oettgen, Effects of levamisole on delayed hypersensitivity reactions in cancer patients. *Proc. Am. Ass. Cancer Res.* **14**, 109 (1973).
9. H. Verhaegen, J. De Cree, W. De Cock and F. Verbruggen, Levamisole and the immune response. *New Engl. J. Med.* **289**, 1148 (1973).
10. M. Biniaminov and B. Ramot, *In-vitro* restoration by levamisole of thymus-derived lymphocyte function in Hodgkin's disease. *Lancet* **1**, 464 (1975).
11. H. Verhaegen, W. De Cock, J. De Cree, F. Verbruggen, M. Verhaegen-Declerq and J. Brugmans, *In-vitro* restoration by levamisole of thymus-derived lymphocyte function in Hodgkin's disease. *Lancet*, **1**, 978 (1975).
12. J. Hoebeke and G. Franchi, Influence of tetramisole and its optical isomers on the mononuclear phagocytic system. Effect on carbon clearance in mice. *Res. J. Reticuloendothel. Soc.* **14**, 317 (1973).
13. N.H. Slack, Bronchogenic carcinoma: nitrogen mustard as a surgical adjuvant and factors influencing survival. University surgical adjuvant lung project. *Cancer*, 987 (1970).
14. W. Amery, Levamisole. *Lancet,* **1,** 574 (1975).
15. J.M. Debois, Trends in survival of patients with breast cancer treated with levamisole. Personal communication.
16. UICC, *TNM Classification of Malignant Tumors*, 2nd edition. International Union Against Cancer, Geneva, 1974.

MEDIATION OF IMMUNE RESPONSES TO HUMAN TUMOR ANTIGENS WITH "IMMUNE" RNA

YOSEF H. PILCH, DIETER FRITZE* and DAVID H. KERN

Department of Surgery, Harbor General Hospital,
1000 West Carson Street, Torrance, California, 90509
and
The UCLA School of Medicine, Los Angeles, California, 90024, U.S.A.

ABSTRACT

Ribonuclei acids extracted from specifically sensitized lymphoid cells (I-RNA) have been shown to transfer specific immunoreactivity to normal, non-immune lymphoid cells. Evidence for the transfer by I-RNA of immune responses to human tumor-associated antigens is reviewed. Lymphocytes from normal donors as well as from cancer patients, when incubated with xenogeneic or allogeneic I-RNA, become specifically cytotoxic for human tumor cells, *in vitro*, with cross-reactivity among tumors of the same histologic type but no cross-reactivity with tumors of other histologic types. I-RNA's directed against "self" normal cell surface antigens appear to be recognized as self by lymphocytes and immune responses against these self antigens are not elicited, whereas I-RNA's directed against "non-self", tumor-associated antigens induce lymphocytes to effect specific anti-tumor immune responses. Preliminary results of a clinical trial of immunotherapy with xenogeneic I-RNA in selected cancer patients are presented. A few encouraging clinical responses have been noted. No local or systemic toxicity has been observed.

INTRODUCTION

Nuclei acids extracted from specifically sensitized lymphoid cells have been shown to transfer specific immune responses to normal, non-immune lymphoid cells. In 1961 Dr. Marvin Fishman reported the first of a series of such experiments [1, 2]. Normal rat macrophages were sensitized to T-2 phage, *in vitro*, and then homogenized. When normal, non-immune rat lymph node cells were incubated, *in vitro*, with a cell-free filtrate of this homogenate, antibody specific for T-2 phage was elaborated into the medium. Enzymatic treatment of the macrophage extract with ribonuclease (RNase) prior to incubation with lymph node cells abrogated this immune response, but treatment of the extract with other enzymes did not. These experiments suggested that the active moiety was one or more species of RNA. Since the active moiety in the macrophage extract was specifically

---

* Present address: Medizinische Universitätsklinik (Director Prof. Dr. med G. Schettler), D-69 Heidelberg, Bergheimerlandstr. 58, West Germany.

digested by RNase and was shown to transfer immune responses, it was referred to as "Immune" RNA (I-RNA). The observations of Fishman and his colleagues were later confirmed by other investigators using a variety of bacterial and other antigens in different experimental test systems. In addition to specific antibody production, normal non-immune lymphoid cells were shown to be converted to specific effector cells of cellular immunity. In 1962 Mannick and Egdahl reported the transfer of immune responses to cell-surface (transplantation) antigens [3]. They transferred immunity to skin allografts in rabbits by incubation of autologous spleen cells, *in vitro*, with allogeneic I-RNA extracted from the lymphoid organs of specifically immunized rabbits. Reinfusion of the RNA-incubated lymphoid cells produced accelerated rejection of skin allografts taken from the same rabbit used to immunize the I-RNA donor [3–5]. The successful transfer of immunity to normal transplantation antigens by I-RNA was confirmed *in vitro* [6–8] and *in vivo* [9–12].

TRANSFER OF TUMOR IMMUNITY BY XENOGENEIC I-RNA IN ANIMALS

Since immunity to a variety of antigens, including normal histocompatibility antigens, had been transferred to non-immune lymphoid cells by I-RNA, it was reasonable to assume that I-RNA could also mediate immune responses to tumor-associated antigens. In 1967 Alexander *et al.* showed that footpad injections of crude RNA-rich extracts prepared from the lymphoid cells of immunized sheep resulted in occasional tumor regressions of rat sarcomata. The transfer of this anti-tumor immune response by crude RNA-rich extracts was specific for a given tumor [13–15].

Ramming and Pilch later reported that transplantation resistance against one or the other of two carcinogen-induced murine sarcomata could be induced in inbred mice by the administration of syngeneic lymphoid cells pre-incubated, *in vitro*, with specific xenogeneic I-RNA extracts [16–18]. In these experiments, the I-RNA was extracted from the lymphoid organs of guinea pigs that had been immunized to either of two anti-genetically distinct murine sarcomata. Normal mice were resistant only to sarcoma cell transplants when injected intraperitoneally with syngeneic spleen cells that had been pre-incubated, *in vitro*, with the I-RNA extract made against that particular tumor. Extract A protected only against challenge with cells from sarcoma A but did not protect against challenge with cells from sarcoma B, and vice versa. Tumor transplantation resistance was not elicited when the extracts were exposed to RNase prior to use. However, the mice resisted sarcoma transplants when the extracts were exposed to DNase or the proteolytic enzyme pronase. Moreover, injections of syngeneic lymphoid cells not treated with I-RNA or treated with anti-normal tissue I-RNA failed to induce resistance to murine sarcoma transplants. These experiments clearly indicated that xenogeneic I-RNA extracts induced an anti-tumor immune response, *in vivo*, which was specific for the immunizing tumor. Since murine sarcoma cells are known to contain normal trans-plantation antigens as well as tumor-specific antigens, the immunization of guinea pigs with mouse sarcoma cells must have resulted in sensitization against many antigens present on mouse sarcoma cells. Consequently, xenogeneic I-RNA extracts could be expected to transfer immune responses against a variety of mouse tissue antigens including normal and histocompatibility antigens. Injections of lymphoid cells activated by such xenogeneic I-RNA extracts might have induced a graft versus host (GvH) reaction.

However, neonatal as well as adult mice which received intraperitoneal injections of syngeneic spleen cells pre-incubated, *in vitro*, with xenogeneic I-RNA failed to evidence any GvH reaction. These findings supported the hypothesis that lymphoid cells recognize as "self" I-RNA's directed against "self" antigens and do not effect immune responses against these antigens. By contrast, the only reactions mediated by xenogeneic I-RNA, which were not directed against "self" antigens, were those directed against tumor-associated antigens and, therefore, tumor-specific immune responses were induced.

MEDIATION OF IMMUNE RESPONSES AGAINST RODENT TUMOR CELLS, *IN VITRO*, BY I-RNA

Using a semiquantitative "plaque assay", Ramming and Pilch [19] reported that syngeneic guinea-pig spleen cells pre-treated with syngeneic anti-tumor I-RNA specifically lysed syngeneic tumor target cells, *in vitro*, but failed to mediate immune cytolysis of normal syngeneic epithelial cells. This observation provided further evidence that the anti-tumor immunoreactivity of I-RNA extracts could be directed specifically against tumor-associated antigens. More recently, Kern *et al.* have demonstrated that incubation of normal, non-immune rodent lymphoid cells with either xenogeneic or syngeneic anti-tumor I-RNA converts them into specific effector cells which mediate immune cytolysis of mouse or rat sarcoma cells, *in vitro* [20, 21].

MEDIATION OF IMMUNE CYTOLYSIS OF HUMAN TUMOR CELLS, *IN VITRO*, BY XENOGENEIC "IMMUNE" RNA

Confirmation of the capacity of xenogeneic "Immune" RNA to mediate cellular immune responses using human lymphoid cells was provided in 1972 by Paque and Dray [22]. They incubated xenogeneic "Immune" RNA, extracted from the lymphoid organs of monkeys immunized with complete Freund's adjuvant or with the H37RA strain of *M. tuberculosis*, with normal, non-immune human leukocytes, and demonstrated that these leukocytes would then mediate the inhibition of migration of guinea-pig peritoneal exudate cells when tuberculin was added to the medium. This was the first report of the interspecies transfer of a cellular immune response from animal to man with "Immune" RNA. In recent studies conducted in our laboratory, we succeeded in mediating immune cytolysis of human tumor cells, *in vitro*, with xenogeneic "Immune" RNA. In these studies, normal, non-immune human peripheral blood lymphocytes were converted into "killer cells", which effected immune cytolysis of human tumor cells, by incubation with "Immune" RNA extracted from the lymph nodes and spleens of sheep or guinea pigs which had previously been immunized with cells from the particular human tumor being studied. The human tumors employed were: (1) a human gastric adenocarcinoma, RI-H, established in tissue culture in our laboratory by primary explant from a surgical specimen, and studied in its 12th to 14th passage; (2) a human adenocarcinoma of the breast, BT-20, obtained from Dr. E. Lasfargues, and studied in its 300th–310th passage; (3) a human malignant melanoma, ED-H, explanted from a surgical specimen in our laboratory and studied in its 18th–25th passage; and (4) a human melanoma, RO-H, established from a primary explant, in its 10th–15th passage. These cells were maintained in RPMI 1640 supplemented with 20% fetal calf serum or 20% agamma human serum,

2

CLINICAL TUMOR IMMUNOLOGY

0.15% glutamine, 0.25 mg/ml amphotercin B and 100 I.U./ml penicillin and 100 μg/ml streptomycin. When cells from the 13th passage of the RI-H line were injected into the cheek pouch of an immunosuppressed hamster, a tumor developed which was histologically similar to the original tumor.

Between 10^7 and 10^8 viable tumor cells in 3 ml RPMI 1640 were emulsified in an equal volume of complete Freund's adjuvant and injected intradermally into all four extremities of sheep at weekly intervals for three consecutive weeks. In some instances, tumor cells for immunization were harvested from monolayer cultures with trypsin, in most instances tumor cells were obtained from a fresh surgical specimen. Ten days after the last injection, the sheep were sacrificed and spleen and mesenteric lymph nodes were harvested and immediately frozen in dry ice. Hartley guinea pigs were also immunized by the injection of 10^7 tumor cells emulsified in an equal volume of complete Freund's adjuvant into each footpad. A simultaneous intraperitoneal injection of 10^7 tumor cells without adjuvant was also given. These animals were sacrificed 10 days later, and the axillary and inguinal lymph nodes and spleens frozen in dry ice. "Immune" RNA was extracted from the frozen lymphoid tissues. Control RNA preparations were also extracted from the spleens and lymph nodes of other guinea pigs and other sheep immunized with complete Freund's adjuvant only. In some experiments "Immune" RNA was treated with ribonuclease, deoxyribonuclease, or pronase as previously described.

In early experiment peripheral blood leukocytes from normal human volunteers were isolated from specimens by sedimentation in 10% Plasmagel (Roger Bellon Laboratories, Neuilly, France). Red blood cells were lysed with 0.85% ammonium chloride. The leukocytes were washed twice with RPMI 1640, counted and then used for incubation with RNA. In subsequent experiments, purified lymphocyte populations were prepared from heparinized blood specimens on Ficol-Isopaque gradients, suspended in RPMI 1640 with 40% agamma human serum and 10% dimethysulfoxide (DMSO) frozen in liquid nitrogen at $1°C$ min, and thawed at $37°C$ prior to use. One ml RPMI 1640 containing 1.5×10^7 lymphocytes was incubated with 1 ml of the appropriate RNA preparation at a concentration of 2 mg/ml for 20 min at $37°C$. The cells were washed twice and diluted to the appropriate cell concentration for addition to target cells. The assay for immune cytolysis employed was a modification of the microcytotoxicity assay of Cohen et al. (23), described above, in which tumor target cells are pre-labeled with ^{125}I-iododeoxyuridine.

Immune Cytolysis of RI-H Tumor Cells

The results of three typical early experiments using buffy coat leukocytes as effector cells are presented in Table 1. In experiments 1 and 2 xenogeneic "Immune" RNA extracted from the lymphoid organs of sheep immunized with RI-H tumor cells were incubated with normal human leukocytes, and in experiment 3 the "Immune" RNA was extracted from the lymph nodes and spleens of immunized guinea pigs. The optimal leukocyte to tumor cell ratio was found to be 500:1. Higher ratios resulted in an unacceptable degree of nonspecific lysis, and lower ratios were usually less effective or ineffective. In experiment 1, the cytotoxicity index (CI) obtained with leukocytes incubated with RNA extracted from the lymphoid organs of immunized sheep ("Immune" RNA) was 0.45 ± 0.08. The CI for leukocytes incubated with no RNA was 0 + 0.14. The difference was significant at p value < 0.01. Leukocytes incubated with RNA extracted from the lymphoid organs of a sheep immunized with complete Freund's

Table 1. *Immune Cytolysis of RI-H Tumor Cells Mediated by "Immune" RNA*

Only leukocyte to target cell ratios of 500:1 are included in the table. Six replicate wells were used for each determination and mean cytoxicity indices with their standard deviations are presented. The p values were calculated by Student's t-test for unpaired data and represent differences between "Immune" RNA and the various control groups.

| Experiment number: | 1 | | 2 | | 3 | |
RNA donor:	Sheep		Sheep		Guinea pig	
	Cytotoxicity index	p	Cytotoxicity index	p	Cytotoxicity index	p
Leukocytes incubated with:						
"Immune" RNA[a]	0.45 ± .08		0.30 ± .05		0.41 ± .13	
"Immune" RNA + ribonuclease[b]	0.18 ± .14	< .05	0.38 ± .05	< .005	−0.37 ± .03	< .005
Freund's Adjuvant RNA[c]	−0.10 ± .18	< .005	−0.30 ± .05	< .005	−0.20 ± .10	< .005
No RNA	0.0 ± .14	< .01	0.0 ± .15	< .01	0.0 ± .07	< .025

[a] RNA from the lymphoid organs of animals immunized with RI-H tumor cells.
[b] "Immune" RNA treated with ribonuclease prior to incubation with leukocytes.
[c] RNA from the lymphoid organs of animals immunized with Freund's adjuvant only.

adjuvant only (Freund's Adjuvant RNA) gave a CI for − 0.10 ± 0.18, a value significantly different ($p < 0.005$) from "Immune" RNA but not different from the leukocyte preparation incubated with no RNA. When the same "Immune" RNA preparation was treated with ribonuclease prior to incubation with leukocytes, a CI of 0.18 ± 0.14 was obtained. This value was significantly different from the CI obtained with untreated "Immune" RNA ($p < 0.05$) but not different from the other two control leukocyte preparations. In this particular experiment, the ribonuclease used did not completely degrade the "Immune" RNA. This was evident from the profile obtained upon analysis of this RNA preparation on a sucrose density gradient. When a fresh preparation of ribonuclease was utilized in experiments 2 and 3, complete degradation of the "Immune" RNA resulted and all immunologic activity was abrogated. In experiment 2, again using sheep "Immune" RNA, results similar to those of experiment 1 were obtained. The leukocytes incubated with "Immune" RNA gave a CI of 0.30 ± 0.05. This was a significantly greater cytotoxicity index than those obtained with leukocytes incubated without RNA (CI = 0 ± 0.15; $p < 0.01$), leukocytes incubated with Freund's Adjuvant RNA (CI = 0.30 ± 0.05; $p < 0.005$). Again the CI of the three control leukocytes preparations were not statistically different from each other. In experiment 3, guinea-pig "Immune" RNA was employed instead of sheep RNA but all other parameters were the same. The CI for leukocytes incubated with guinea-pig "Immune" RNA was 0.41 ± 0.13. This was a significantly higher cytotoxicity index than those obtained with leukocytes incubated without RNA (CI of 0 ± 0.07; $p < 0.025$), leukocytes incubated with Freund's Adjuvant RNA (CI of − 0.20 ± 0.1; $p < 0.0005$) and leukocytes incubated with "Immune" RNA treated with ribonuclease (CI = − 0.37 ± 0.08; $p < 0.005$). The cytotoxicity indices for control leukocyte preparations were not statistically different from one another. Note that in all three experiments there was no significant difference between the cytotoxicity indices obtained with control RNA preparations.

When purified lymphocyte populations, prepared on Ficol-Isopaque gradients [24], were incubated with the RNA instead of buffy coat leukocytes, the magnitude of the

Table 2. *Immune Cytolysis of RI-H Tumor Cells Mediated by "Immune" RNA from the Lymphoid Organs of Immunized Sheep*

Six replicate wells were used for each determination and mean cytotoxicity indices with their standard deviations are presented. The p values were calculated by Student's t-test for unpaired data and represent differences between "Immune" RNA and the various control groups. In these experiments purified lymphocyte populations were employed rather than buffy coat leukocytes.

| Experiment number: | 4 | | 5 | | 6 | | 7 | |
| Lymphocyte to target cell ratio: | 100:1 | | 200:1 | | 100:1 | | 100:1 | |
	Cytotoxicity index	p	Cytotoxicity index	p	Cytotoxicity index	p	Cytotoxicity index	p
Lymphocytes incubated with:								
"Immune" RNA[a]	0.60 ± .06		0.84 ± .02		0.69 ± .07		0.60 ± .06	
"Immune" RNA + ribonuclease[b]	N.D.[f]		N.D.		−0.08 ± .14	< .005	0.05 ± .02	< .005
"Immune" RNA + deoxyribonuclease[c]	N.D.		0.08 ± .03	N.S.[g]	N.D.		N.D.	
"Immune" RNA + pronase[d]	N.D.		N.D.		N.D.		0.53 ± .06	N.S.
Freund's Adjuvant RNA[e]	0.22 ± .05	< .005	0.22 ± .13	< .005	0.12 ± .24	< .05	N.D.	
No RNA	0.0 ± .10	< .005	0.0 ± .19	< .005	0.0 ± .14	< .005	0.0 ± .04	< .005

(a) RNA from the lymphoid organs of sheep immunized with RI-H tumor cells.
(b) "Immune" RNA treated with ribonuclease prior to incubation with lymphocytes.
(c) "Immune" RNA treated with deoxyribonuclease prior to incubation with lymphocytes.
(d) "Immune" RNA treated with pronase prior to incubation with lymphocytes.
(e) RNA from the lymphoid organs of animals immunized with Freund's Adjuvant only.
(f) Not done.
(g) Not significant.

cytotoxicity observed was increased and the lymphocyte to target cell ratio could be significantly reduced (from 500:1 to 100:1 or 200:1). These data are presented in Table 2. From these results, it may be seen that at a lymphocyte to target cell ratio of 100:1 CI's of from 0.60 to 0.69 were obtained in a very consistent fashion. Since lymphocytes account for 20–40% of the total peripheral white blood cells in man, this result is quite consistent with what would be expected assuming that one or more populations of lymphocytes are the active effector cell population. By effecting approximately a five-fold increase in lymphocyte concentration, the leukocyte to target cell ratio could be reduced by a factor of 5 with no loss (or even an increase) in cytotoxicity.

When the active "Immune" RNA preparations were pretreated with deoxyribonuclease (experiment 5) at an enzyme to substrate ratio of 1:50 (based on the actual amount of DNA in the sample) or with pronase (experiment 7) at an enzyme to substrate ratio of 1:20 (based on the actual amount of protein in the sample) and then incubated with lymphocytes the resultant cytotoxicity index was not significantly altered. The fact that deoxyribonuclease and pronase treatment of the "Immune" RNA preparations did not affect the transfer of immunity and that ribonuclease treatment of the "Immune" RNA abrogated the response offers strong evidence that one or more moieties of RNA were responsible for the immunological activity of these preparations.

Attempts were then made to determine the effect of varying the RNA concentration upon the magnitude of the immune response observed. The concentration of RNA in which the lymphocytes were incubated was progressively reduced so that a dose–response curve might be established and a threshold RNA concentration determined. The results of these experiments are depicted in Table 3. From these data it can be seen that reducing the RNA concentration from 2.0 mg/ml to 1.0 mg/ml or even to 0.5 mg/ml had little effect on the response but reducing the concentration still further to 0.25 mg/ml resulted in approximately 50% decrease in cytotoxicity. Further reducing the RNA concentration to 0.10 mg/ml reduced cytotoxicity still further but this result remained significantly

Table 3. *Immune Cytolysis of RI-H Tumor Cells Mediated by "Immune" RNA from the Lymphoid Organs of Immunized Sheep*

Six replicate wells were used for each determination and mean cytotoxicity indices with their standard deviations are presented. The p values were calculated by Student's t-test for unpaired data and represent differences between no RNA and the various other groups. In these experiments purified lymphocyte populations were employed rather than buffy coat leukocytes.

| Experiment number: | 8 | | 9 | |
Lymphocyte to target cell ratio:	100:1		100:1	
	Cytotoxicity index	p	Cytotoxicity index	p
Concentration of "Immune" RNA[a]				
No RNA	0.0 ± .14		0.0 ± .06	
2.0 mg RNA/ml	0.69 ± .07	< .005	0.53 ± .06	< .005
1.0 mg RNA/ml	0.79 ± .02	< .005	0.36 ± .02	< .005
0.5 mg RNA/ml	0.62 ± .03	< .005	N.D.[b]	
0.25 mg RNA/ml	N.D.		0.21 ± .05	< .05
0.10 mg RNA/ml	N.D.		0.17 ± .07	< .05

[a] RNA from the lymphoid organs of sheep immunized with RI-H tumor cells.
[b] Not done.

Table 4. *Immune Cytolysis of BT-20 Tumor Cells Mediated by "Immune" RNA from the Lymphoid Organs of Immunized Guinea Pigs*

Six replicate wells were used for each determination and mean cytotoxicity indices with their standard deviations are presented. The p values were calculated by Student's t-test for unpaired data and represent differences between "Immune" RNA and the various control groups. In these experiments purified lymphocyte populations were employed as effector cells.

Experiment number: Lymphocyte to target cell ratio:	1 200:1		2 200:1		3 200:1		4 200:1	
	Cytotoxicity index	p	Cytotoxicity index	p	Cytotoxicity index	p	Cytotoxicity index	p
Lymphocytes incubated with:								
"Immune" RNA[a]	0.57 ± .10		0.54 ± .05		0.73 ± .06		0.71 ± .08	
"Immune" RNA + ribonuclease[b]	N.D.[f]		0.11 ± .09	$< .005$	$- 0.2 ± .06$	$< .005$	$-0.02 ± .06$	$< .005$
"Immune" RNA + deoxyribonuclease[c]	N.D.		N.D.		N.D.		0.48 ± .06	N.S.[c]
"Immune" RNA + pronase[d]	N.D.		N.D.		N.D.		0.68 ± .03	N.S.
Freund's Adjuvant RNA[e]	0.21 ± .30	$< .05$	N.D.		0.17 ± .04	$< .005$	N.D.	
No RNA	0.0 ± .36	$< .05$	0.0 ± .05	$< .005$	0.0 ± .04	$< .005$	0.0 ± .05	$< .005$

[a] RNA from the lymphoid organs of guinea pigs immunized with BT-20 tumor cells.
[b] "Immune" RNA treated with ribonuclease prior to incubation with lymphocytes.
[c] "Immune" RNA treated with deoxyribonuclease prior to incubation with lymphocytes.
[d] "Immune" RNA treated with pronase prior to incubation with lymphocytes.
[e] RNA from the lymphoid organs of animals immunized with Freund's Adjuvant only.
[f] Not done.
[g] Not significant.

different from that obtained with no RNA. A number of the experiments described above have been reported in detail elsewhere [25–27].

Immune Cytolysis of BT-20 Tumor Cells

Experiments similar to those described above for the RI-H cell line were performed utilizing the BT-20 cell line. In these experiments guinea-pig RNA was used. The results are depicted in Table 4. Again, xenogeneic "Immune" RNA induced normal, non-immune human lymphocytes to become cytotoxic to BT-20 cells in a consistent and reproducible fashion. RNA from guinea pigs immunized with Freund's Adjuvant only was inactive. The activity was abolished by treatment of the "Immune" RNA preparations with RNase but was not affected by treatment with DNAse or pronase.

Immune Cytolysis of Melanoma Cells (ED-H and RO-H)

In these experiments two types of "Immune" RNA preparations were studied: (1) RNA from the lymphoid organs of guinea pigs immunized with ED-H cells, and (2) RNA from the lymphoid organs of a sheep immunized with melanoma cells from a fresh surgical specimen obtained from a third melanoma patient HO. The results of these experiments are tabulated in Table 5. Of particular interest is the fact that RNA from the lymphoid organs of a sheep immunized with melanoma cells from one patient, HO, was effective in mediating cytotoxic immune responses against melanoma cells from two other patients, RO and ED.

Table 5. *Immune Cytolysis of Melanoma Cells Mediated by "Immune" RNA*

Only lymphocyte to target cell ratios of 500:1 are included in the table. Six replicate wells were used for each determination and mean cytotoxicity indices with their standard deviations are presented. The p values were calculated by Student's t-test for unpaired data and represent differences between "Immune" RNA and the various control groups. Purified lymphocyte populations were employed as effector cells.

Experiment number: Target cell line: RNA donor:	1 RO-H Sheep		2 ED-H Sheep		3 ED-H Guinea pig	
	Cytotoxicity index	p	Cytotoxicity index	p	Cytotoxicity index	p
Lymphocytes incubated with:						
"Immune" RNA[a]	0.53 ± .12		0.37 ± .05		0.30 ± .02	
Freund's Adjuvant RNA[b]	−0.20 ± .08	< .005	−0.30 ± .10	< .005	0.07 ± .04	< .05
No RNA	0.0 ± .08	< .005	0.0 ± .08	< .005	0.0 ± .03	< .005

[a] RNA from the lymphoid organs of animals immunized with melanoma cells.
[b] RNA from the lymphoid organs of animals immunized with Freund's Adjuvant only.

The Specificity of Immune Reactions against Human Tumors
Mediated by Xenogeneic I-RNA

A critical experiment was then performed in an autologous system using autologous lymphocytes obtained from the same patient from whom the ED-H cell line originated. These lymphocytes were incubated with the sheep anti-melanoma "Immune" RNA and reacted with cells from the patient's own tumor, *in vitro*. The patient's lymphocytes incubated without RNA served as a control. The results of this experiment are presented in Fig. 1. When incubated with no RNA, the patient's lymphocytes were very slightly cytotoxic to his tumor cells (CI = 0.22 ± 0.05) as might be expected. However, when this patient's lymphocytes were incubated with "Immune" RNA, the cytotoxicity index of his lymphocytes more than doubled (CI = 0.45 ± 0.02). This increase was significant at $p < 0.005$. At the same time, lymphocytes from a normal volunteer were incubated with this RNA. The resulting CI was 0.49 ± 0.05. It can be seen that the effect of "Immune" RNA upon *autologous* lymphocytes (autologous with respect to the tumor target cells) was equal in magnitude to its effect on normal, non-immune responses directed specifically against melanoma-associated antigens where mediated by the "Immune" RNA. Again, it is important to remember that the anti-melanoma "Immune" RNA was extracted from the lymphoid organs of a sheep immunized with melanoma cells from a *different* melanoma patient.

To derive additional evidence that immune responses directed specifically against tumor-associated antigens could be mediated by "Immune" RNA, a second experiment was performed which included additional controls. "Immune" RNA was extracted separately from the lymphoid organs of two groups of guinea pigs. One group had been immunized with ED's autologous skin fibroblasts (anti-Ed-Fib RNA). Each "Immune" RNA preparation was incubated separately with normal, allogeneic lymphocytes (from a

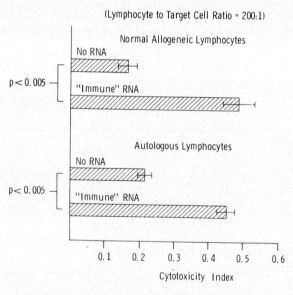

Fig. 1. Immune cytolysis of ED-H melanoma cells by autologous lymphocytes and by allogeneic lymphocytes (from a normal donor) following incubation with "Immune" RNA extracted from the lymphoid tissue of a sheep immunized with melanoma cell.

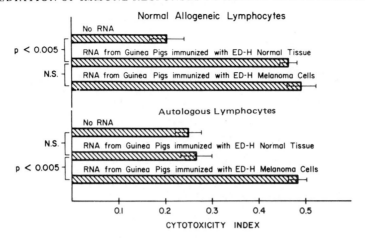

Fig. 2. Immune cytolysis of ED-H melanoma cells by autologous lymphocytes and by allogeneic lymphocytes (from a normal donor) following incubation with "Immune" RNA extracted from the lymphoid organs of guinea pigs immunized with ED-H melanoma cells or with ED's autologous skin fibroblasts.

healthy donor) and with ED's own autologous lymphocytes. Following incubation each lymphocyte sample was tested for cytotoxic effect upon ED's own melanoma target cells. The results of this experiment are depicted in Fig. 2. Note that when effector cells which were allogeneic with respect to the target cells were used, both anti-ED-Fib RNA and anti-Mel RNA were equally effective in mediating cytotoxic immune responses to ED-H melanoma target cells. However, when autologous lymphocytes were used as effector cells, only anti-ED-Mel RNA was active, and anti-ED-Fib RNA did not cause any increase in the cytotoxic activity of ED's lymphocytes for autologous melanoma cells. We interpret these results as follows: Both anti-Ed-Mel RNA and anti-ED-Fib RNA induced allogeneic lymphocytes to effect immune responses directed against normal transplantation antigens (primarily HL-A antigens). When these "Immune" RNA were incubated with autologous lymphocytes "Immune" RNA's directed against normal transplantation antigens were recognized as "self" by the lymphocytes and no immune responses against these antigens were elicited. Therefore, anti-ED-Fib RNA was inactive when incubated with autologous lymphocytes, however, since anti-ED-Mel RNA contained "Immune" RNA's directed against tumor associated antigens which were not recognized as "self" by autologous lymphocytes, this RNA preparation was effective in inducing ED's lymphocytes to become cytotoxic to ED's autologous melanoma cells.

We then looked for additional evidence to confirm that "Immune" RNA could mediate immune responses directed specifically against melanoma-associated antigens. Allogeneic "Immune" RNA was extracted separately from the peripheral blood lymphocytes of five "cured" melanoma patients (collected on the continuous flow blood cell separator), one patient with colon carcinoma, one patient with hypernephroma and five normal volunteers. Each "Immune" RNA preparation was incubated separately with aliquots of a single sample of normal lymphocytes collected on the continuous flow blood cell separator from another healthy volunteer and each aliquot was then tested for cytotoxic activity against ED-H melanoma target cells. The results are depicted in Fig. 3. From these data it is apparent that only "Immune" RNA from the lymphocytes of

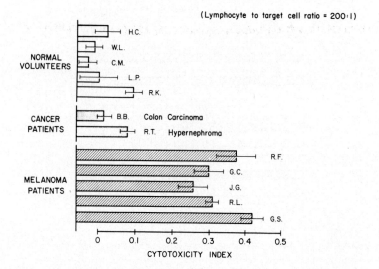

Fig. 3. Immune cytolysis of ED-H melanoma cells mediated by allogeneic "Immune" RNA extracted from the peripheral blood lymphocytes of "cured" colon cancer patients.

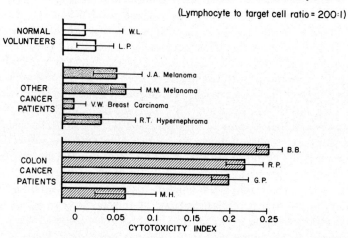

Fig. 4. Immune cytolysis of colon cancer cells mediated by allogeneic "Immune" RNA extracted from the peripheral blood lymphocytes of "cured" colon cancer patients.

melanoma patients was effective in mediating a cytotoxic immune response against melanoma target cells. RNA from the lymphocytes of normal volunteers was invariably inactive, as was RNA from the lymphocytes of the colon cancer patient and the hyper-nephroma patient. Presumably, the melanoma patients had been sensitized to melanoma associated antigens *in vivo*, but not to normal histocompatibility antigens (all were male and none had been multiply transfused), and "Immune" RNA was synthesized against these melanoma-associated antigens.

Many of these same allogeneic I-RNA preparations and three additional preparations of I-RNA extracted from the peripheral blood lymphocytes of three additional "cured" colon cancer patients were studied in another experiment. Aliquots of a single sample of human lymphocytes from a normal donor were incubated separately with each of the various preparations of allogeneic I-RNA and each aliquot was then tested for cytotoxicity activity against colon cancer target cells. The results are depicted in Fig. 4. It is apparent that three out of four I-RNA preparations from the lymphocytes of colon cancer patients was effective in mediating cytotoxic immune responses against colon cancer target cells. RNA extracted from the lymphocytes of normal volunteers was inactive, as were RNA preparations from the lymphocytes of patients with malignancies of other histologic types (melanoma, hypernephroma and breast cancer). Again all the colon cancer patients were male and none had been multiply transfused.

INITIAL CLINICAL TRIALS OF IMMUNOTHERAPY WITH "IMMUNE" RNA

"Immune" RNA offers several theoretical advantages over other methods of adoptive immunotherapy. (1) There is no need to give serum or plasma which has been shown in some instances to contain blocking factors *in vitro*, and which may facilitate tumor growth, *in vivo*. (2) Since it is not necessary to transfuse foreign leukocytes, there is no sensitization of the recipient to foreign histocompatibility (HL-A antigens). Repeated transfusion of allogeneic leukocytes can result in significant toxicity. "Immune RNA itself does not contain transplantation antigens. (3) The danger of inducing a graft-versus-host reaction in immunodeficient or immunosuppressed individuals is eliminated. (4) Since "Immune" RNA itself is not a strong antigen, repeated injections of human or even animal RNA would not be expected to sensitize the recipient, cause secondary syndromes, or result in immune elimination of subsequent doses of RNA. "Immune" RNA does not require the simultaneous administration of adjuvants. "Immune" RNA would probably be more immunogenic than immunization with tumor antigens alone, assuming that good preparations of human tumor antigens eventually become available. "Immune" RNA could conceivably make purification and isolation of human tumor specific transplantation antigens unnecessary for effective immunotherapy. Finally, "Immune" RNA might be effective despite certain types of host energy (defects in the afferent arc of the immune response, i.e. antigen recognition or processing).

Two sources of "Immune" RNA for the immunotherapy of cancer have been proposed: allogeneic "Immune" RNA derived from the lymphocytes of "cured" cancer patients, and xenogeneic "Immune" RNA derived from animals which have been specifically immunized with either autologous tumor cells or with allogeneic tumor cells from a tumor of the same histogenic type. There are also two methods by which "Immune" RNA may be administered: (1) by direct injection intradermally, or (2) by collecting autologous peripheral blood lymphocytes from the patient utilizing the continuous-flow blood-cell separator, incubating these lymphocytes, *in vitro*, with "Immune" RNA and then reinfusing them intravenously.

The transfer of anti-tumor immunity *in vitro* by human allogeneic "Immune" RNA has been demonstrated. As described above, lymphocytes from patients who had undergone successful excision of primary malignant melanoma and who had been free of disease for more than 9 months provided the source of "Immune" RNA. Control RNA was extracted from peripheral blood lymphocytes of normal volunteers. Each RNA fraction was incubated with non-immune peripheral blood lymphocytes of normal donors. The normal (allogeneic) lymphocytes were rendered cytotoxic against human melanoma cells, *in vitro*, by the "Immune" RNA extracted from the lymphocytes of the "cured" patients. RNA from normal volunteers did not cause these lymphocytes to become cytotoxic to melanoma cells.

Extension of this laboratory model for the adoptive transfer of tumor-specific immunity to clinical immunotherapy has been greatly facilitated by the development of the continuous blood-flow cell separator. This technique provides a method for the continuous collection of lymphocytes from the peripheral blood and the reinfusion of remaining blood elements. Waldman et al. detected no clinically significant changes in hematocrit, and no evidence of systemic toxicity, following leukapheresis of both normal volunteers and in melanoma patients. The peripheral blood leukocyte and lymphocyte counts fell transiently, but returned to normal within 3 days [28]. A potential danger of leukapheresis in cancer patients was the possibility of decreased cellular immuno-competence in the donor following removal of the large number of peripheral lymphocytes. However, Waldman et al. detected no change in skin-test reactivity to DNCB or common skin-test antigens following leukapheresis. Lymphocyte mediated cytotoxicity to melanoma cells decreased transiently in one melanoma patient following leukapheresis, but cytotoxicity indices returned to normal within 24 hr [29].

Allogeneic "Immune" RNA, like transfer factor, requires a human donor and, therefore, involves a number of inherent disadvantages. (1) The problem of donor selection. (2) The problem of donor availability. (3) The question of whether any human can provide lymphocytes which will yield an optimally immunoreactive extract. Human tumors may be more immunogeneic when inoculated into animals than they are in their host of origin. (4) Will immunization of human donors be required or will "cured" cancer patients be adequate donors? (5) Will repeated removal of lymphocytes from "cured" cancer patient donors result in sufficient immunosuppression to cause exacerbation of the donor's malignant disease? Due to these practical and theoretical problems with allogeneic "Immune" RNA as an immunotherapeutic reagent, initial clinical trials have utilized xenogeneic rather than allogeneic "Immune" RNA.

The successful interspecies transfer of cell-mediated immunity to human tumors, in vitro (see above), provided a logical basis for the immunotherapy of human cancer with "Immune" RNA extracted from the lymphoid tissues of animals specifically immunized with the type of human tumor to be treated. There are several obvious advantages to this form of immunotherapy. First, large quantities of "Immune" RNA could be readily produced without dependence upon human donors. Secondly, since histologically similar human tumors appear to contain common tumor-associated antigens, many patients with the same tumor type could be treated with RNA from a sheep sensitized with a single patient's tumor. However, there are also some potential dangers associated with xenogeneic "Immune" RNA; we have recently undertaken a preliminary trial of immunotherapy of human cancer with xenogeneic "Immune" RNA. At the time of this writing thirty-five patients have been treated. The main intent of this study was to determine the safety and feasibility of immunotherapy with xenogeneic "Immune" RNA. However, some interesting observations have been made regarding the effects of "Immune" RNA therapy on certain anti-tumor immune responses assessed in vitro and some indications of possible therapeutic benefit have been observed.

Two types of patients were studied: patients with grossly detectable and measurable metastatic disease, and patients with "minimum residual disease". Patients in the latter category had no clinically detectable disease following surgical resection of all gross tumor but had a greater than 50% likelihood of developing recurrent and/or metastatic disease within 24 months. The histologic types of tumors treated included malignant melanoma, hypernephroma, sarcoma, breast carcinoma and carcinoma of the stomach.

Table 6. *Number of Patients Treated with "Immune" RNA Grouped According to Tumor Type and Extent of Disease*

Tumor types treated	Gross disease	Minimum residual disease	Total
Malignant melanoma	11	4	15
Hypernephroma	11	1	12
Sarcoma	3	0	3
Breast carcinoma	0	2	2
GI carcinoma	1	1	2
Cholangiocarcinoma	1	0	1
Total	27	8	35

The number of patients within each disease category and of each tumor type are given in Table 6. Of the three sarcoma patients, one had an alveolar soft part sarcoma, one a liposarcoma and one an osteogenic sarcoma. Patients with gross disease were accepted for treatment only if (1) they had failed all standard therapy (including standard chemotherapy) or (2) no standard therapy of proven efficacy existed or (3) they had relatively stable disease and standard therapy could be interrupted or withheld for 8 weeks (the minimum duration of the study).

Tumor tissue obtained from surgical specimens (either fresh or frozen in liquid nitrogen) was used. A thick suspension of viable tumor cells, emulsified in an equal volume of complete Freund's adjuvant, was injected intradermally into all four extremities of a sheep at weekly intervals for 3 consecutive weeks. Ten days after the last injection the animals were sacrificed and "Immune" RNA was extracted from the spleens and mesenteric lymph nodes. The RNA was reprecipitated twice from solutions made 2 M with respect to potassium acetate, treated with pronase (to remove contaminating protein), and again reprecipitated from 2 M potassium acetate. The RNA was then dialyzed against sterile distilled water, sterilized by passage through a 0.22 micron millipore filter and lyophylized. The RNA was resuspended in normal saline prior to injection. Aliquots were cultured to assure sterility.

Initially the "Immune" RNA was administered at a concentration of 1 mg RNA/ml. Later the concentration was increased to 2 mg RNA/ml. At higher concentrations the RNA was administered intradermally, in 0.1-ml aliquots, in the skin of the upper anterior chest near the axillae and lower abdomen near the groins. Usually the RNA was given at weekly intervals rotating injection sites. Initially the weekly dose of RNA was 1 mg. Later the 2 mg/week was given and most recently 4 mg/week has been the usual dose. A few patients have received up to 12 mg/week. Whenever possible, each patient received "Immune" RNA against allogeneic tumor tissue followed by RNA against autologous tumor tissues when it became available. Treatment was given for 8 weeks following which initial responses were evaluated. If progression of disease was noted, "Immune" RNA therapy was discontinued and alternative therapy instituted.

No significant local or systemic toxicity related to "Immune" RNA therapy was noted with "Immune" RNA therapy administered weekly for up to 15 months. "Burning" on injection was minimal. Local irritation as evidenced by erythema, induration or swelling was absent or very minimal. No febrile reactions of any kind occurred and no allergic or anaphylactoid reactions resulted.

The thirty-four patients treated with "Immune" RNA ranged in age from 10 to 69. All were sensitized and skin tested with DNCB and a battery of four common skin-test antigens (PPD, monilia, mumps and streptokinase/streptodornase) prior to the initiation of immunotherapy and all were immunocompetent.

The duration of therapy to date ranges from 6 months to less than 2 months. Responses to therapy in patients with gross disease were evaluated by the following criteria: (1) Patients were considered "improved" if grossly detectable (and measurable) lesions objectively regressed (i.e. decreased in area) and, following regression, did not increase in size for at least 2 months. (2) Patients were considered treatment "failures" if gross lesions significantly increased in area of new lesions appeared. (3) Patients were considered as having achieved "stability" if lesions which had been growing progressively prior to the initiation of therapy ceased all growth and remained stable for at least 2 months. (4) A few patients were classified as having achieved "possible benefit" when transitory regressions occurred or when prolonged stability was later followed by regrowth while on therapy. (5) Patients with minimum residual disease were considered "stable" as long as no recurrence or metastases developed. If recurrence occurred, this was considered a treatment failure. When progression occurred, "Immune" RNA therapy was discontinued.

The clinical results are summarized in Table 7. The first twenty-six patients are being reported, in detail, elsewhere [30–31]. In reviewing the results of this study to date, it must be remembered that clinical remissions were not expected at this stage of our work and any clinical responses reported must be considered anecdotal. In this initial Phase I trial, the objectives were: (1) to establish the safety (or toxicity) of sheep "Immune" RNA, (2) to evaluate dosage schedules and routes of administration and (3) to monitor any possible effects of "Immune" RNA treatment on immunologic parameters, both tumor-specific and non-specific. The optimum dosage and route and frequency of

Table 7. *Summary of Clinical Results*

Tumor types	Improvement	Stability or possible improvement	Failure	Indeterminate	Total
Malignant melanoma					
Gross	0	4	6	1	11
Minimum residual		3	0	1	4
Hypernephroma					
Gross	3	3	2	3	11
Minimum residual		1	0	0	1
Sarcoma					
Gross	1	0	1	1	3
Breast carcinoma					
Minimum residual		1	0	0	1
Cholangiocarcinoma					
Gross	0	0	0	1	1
GI carcinoma					
Minimum residual		0	1	1	2
Total	4	12	10	8	34

administration of "Immune" RNA is not known. Certainly, we have not as yet approached a toxic dose of RNA.

In our previous animal experiments, it appeared desirable to administer "Immune" RNA in a medium containing a strong ribonuclease inhibitor (the polyanion sodium dextran sulfate). However, since we have not as yet received approval from the Food and Drug Administration to administer dextran sulfate experimentally in man, we have not incorporated a ribonuclease inhibitor into our RNA preparations. Perhaps by so doing we might significantly increase the efficacy of "Immune" RNA therapy.

Although treatment of lymphocytes *in vitro* with "Immune" RNA has been shown to induce such lymphocytes to effect antitumor responses *in vivo* and *in vitro*, we have not as yet treated any patients by the intravenous infusion of autologous lymphocytes pre-incubated *in vitro* with "Immune" RNA. This reluctance has been due to the fear of inducing untoward allergic reactions related to small amounts of sheep protein which contaminate the RNA and might be expected to remain with the lymphocytes even after several washes. However, this method of utilizing "Immune" RNA therapeutically may offer promise of greater efficacy.

Many of our patients had large tumor burdens and may not have been good candidates for immunotherapy of any kind. Perhaps (and this may be true for all types of immunotherapy) the primary usefulness of "Immune" RNA proved to be in the therapy of minimum residual disease. Our number of patients with minimum residual disease is small. The follow-up period for most of these patients is very short, and we have no concomitantly generated control population. Therefore, few if any conclusions can be drawn at the present time from the results observed in these patients.

In a number of instances, lymphocytes obtained from patients prior to the onset of treatment were incubated, *in vitro*, with the "Immune" RNA which they were to receive. Following incubation of the lymphocytes with "Immune" RNA for 20 min at 37°C, the lymphocytes were tested for cytotoxic effect, *in vitro*, of alogeneic tumor target cells of the same histologic type.

One example is presented in the experiment illustrated in Fig. 5. In this experiment, pre-treatment lymphocytes from melanoma patient CA were tested against allogeneic melanoma cells (ED-H) before and after incubation with I-RNA extracted from the

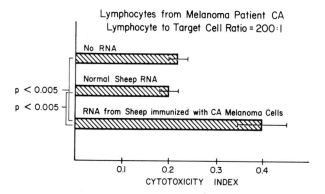

Fig. 5. Cytotoxicity of pretreatment lymphocytes from melanoma patient CA for ED-H melanoma cells prior to and following incubation "Immune" RNA extracted from the lymphoid tissues of a sheep immunized with CA's own autologous tumor tissue and (as a control) "Immune" RNA extracted from the lymphoid organs of a normal sheep.

lymphoid organs of a sheep immunized with CA's own autologous tumor cells and after incubation with I-RNA extracted from the lymphoid organs of an unimmunized sheep. Following incubation with "Immune" RNA from a sheep immunized with CA's tumor cells, the cytotoxicity of CA's lymphocytes for melanoma cells was greatly increased while incubation with I-RNA from an unimmunized sheep was ineffective.

In fourteen of the thirty-four patients treated with "Immune" RNA, peripheral blood lymphocytes, from serial bleedings obtained prior to an infection weekly during "Immune" RNA therapy, were tested for cytotoxicity against allogeneic target cells of the same histologic type. Of five patients in whom significant increases in cytotoxicity were noted four evidenced stability or possible benefit in their clinical course. One was a treatment failure. Of eight patients in whom no change in lymphocyte-mediated cytotoxicity was noted, four evidenced stability or possible benefit while four failed treatment. In one patient, a decrease in cytotoxicity was noted and this patient was a treatment failure. Table 8 presents a correlation between changes in lymphocyte-mediated cytotoxic responses, assessed *in vitro,* and clinical response. There does appear to be a possible correlation between increases in lymphocyte-mediated cytotoxicity, assessed *in vitro*, and clinical response.

Table 8. *Correlation Between Changes in Lymphocyte-mediated Cytotoxicity* in vitro *and Clinical Response*

Cytotoxicity	Stability or possible benefit	Failure	Total
Increase	4	1	5
No change	4	4	8
Decrease	0	1	1

The results of experiments performed in three of these patients is presented in detail in Figs. 6–9. In Fig. 6, the results of testing the cytotoxicity of lymphocytes from gastric carcinoma patient KI on RI-H gastric carcinoma

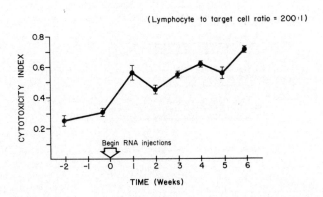

Fig. 6. Cytotoxicity for RI-H gastric carcinoma target cells of lymphocytes from gastric carcinoma patient KI prior to and following the initiation of treatment with "Immune" RNA extracted from the lymphoid organs of a sheep immunized with KI's own tumor tissue.

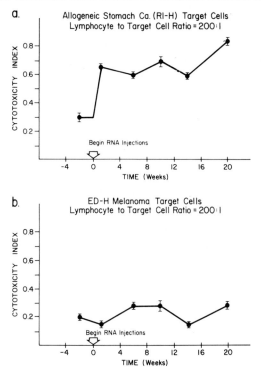

Fig. 7. Cytotoxicity for RI-H gastric carcinoma target cells (Fig. 7a) and for ED-H melanoma cells (Fig. 7b) of lymphocytes from gastric carcinoma patient KI prior to and following the initiation of treatment with xenogeneic "Immune" RNA extracted from the lymphoid organs of a sheep immunized with KI's own tissue.

target cells is presented, while Fig. 7 depicts the results of testing aliquots of the same lymphocyte samples on RI-H gastric carcinoma cells and on ED-H melanoma target cells. It is evident that, while the cytotoxicity of KI's lymphocytes for RI-H cells increased substantially following the initiation of therapy with "Immune" RNA, no significant cytotoxic activity was evidenced against ED-H melanoma target cells. Figures 8 and 9 illustrate the results of testing lymphocytes from two different melanoma patients for cytotoxic activity on ED-H melanoma target cells. Again, significant increases in cytotoxicity were observed following the initiation of "Immune" RNA therapy.

These data suggest that treatment with "Immune" RNA *does* effect at least certain immunologic parameters. This implies that these RNA preparations *are*, at least to some extent, immunologically active in man when administered in the dose and manner described above. These data also provide some evidence to suggest that the immune responses effected by "Immune" RNA may, at least in part, be specific for the particular tumor type used to immunize the sheep from whose lymphoid tissues the RNA was extracted.

The results of the *in vitro* microcytotoxicity tests performed in the lymphocytes of our patients do appear encouraging. When pretreatment lymphocytes were incubated with "Immune" RNA, cytotoxicity responses were significantly increased. Moreover, in most of the patients tested, the cytotoxicity of peripheral blood lymphocytes for tumor cells increased substantially following "Immune" RNA therapy and we have some evidence

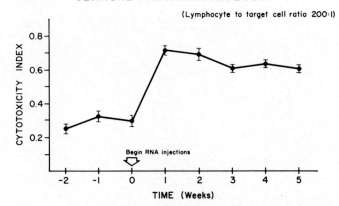

Fig. 8. Cytotoxicity for ED-H melanoma cells of lymphocytes from melanoma patient SM prior to and following initiation of therapy with "Immune" RNA extracted from the lymphoid organs of a sheep immunized with melanoma cells.

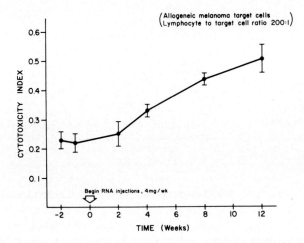

Fig. 9. Cytotoxicity for ED-H melanoma cells of lymphocytes from melanoma patient VE prior to and following initiation of therapy with "Immune" RNA extracted from the lymphoid organs of a sheep immunized with melanoma cells.

that this increase is specific for the particular type of tumor used to immunize the RNA donor sheep. It therefore appears that "Immune" RNA treatment *does* effect host immune responses. We do not know if the nature or magnitude of this effect is relevant to the clinical course of human cancer or if it can result in therapeutic benefit. However, we have some evidence that these cytotoxic responses, assessed *in vitro*, may correlate with clinical responses to therapy.

Finally, it is clear that sheep "Immune" RNA, when prepared as described above and administered intradermally in the doses and schedules described, is completely free of significant local and systemic toxicity and is very well tolerated. "Immune" RNA offers several practical and theoretical advantages as a new modality for the immuno-therapy of cancer. Much further study will be required to determine its potential immunotherapeutic efficacy.

REFERENCES

1. M. Fishman, Antibody formation *in vitro*. *J. Exp. Med.* **114**, 837 (1961).
2. F.L. Adler and M. Fishman, Antibody formation initiated *in vitro*: II. Antibody synthesis in X-irradiated recipients of diffusion chambers containing nucleic acid derived from macrophages incubated with antigen. *J. Exp. Med.* **117**, 595 (1963).
3. J.A. Mannick and R.H. Egdahl, Transformation of nonimmune lymph node cells to state of transplantation immunity by RNA. A preliminary report. *Ann. Surg.* **156**, 356 (1962).
4. J.A. Mannick and R.H. Egdahl, Transfer of heightened immunity to skin homografts by lymphoid RNA. *J. Clin. Invest.* **43**, 2166 (1964).
5. J.A. Mannick, In: *Nucleic Acids in Immunology*, edited by O.J. Plescia and W. Braun, p. 547. Springer-Verlag, New York, 1968.
6. H. Bondevik and J.A. Mannick, RNA-mediated transfer of lymphocyte vs. target cell activity. *Proc. Soc. Exp. Biol.* **129**, 264 (1968).
7. D.B. Wilson and E.E. Wecker, Quantitative studies on the behavior of sensitized lymphoid cells *in vitro*. III. Conversion of normal lymphoid cells to an immunologically active status with RNA derived from isologous lymphoid tissues of specifically immunized rats. *J. Immunol.* **97**, 512 (1966).
8. K.P. Ramming and Y.H. Pilch, RNA-mediated immune cytolysis to transplantation antigens, *in vitro*. *Surg. Forum* **21**, 267 (1970).
9. K.P. Ramming and Y.H. Pilch, Transfer of transplantation immunity by ribonucleic acid. *Transplantation* **7**, 296 (1969).
10. E. Sabbadini and A.H. Sehon, Acceleration of allograft rejection induced by RNA from sensitized donors. *Int. Arch. Allerg. Appl. Immunol.* **32**, 55 (1967).
11. E. Sabbadini and A.H. Sehon, In: *Advance in Transplantation*, edited by J. Dausset, J. Hamburger and G. Mathé, p. 55. Williams & Wilkins, Baltimore, 1968.
12. E. Sabbadini and A.H. Sehon, In: *Nucleic Acids in Immunology*, edited by O.J. Plescia and W. Braun, p. 560. Springer-Verlag, New York, 1968.
13. P. Alexander, E.J. Delorme, L.D. Hamilton and J.G. Hall, Effect of nucleic acids from immune lymphocytes on rat sarcomata. *Nature*, **213**, 569 (1967).
14. P. Alexander, E.J. Delorme, L.D. Hamilton and J.G. Hall, Stimulation of anti-tumor activity on the host with RNA from immune lymphocytes. In: *Nucleic Acids in Immunology*, edited by O.J. Plescia and W. Braun, p. 527. Springer-Verlag, New York, 1968.
15. P. Alexander and J.G. Hall, The role of immunoblasts in host resistance and immunotherapy of primary sarcomata. *Adv. Cancer Res.* **12**, 1 (1970).
16. Y.H. Pilch and K.P. Ramming, Transfer of tumor immunity with ribonucleic acid. *Cancer*, **26**, 630 (1970).
17. K.P. Ramming and Y.H. Pilch, Mediation of immunity to tumor isografts in mice by heterologous ribonucleic acid. *Science*, **168**, 492 (1970).
18. K.P. Ramming and Y.H. Pilch, Transfer of tumor-specific immunity with RNA: Inhibition of growth of immune tumor isografts. *J. Nat. Cancer Inst.* **46**, 735 (1971).
19. K.P. Ramming and Y.H. Pilch, Transfer of tumor specific immunity with RNA: Demonstration by immune cytolysis of tumor cells *in vitro*. *J. Nat. Cancer Inst.* **45**, 543 (1970b).
20. D.H. Kern, C.R. Drogemuller and Y.H. Pilch, Immune cytolysis of rat tumor cells mediated by syngeneic "Immune" RNA. *J. Nat. Cancer Inst.* **52**, 299 (1974).
21. D.H. Kern and Y.H. Pilch, Immune cytolysis of murine tumor cells mediated by xenogeneic "Immune" RNA. *Int. J. Cancer*, **13**, 679 (1974).
22. R.E. Paque and S. Dray, Monkey to human transfer of delayed hypersensitivity *in vitro* with RNA extracts. *Cell. Immunol.* **5**, 30 (1972).
23. A.M. Cohen, J.R. Burdick and A.S. Ketcham, Cell mediated cytotoxicity: an assay using ^{125}I-Iododeoxyuridine labeled target cells. *J. Immunol.* **107**, 895 (1971).
24. A. Boyum, Separation of leukocytes from blood and bone marrow. *Scand. J. Clin. Lab. Invest. (Suppl.)* **21**, 97 (1968).
25. L.L. Veltman, D.H. Kern and Y.H. Pilch, Immune cytolysis of human tumor cells mediated by xenogeneic "Immune" RNA. *Cell. Immunol.* **13**, 367 (1974).
26. Y.H. Pilch, L.L. Veltman and D.H. Kern, Immune cytolysis of human tumor cells mediated by xenogeneic "Immune" RNA. *Arch. Surg.* **109**, 30 (1974).
27. Y.H. Pilch, L.L. Veltman and D.H. Kern, Immune cytolysis of human tumor cells mediated by xenogeneic "Immune" RNA: implications for immunotherapy. *Surgery*, **76**, 23 (1974).
28. S.R. Waldman, J.A. Roth, D.H. Kern and Y.H. Pilch, Effects on cancer patients of leukapheresis using the continuous flow blood cell separator. II. Immunologic parameters, *in vitro*. *J. Lab. Clin. Med.* (in press).

29. S.R. Waldman, J.A. Roth, L.L. Veltman, M.J. Silverstein and Y.H. Pilch, Effects on cancer patients of leukapheresis using the continuous flow blood cell separator. I. Hematologic and immunologic parameters, *in vivo. J. Lab. Clin. Med.* (in press).
30. Y.H. Pilch, J.B. deKernion, D.G. Skinner, K.P. Ramming, P.M. Schick, D. Fritze, P. Brower and D.H. Kern, Immunotherapy of cancer with "Immune" RNA: preliminary report. *Cancer* (in press).
31. D.G. Skinner, J.B. deKernion and Y.H. Pilch, Advanced renal cell carcinoma: treatment with xenogeneic immune ribonucleic acid (RNA) and appropriate surgery. *J. Urol.* (in press).

TRANSFER FACTOR: THE CURRENT PICTURE, WITH SPECIAL REFERENCE TO HUMAN CANCER*

H. HUGH FUDENBERG

*Department of Basic and Clinical Immunology and Microbiology,
Medical University of South Carolina, Charleston, South Carolina 29401, U.S.A.*

INTRODUCTION

Several young students here have asked me "Why is it taking so long for cancer immunology to provide the answers to human disease?" An intelligent answer requires that facts be put in perspective: cancer immunology can move only as rapidly as data are provided by basic immunology laboratories. For those students and for those who may be unfamiliar with the story, a few words of historical background seem warranted.

Although back as early as 1911 certain Italian surgeons noted that patients with tumors that had many lymphocytes in them lived much longer than those whose tumors lacked such cells [reviewed in ref. 1], immunology as such in terms of a modern discipline, particularly cancer immunology, really was in a sad state until very recently. In his classic textbook on the lymphatic system, published in 1941, Professor Yoffey [2] of Bristol asked three questions about lymphocytes: (a) Where do they come from? (b) Where do they go? and (c) What do they do? And as late as 15 years ago, 1960, the lymphocyte was considered a small, nondividing, end-stage cell with no function.

Figure 1, revised from a 1970 paper of the World Health Organization Expert Committee on Immunology [3], shows how little we knew in 1970 and how much we have learned since then, along with how much we still do not know. In 1970, cells important in immune response were divided by the WHO Committee into T- and B-cells. As you know, B-cells become sensitized by antigens, and after further antigenic stimulation they differentiate into plasma cells, which synthesize and secrete the antibodies that protect us from pneumococcal, streptococcal and meningococcal infections. The other cell type listed as important, the T-cell, protects us against atypical bacteria, parasites, fungi and viruses (including presumably oncogenic viruses); these functions, which collectively are termed "cell-mediated immunity", also include rejection of foreign tissue (e.g. kidney transplants) and prevention of growth of mutant cells.

* This is publication no. 22 from the Department of Basic and Clinical Immunology and Microbiology, Medical University of South Carolina. Research supported by grants from the U.S. Public Health Service (HD-05894) and (AI-09145).

B-cell products are easily measurable in serum, for example by hemagglutination, complement fixation, etc.; but T-cell products are very difficult to measure—at present they are detectable only with the aid of complicated *in vitro* assays. When there is a marked aberration in T-cells, the response in terms of blast transformation by the non-specific plant extract phytohemagglutinin is decreased, but a significant aberration is required and small decreases in function are not detected by the assay. A whole host of "soluble lymphocyte factors", produced by sensitized T-cells after exposure to antigen in a test tube under standard conditions, have been described [4]; about two dozen, none yet purified, have been identified, some of which may be identical to each other, while others may represent several active substances.

The 1970 WHO Committee report stated that, for some B-cells, T-cell cooperation is necessary for maximal antibody synthesis. However, our laboratory had evidence at that time that "suppressor T-cells" also existed [5, 6] and that probably a deficiency thereof was important in autoimmune diseases. The Committee preferred to reject this concept and did not bother to list the macrophage—which I think is the most important immune cell—as immunologically important. Nor, among other sins of omission, did they list the lymphopoietic stem cell, which gives rise to the stem cells of both B and T pre-cursors. Further, the Committee statement implied that only one kind of T-lymphocyte existed, although our laboratory had evidence at that time that different cells were responsible for different phenomena, and we felt that many of these were separable [7]. Nonetheless, 5 years ago the Committee felt that there was only one T-cell population. In fact, 5 years ago we could not even measure the number of T- or B-cells in peripheral blood.

What have we learned since then? In the last 5 years we have learned a lot about soluble lymphocyte factors. We have learned how to quantitate T- and B-cells [8]:

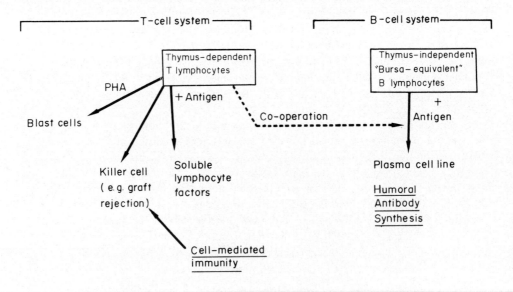

Fig. 1. Cellular basis of the immune response as outlined by the WHO Committee in 1970. (Adapted from ref. 4 by permission of Academic Press.)

Dr. Wybran spoke at some length about the nonspecific binding of sheep red blood cells to T-cells, which is the basis for the T-cell assay that was developed in 1972. B-cells, which do not bind sheep erythrocytes, are now usually identified by the presence of surface immunoglobulins [8].

Table 1. *Mediators of Cellular Immunity Elaborated by Sensitized Lymphocytes after Addition of Antigen* *

1. Skin permeability factor
2. Chemotactic factors for macrophages
3. Macrophage migration inhibitory factor (MIF)
4. Macrophage activating factor (same as MIF?)
5. Chemotactic factors for other leukocytes (neutrophils, eosinophils, basophils, lymphocytes)
6. Granulocytic migration inhibitory factor (LIF)
7. Growth inhibitory factors (clonal inhibitory factor, proliferation inhibitory factor)
8. Lymphocytotoxin (toxic for all cells other than lymphocytes)
9. Osteoclast activating factor
10. Collagen synthesizing factor
11. Interferon
12. Mitogenic factor(s) for lymphocytes

* Two to three dozen mediators have been tentatively identified in studies of lymphocytes in cell culture. It appears that many of these substances might be isolated and, perhaps, used for therapy of a number of different diseases. However, further basic research will be required.

A heuristic explanation for the roles of some of the factors listed is as follows: (1) skin permeability factor dilates the capillaries in the skin, making it easier for cells involved in the immune response to reach foreign substances (antigens) that have entered the body tissues; (2) chemotactic factors attract macrophages (which engulf and destroy foreign cells or parasites, or break them into pieces small enough for the immune system to handle); (3, 4) MIF prevents the macrophages from migrating away from the foreign cells while they are being engulfed; (5) chemotactic factors attract other blood cells which break down and release enzymes that attack viruses, proteins, etc.; (6) LIF prevents those cells from moving away; (7) growth inhibitory factors prevent "transformed" (cancer) cells or foreign organisms from dividing and thus increasing in mass; (8) lymphocytotoxin kills "transformed cells" and foreign organisms; (11) interferon inhibits, at least in animals, the growth of viruses, both those that cause cancer and those that do not; (12) mitogenic factors cause lymphocytes to divide and thus start the process over again—i.e. this is an amplification mechanism.

Adapted from ref. 4.

Table 1 shows what we think we know about soluble lymphocyte factors, which I mention only because they apparently are mediators of cellular immunity, and thus provide one means of measuring the effects of boosting cellular immunity. These presumably act in sequence, but none has been purified, and nobody knows their *in vivo* actions or sequence of action. One of these is the macrophage migration inhibitory factor (MIF). A test has been developed for determining whether cells from a given subject, either normal or abnormal, produce MIF. For this test, either monocytes from human peripheral blood or peritoneal macrophages from guinea pigs are placed in a capillary tube. Then the subject's lymphocytes, which have been presensitized to an antigen (e.g. PPD), are cultured, and the antigen is added to the cell culture. After a standard time under standard conditions of incubation, the supernatant when added to the monocytes or macrophages will inhibit their migration if the subject has cellular immunity to the antigen. If instead one uses a different antigen (e.g. coccidiomycosis), to which the subject has not been presensitized and thus has no cellular immunity, migration will not be inhibited. MIF is a much more sensitive indicator of cellular immunity than skin tests, but is less sensitive than the leukocyte migration inhibition factor (LIF), at least in our hands [9].

By definition, these mediators of cellular immunity are detectable (at least by current methods) only in supernatants after incubation of sensitized cells with antigen, and not in the cells themselves. There are two other factors, which I call "intracellular" mediators of cellular immunity. One is the "killing factor" that Cerottini and Brunner have shown to be present directly within the cell [10]. The other is transfer factor [11].

THE QUESTION OF TRANSFER FACTOR

The past 5 years have also seen a resurgence of interest in transfer factor. When we talk about transfer factor six questions usually occur to the audience: (a) Does it exist? (b) If it exists, does it have any immunologic effect? (c) If it has an immunologic effect, does it have any clinical effect? (d) If it has either of these effects, what is the mechanism of action? (e) Are the effects specific or nonspecific? and (f) What is it? I shall present some data to you to try to answer some of these questions and let you draw your own conclusions as to the answers.

In 1955, Dr. Sherwood Lawrence of New York University took 10 cm^3 of blood from a tuberculin-positive normal subject, positive by a skin test. He separated the white cells and ground them up, and injected an extract of the lysate into a normal tuberculin-negative recipient. That recipient became tuberculin positive by skin test. After 6 months, the recipient was still tuberculin-positive by skin test. Dr. Lawrence then took 10 cm^3 of blood from the primary recipient, isolated the white cells, lysed them, and injected the lysate into a secondary, tuberculin-negative, normal recipient; this secondary recipient also became tuberculin-positive by skin test. Since the material transferred positive skin tests, Lawrence called the factor present in the lysates "transfer factor" [11]. During the next 15 years, he repeatedly demonstrated transfer from normals to normals. In the meantime he showed that treatment of the leukocyte lysate with DNase did not destroy the activity; furthermore, on passage through a dialysis tubing that retained molecules of molecular weight greater than 20,000, the material coming through the bag (i.e. the dialysate) had all the properties of the parent material, including specificity [12]. (The material retained within the bag had some nonspecific booster effects.) I will direct my remarks to the dialyzable transfer factor (the material that comes out of the bag), designated "TFd".

Between 1955 and 1970, few immunologists paid any attention to Lawrence; for several reasons. First, no one knew what skin tests meant. For example, a person who had never knowingly been exposed to tuberculosis might have a positive skin test. On the other hand, patients who were very sick with tuberculosis most often were positive, but some were negative by skin tests. Thus, there was no clinical correlation. It was also generally felt that a reaction measured by skin tests, a nonquantitative parameter, was not very "scientific". That was something that allergists used, and immunologists and allergists, at least at that particular time in our country, did not get along very well. The last point, and probably the most important, was that TFd could only be shown to work in man and not in any laboratory animals e.g. guinea pig, mouse or rabbit. Thus TFd was largely ignored until 1970.

In 1970 we were trying to demonstrate that different functional subpopulations of T-cells existed. We had shown in guinea pigs, using two different antigens, that the population of cells responsible for DNA synthesis in response to antigen was different from the population responsible for MIF production and conversion of skin tests [6]. At that time we were seeing many cases at our immunodeficiency clinic, including some patients with Wiskott-Aldrich syndrome (WAS). These patients are defective in DNA synthesis in response to PHA or mitogens, they do not make MIF to relevant antigens, and they are negative by skin tests for the standard battery of six antigens we use. WAS presents a classical clinical picture, sex-linked (i.e. it occurs only in males), with a triad of symptoms (recurrent infections, a characteristic eczema, and thrombocytopenia, often with bleeding). Half of the victims also have enlarged spleens and half of them have partial baldness. They all die before puberty, either because of recurrent infections or because of bleeding. Since to make a biological generalization one cannot use data from just one species, we decided to use man, specifically patients with WAS, as another species to test our hypothesis that subpopulations of T-cells exist. We thought we might try to use this population to restore one or two of the three parameters of cellular immunity, thus demonstrating the existence of functionally distinct T-cell subpopulations; but rather than using 0.1 cm^2 of white cells, we used the white cells from 250 cm^3 of blood, since we also wanted to try to help the patients by perhaps restoring some of these functions so that they would not die from recurrent infection.

The first patient we treated was a 9-year-old boy who had had 28 documented episodes of pneumonia and on the average lost 56 days a year from school due to pyroderma, otitis and other infections (Fig. 2). When he was given TFd, his skin tests converted, MIF converted, but lymphocyte stimulation did not change. Eczema disappeared, splenomegaly disappeared, and he did well for 6 months. At the end of 6 months he lost his MIF, he lost his skin test reactivity, and his eczema returned [13]. We began wondering whether it would be safe to give him another dose of TFd. All we knew then

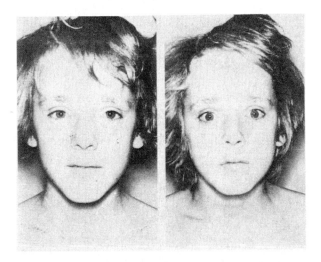

Fig. 2. Nine-year-old WAS patient who was the first to receive TFd therapy. Before treatment (left), he had extensive purpura, which disappeared with treatment. (Taken from ref. 14, by permission from the editors.)

was that its molecular weight was less than 20,000. [Now, in our hands, it has at least 3 separate components: one (MW ≈ 1500) responsible for conversion of skin tests, another (MW ≈ 10,000) responsible for increased DNA synthesis, and a third (intermediate MW) responsible for LIF conversion. Presumably, each acts on a different subpopulation of T-cells.] It seemed that reinjection of TFd would be safe, but we spent the next few months busily injecting rabbits to see whether they formed antibodies, since if they did it was possible that he might. While this was going on, about 2 months after his laboratory signs became bad, he developed within 3 days ear infection, then pneumonia, then meningitis. He was treated by his local pediatrician with appropriate antibodies, and the infections subsided. Then we decided, since the rabbits had not formed antibodies, that it was safer to treat him, even with the remote risk of an adverse immunologic reaction, than to let him risk further severe infections. Again, his splenomegaly went away, his eczema went away, and MIF came back. (Incidentally, the active T-cells, as Dr. Wybran pointed out, for these patients are 3 or 4% instead of 28%; after one "unit" of transfer factor–i.e. TFd from 10^9 leukocytes–active T-cells rise to about 12%, or about half of what is normally present.) This pattern continued for 6 months [14].

The MIF of the donor and recipient in that first trial are shown in Fig. 3 for the six antigens we use (PPD, candida, coccidiomycosis, streptococcal antigen, mumps and trichophyton). The donor was positive by MIF for five of the antigens but not for coccidiomycosis; after he received the TFd injections, the boy's reactivity was converted to match that of the donor. Of the thirty-four WAS patients subsequently treated with TFd, about 60% responded with absence of infection and bleeding for 6 months. Those who showed a clinical response had an increase in active T-cells, skin test conversion, and induction of MIF production, but lymphocyte stimulation did not change [15]. In those who did not respond clinically, MIF was not induced, the level of active T-cells did not rise, and the skin tests did not change.

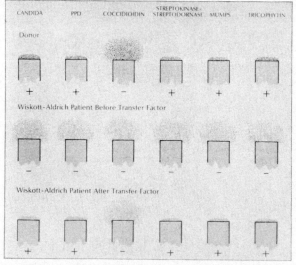

Fig. 3. Conversion of MIF assay after administration of TFd. The donor (top) was positive for five of the six antigens tested. Before receiving transfer factor (middle), the recipient, a WAS patient, was negative for all six antigens. After receiving transfer factor (bottom), the recipient became positive for the five antigens to which the donor was reactive and remained negative for coccidiodin. (Taken from ref. 14, by permission from the editors.)

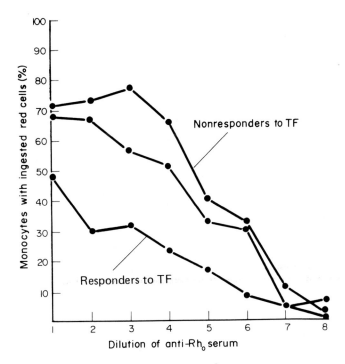

Fig. 4. Differentiation of responders and nonresponders among WAS patients treated with TFd, based on deficiency of monocyte IgC receptors. The center line shows the curve for control subjects. (Taken from ref. 14, by permission from the editors.)

Why do only about 60% of these patients respond? We believe that there are two types of WAS [14, 16]. I stated earlier that the macrophage is probably the most important cell immunologically. Several years ago Hans Huber, now at Innsbruck, was working in our laboratory, trying to find biologic parameters for identifying macrophages. He showed that macrophages and monocytes have receptors for IgC [17]. Now, when we examine WAS patients who do and do not respond to TFd, the latter (nonresponders) show a paucity of normal monocytes (Fig. 4) [14, 15]. Their mothers have intermediate numbers of monocytes (this is an X-linked disease); thus, this parameter appears to be genetically controlled. This is similar to the two kinds of hemophilia: both are X-linked, and both have the same clinical manifestations and severity, but we know they are two different conditions. We think that perhaps one kind of WAS is due to a macrophage—monocyte defect and the other kind is not.

What about selective defects? The first one we looked at was chronic mucocutaneous candidiasis, a disease that causes terrible lesions of the hands, feet, and mouth. We began by treating a patient who was resistant to amphotericin, the antifungal drug, which had been given until he had developed renal toxicity. We used TFd from individuals who had high cellular immunity to candida, but still it took *many* injections of TFd to bring about an improvement, since the patient had a huge amount of antigen on board. We gave him about eight injections in the first 2 months; after that the lesions cleared up, and he needed injections about every 6 months thereafter [18]. (It seems that the effect of TFd, if there is no antigen on board, lasts about 6 months. This is one of the things that makes it so interesting to molecular biologists; i.e. how does such a small molecule exert its effect for 6 months?) When we first used TFd, I also suggested that it would be useful in many disorders of cellular immunity, provided thymus function was present. Severe dual immunodeficiency is really several different diseases. TFd has been effective clinically in three out of eight patients whom we have treated in collaboration with several groups [18, 19]. Since these patients are lymphopenic, this too may indicate that TFd works through the monocyte–macrophage series rather than directly on T-cells. [It does act on T-cells; it appears to act indirectly via adherent cells (e.g. monocytes) (H.H. Fudenberg, J.M. Goust, M.P. Arala-Chaves, and G.B. Wilson, *Folia Allerg. Clin. Immunol.*, to be published, 1976).] TFd should also work for disseminated fungal infections, which are handled by T-cells, and in massive doses it should work on leprosy. It should also work in autoimmune disease if one accepts my hypothesis, first presented in 1967 [5], that in autoimmune diseases the primary defect is a deficiency in suppressor T-cells: that is, we all make autoantibodies all the time to remove aged and damaged tissues (this is in contrast to Burnet's clonal selection hypothesis), and the auto-antibody-producing cells are monitored by suppressor T-cells; if suppressor T-cells become deficient in number or function, the level of autoantibodies rises and disease results.

We have now treated about 150 patients with a variety of conditions [14, 20]. When these data were first presented, a good friend of mine opened the discussion with the question, "Where did you ever get the courage to do this imaginative quackery?" I think it is very fortunate that he made that remark, because it was soon carried by word of mouth around the entire immunologic world, and it got many people interested in transfer factor who otherwise would not have been. At my last count, there were 400 laboratories working with one or another aspect of transfer factor. (My own answer to his remark was, "Think of all the beautiful princesses who will never be able to marry a handsome prince simply because they lack the courage to kiss a frog.")

TRANSFER FACTOR AND HUMAN CANCER

In 1971 we began our first trial of "tumor-specific transfer factor" (TS-TFd) in a cancer patient [21]. (TS-TFd may be better defined as TFd from donors with high T-cell-mediated cytotoxicity to a given tumor cell line, e.g. osteosarcoma.) We started with osteosarcoma, for several reasons, the most important being that osteosarcoma is the human tumor for which the best evidence has been found of viral etiology, and transfer factor apparently works on T-cells, which monitor virus infections. Furthermore, at the time we started these trials there was no effective therapy after surgery; i.e. radiation therapy, chemotherapy, and endocrine therapy, singly or in combination, were ineffective. So the surgeons let us treat these patients.

We found that the most important principle was to select the right donor for TS-TFd. We do this by a chromium-51 release assay for cytotoxicity [22]. Several long-term cultured osteosarcoma cell lines are used, and each has a companion skin fibroblast culture, so that when high cytotoxicity is found—indicating cell-mediated immunity—we can determine whether it is tumor specific or due to a histocompatibility difference. Labeled chromate is incorporated into the tumor cells, and then they are incubated with the donor's lymphocytes. Cell killing is determined from the release of radioactivity into the medium. We have found that lymphocytes from people without tumor-specific immunity (i.e. lymphocytes with low T-cell-mediated cytotoxicity) usually cause the release of 6 to 7% of the total bound chromium (never more than 20%), whereas those from "immune" donors cause more than 35% (up to 95%) of the label to enter the medium. To confirm tumor specificity, the cytotoxic lymphocytes are simultaneously tested against skin fibroblasts and against fibrosarcoma tumor cells (a closely related tumor cell line). Donor selection is based on the demonstration that the lymphocytes are cytotoxic against the several osteosarcoma tumor lines but not against fibroblasts or fibrosarcoma cells; and to assure maximum anti-tumor activity, only those donors are selected whose lymphocytes cause 50% or higher cell killing [14, 23].

Osteogenic sarcoma has a characteristic clinical course, which we hoped to modify with TFd therapy. After amputation of the primary tumor, sometimes there are already metastases clinically evident but usually not. Within 2 months, the cytotoxicity index (usually about 40 or 50) drops below 20. By approximately another 17 months, the active T-cells drop. Within about 6 weeks thereafter (6 weeks to 3 months), metastases appear, and 90% of the patients die within 6 weeks to 6 months after metastasis [24]. We thought we could interrupt this course by administering TS-TFd at the point where active T-cells drop, i.e. 6 weeks or more before the appearance of overt metastases. We also individualize the therapy, and we monitor patients every 2 weeks by tests for active T-cells, active rosette-forming cells, and lymphocyte cytotoxicity.

Clinically, we divide these patients into four stages (Fig. 5). The first is when the primary tumor has been removed and there is no tumor on board. In the second stage there is only a single small metastasis, or maybe several. The third is when there is a large tumor still on board, and the fourth is when there is a large tumor with multiple metastases. Our goal in stage 1 is to prevent metastases; in stage 2 it is to destroy the existing metastases (we have been able to do this in one case with a very small metastasis) and to prevent new metastases; in stage 3, where the patient has refused operation or where the surgeon has decided because he cannot take the whole tumor out not to take out any of it, we try to prevent metastases; and in the fourth stage, there is essentially no point in attempting therapy. To do optimal work in this area requires intelligent, cooperative, informed surgeons.

In our test system we found that a 3-hr incubation was optimal, with a 40:1 ratio of tumor cells to lymphocytes. Under these conditions, cytotoxicity was below 20% for all the cell lines tested against non-immune lymphocytes. We called donors "immune" if their lymphocytes gave cytotoxicity indices greater than 40, and we preferred donors with values of 50 to 95. In household contacts (parents, siblings, servants, guardians, spouses, etc.) about 25% had very high cytotoxicity indices, whereas in a typical control group a cytotoxicity index above 40 was present in only one of seventy-eight people. I think it is quite clear that the household contacts had significant cytotoxicity by our assay [23, 25].

Interestingly, these results also give some proof for the viral etiology of human osteosarcoma [25]. We believe that there is a genetic predisposition, so that when an individual gets a viral infection that lowers his general cellular immunity, if he is then exposed to the oncogenic virus that causes osteosarcoma at the same time, he is apt to get the disease. In contrast, the household contact who lacks the genetic immune defect has little chance of developing the disease [25]. We have also looked at breast cancer and have found a slightly higher incidence (about 30–40%) of household contacts with tumor-specific immunity; and in husbands it is even higher, almost 45% [23]). It is

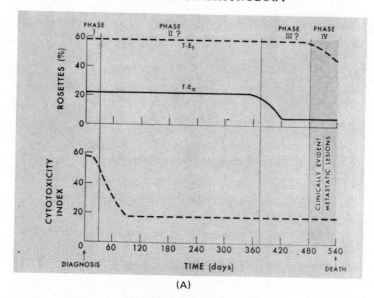

(A)

IMMUNOTHERAPY GOALS

DISEASE STAGE	GOALS
1. Primary surgically removed No demonstrable metastases	Prevent metastases
2. Primary surgically removed Single metastasis	Destroy metastasis (possible if very small?) Prevent new metastases
3. Primary not operable No metastases	Prevent growth of primary Prevent metastases
4. Primary not operable Multiple metastases	Palliation

1.   2.   3.   4.

(B)

Fig. 5. Postulated natural history of osteogenic sarcoma. Although the time varied, the pattern suggested has been observed in all patients referred to our care who had received conventional therapy (amputation, resection, radiation, chemotherapy) and who died with metastatic lesions. Transfer factor appeared to alter the natural course of the disease. (A) Clinical states, in regard to possible benefits of tumor-specific transfer factor. (Taken from H.H. Fudenberg. An admittedly biased view of the role of immunology in human bone cancer. *Front. Radiat. Ther. Oncol.* **10,** in press, by permission from the editors.) (B) Immunologic parameters of the postulated clinical stages. (Taken from ref. 24, by permission from the editors.)

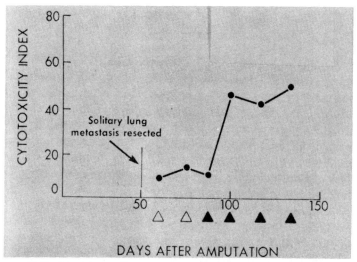

Fig. 6. Tumor-specific cytotoxicity profile for a patient with a primary tumor and a single lung metastasis, before and after administration of transfer factor. Closed triangles show points at which tumor-specific transfer factor was administered; open triangles show administration of nonspecific transfer factor. (Taken from ref. 24, by permission from the editors.)

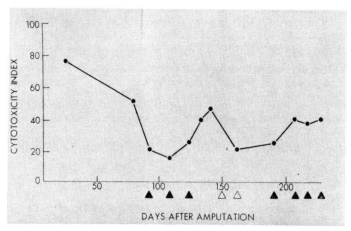

Fig. 7. Tumor-specific cytoxicity profile for a patient with no demonstrable tumor. Closed triangles show administration of tumor-specific transfer factor; open triangles show administration of nonspecific transfer factor. (Taken from ref. 24, by permission from the editors.)

hard for me to imagine that there was a malignant transformation occurring in the male breast, or an asymptomatic transformation, so I think this provides further evidence. We are just beginning trials with breast-tumor-specific transfer factor.

Figures 6 and 7 show a representative sample of osteosarcoma patients [24]. When we first see patients after operation, the cytotoxicity index is usually around 40. The cytotoxicity then usually drops to about 20 between 60 and 90 days after surgery. These people have very poor prognoses. Figure 6 shows the results for a patient who had not only a primary tumor but also a solitary lung metastasis. By 60 days, his cytotoxicity had already dropped below 20. With nonspecific TFd there was no change, but with TS-TFd we were able to boost the level of cell-mediated immunity to the level shown.

Figure 7 shows the data for a patient with no tumor demonstrable by tomogram or by scans of bones and liver. We have six such patients among the eighteen we have treated. Typically, by 20 months approximately 80% of these patients would have pulmonary metastases and would go on to die. Among our six patients, ranging from 10 to 32 months after surgery, no metastases have been detected. Two patients who were maintained on nonspecific TFd followed the typical course of metastasis and death.

Thus, the results of TFd therapy depend on several factors. First, the transfer factor must be tumor specific. Indeed, much of the controversy over transfer factor has arisen because of the failure to select appropriate donors with tumor-specific immunity. Second, the donor must be monitored over the course of therapy. Third, appropriate doses must be given. (We now define "one unit" as the dialysate from 10^9 leukocytes.) Finally, recipients must also be monitored, since individual requirements fluctuate with time. The situation is perhaps analogous to insulin therapy of diabetics. When the treatment was first being tested, all patients were given the same dose. Later it was found that each individual had different requirements, and still later that the requirements of a single patient could vary over the course of time. This explains, I believe, why at present the results of transfer factor therapy are much better in some laboratories for a given type of tumor than in other laboratories where therapy is not individualized—as, for example, in those using "recovered cancer patients" as donors (we find that few such patients have cytotoxicity for more than 3 years after removal of the tumor [26]) or those using TFd preparations that are pooled from randomly chosen normal donors [27] (in our experience, few donors have tumor-specific immunity).

CONCLUSION

One reason for the long delay in finding out how transfer factor works is that human subjects are required for assays. Dr. Welch and Dr. Jean-Michel Goust, who has just joined our laboratory, in double-blind studies have obtained what I believe is convincing evidence that transfer factor does not induce *de novo* specific cellular immunity but greatly amplifies preexisting very low levels thereof [28]. We have partially purified TFd by chromatography on Sephadex G-25, then Sephadex G-10, and then Bio-Gel columns [29, 30], and we plan to further purify this still highly impure preparation for use in further investigations of this possibility. (Results from the purification studies will be reported elsewhere.)

Drs. Ascher and Lawrence have devised an assay in which lymphocytes from individuals who are negative for PPD sensitivity by skin tests are treated with PPD plus TFd, and their DNA synthesis is increased [31]. Interestingly, the individuals whose lymphocytes respond in the assay, even if they are negative by skin tests, do show response to PPD *in vitro*. (In our hands, the magnitude of the rise is proportional to the preexisting immunity as measured by DNA synthesis [32].) Transfer factor will only increase the rise in DNA synthesis. Thus, either Lawrence's hypothesis that TFd is specific is incorrect, or something in the mixture other than TFd is not measured in their assay. My own opinion is that TFd specifically boosts cellular immunity that is present at low levels, not detectable by ordinary means. The one experiment that does suggest *de novo* specificity was performed by the Ohio group, who showed that TFd could transfer immunity to hemocyanin [33]. We were very perturbed by their results and so went to the laboratory to try to find out whether they might have been detecting cross-reacting antigens. We discovered that hemocyanin cross-reacts with penicillin, sheep red blood cells, and a wide range of other antigens [34].

Other investigators have said that TFd is nonspecific because they found that when TFd from donors who were positive by skin tests for PPD and negative for coccidiodin was given to recipients who were negative for both, the recipients became positive for both. However, we often find people who are negative for one or another antigen by skin testing but show a positive response by MIF or LIF assays [35]. Further, all the people who reportedly showed such nonspecific transfer were skin-tested before they received the TFd. Therefore, we went back and did a study to see what happens to cellular immunity as a result of skin testing with first-strength and second-strength antigens. We found that the administration of antigen in small amounts converts about 30% of normals from negative to positive by skin tests and/or *in vitro* tests of cellular immunity [36]. Thus, when appropriate controls are introduced into the experimental design, the argument against specificity is invalidated.

In conclusion, then, I would answer the six questions raised earlier concerning transfer factor as follows: (a) Certainly, as shown by clinical results, it does exist. (b) It does have a definite immunologic effect in humans, boosting cell-mediated immunity, as shown by a rise in the level of active T cells. (c) Its clinical effects have been demonstrated repeatedly, and it should become useful in still other clinical situations as further research provides more effective therapeutic modalities. (d) Its mechanism of action has not been conclusively defined, but I believe that it acts by boosting preexisting low levels of cellular immunity. (e) The best evidence is that the effects are specific. (f) The exact nature of the substance we call "transfer factor" remains to be discovered. In this context it should be mentioned that the crude preparations now being used, which can be separated into at least six fractions, may in fact contain several activities, e.g. one responsible for conversion of skin tests, one that converts MIF activity, etc. Further research should provide more conclusive answers to these questions.

ACKNOWLEDGMENT

Editorial assistance in the preparation of this manuscript was provided by Charles L. Smith.

REFERENCES

1. H.H. Fudenberg, Immune concepts and malignancy. In: *Immunology and Cancer*, edited by R.K. Smiley, p. 2. University of Ottawa Press, Ottawa, 1973.
2. C.K. Drinker and J.M. Yoffey, *Lymphatics, Lymph, and Lymphoid Tissue*, Harvard University Press, Cambridge, Mass., 1941.
3. H.H. Fudenberg, R.A. Good, W.H. Hitzig *et al.,* Primary immune deficiencies: Report of a WHO Committee, *Bull. WHO Comm.* **45,** 125 (1971).
4. H.H. Fudenberg, Are autoimmune diseases and malignancy due to selective T-cell deficiencies? In: *Critical Factors in Cancer Immunology*, edited by J. Schultz and R.C. Leif, Vol. 10, pp. 179–210, Academic Press, New York, 1975.

5. H.H. Fudenberg, Genetically determined abnormalities in antigen–antibody interaction. In: *Proceedings of the Third International Congress on Human Genetics*, edited by J.V. Neel and J.F. Crow, p. 233, Johns Hopkins Press, Baltimore, 1967.

6. H.H. Fudenberg, Genetically determined immune deficiency as the predisposing cause of "autoimmunity" and lymphoid neoplasia. *Amer. J. Med.* **51**, 295 (1971).

7. L.E. Spitler, E. Benjamini, J.D. Young and H.H. Fudenberg, Studies on the immune response to a characterized antigenic determinant of the tobacco mosaic virus protein (TMVP). *J. Exp. Med.* **131**, 133 (1970).

8. F. Aitui, J.-C. Cerottini, R.R.A. Coombs, M. Cooper, H.B. Dickler, S. Froland, H.H. Fudenberg *et al.*, Identification, enumeration, and isolation of B- and T-lymphocytes from human peripheral blood (IUIS Report). *Clin. Immunol. Immunopathol.* **3**, 584 (1975).

9. M. Hsu, T. Welch and H.H. Fudenberg, In preparation.

10. J.-C. Cerottini and K.T. Brunner, Cell-mediated cytotoxicity, allograft rejection, and tumor immunity. *Adv. Immunol.* **18**, 67 (1974).

11. H.S. Lawrence, The transfer in humans of delayed skin sensitivity to streptococcal M. substance and to tuberculin with disrupted leucocytes. *J. Clin. Invest.* **34**, 219 (1955).

12. H.S. Lawrence, Transfer factor and cellular immune deficiency disease. *N. Engl. J. Med.* **283**, 411 (1970).

13. A.S. Levin, L.E. Spitler, D.P. Stites and H.H. Fudenberg, Wiskott-Aldrich syndrome, a genetically determined cellular immunologic deficiency: clinical and laboratory response to therapy with "transfer factor". *Proc. Nat. Acad. Sci. (Wash).* **67**, 821 (1970).

14. H.H. Fudenberg, A.S. Levin, L.E. Spitler, J. Wybran and V. Byers, The therapeutic uses of transfer factor. *Hosp. Pract.* **9**, 95 (1974).

15. L.E. Spitler, A.S. Levin, D.P. Stites, H.H. Fudenberg *et al.*, The Wiskott-Aldrich syndrome. Results of transfer factor therapy. *J. Clin. Invest.* **51**, 3216 (1972).

16. 'L.E. Spitler, A.S. Levin, D.P. Stites, H.H. Fudenberg and H. Huber, The Wiskott-Aldrich syndrome. Immunologic studies in nine patients and selected family numbers. *Cell. Immunol.* (in press).

17. H. Huber and H.H. Fudenberg, Receptor sites of human monocytes for IgC. *Int. Arch. Allerg. Appl. Immunol.* **34**, 19 (1968).

18. H.H. Fudenberg, L.E. Spitler and A.S. Levin, Treatment of immune deficiency disorders. *Amer. J. Pathol.* **69**, 529 (1972).

19. A.S. Levin, L.E. Spitler and H.H. Fudenberg, Transfer factor. I. Results of therapy. In: *Birth Defects–Original Article Series. Primary Immunodeficiency Diseases in Man*, edited by D. Bergsma and R.A. Good, Vol. 11, p. 489, National Foundation, New York, 1975.

20. H.H. Fudenberg, Transfer factor in immunodeficiencies: One man's one-eyed perspective. In *Progress in Immunology II*, edited by L. Brent and J. Holborow, Vol. 5, p. 215, North-Holland Publ. Co., Amsterdam, 1974.

21. A.S. Levin, L.E. Spitler and H.H. Fudenberg, Treatment of osteogenic sarcoma with tumor specific transfer factor. *Clin. Res.* **20**, 568 (1972). (Abstract.)

22. H.H. Fudenberg, V. Byers and A.S. Levin, Immunologic evidence for a viral etiology of certain malignant tumors. In: *Perspectives in Virology*, edited by M. Pollard, Vol. 9, p. 153, Academic Press, New York, 1975.

23. V.S. Byers, A.S. Levin, A.J. Hackett and H.H. Fudenberg, Tumor-specific cell mediated immunity in household contacts of cancer patients. *J. Clin. Invest.* **55**, 500 (1975).

24. A.S. Levin, V.S. Byers, H.H. Fudenberg, J. Wybran, A.J. Hackett and J.O. Johnston, Osteogenic sarcoma: immunologic parameters before and during immunotherapy with tumor-specific transfer factor. *J. Clin. Invest.* **55**, 487 (1975).

25. H.H. Fudenberg, V.S. Byers and A.S. Levin, Viral etiology of human osteosarcoma: evidence based on response to tumor-specific transfer factor and on immuno-epidemiologic studies. In *Fundamental Aspects of Neoplasia*, edited by A.A. Gottlieb, O.J. Plescia, and D.H.L. Bishop, pp. 203–212, Springer-Verlag, New York, 1975.

26. H.H. Fudenberg *et al.*, Unpublished observations.

27. H.F. Oettgen *et al.*, Effects of dialyzable transfer factor in patients with breast cancer. *Proc. Nat. Acad. Sci. (Wash.)* **71**, 2319 (1974).

28. T. Welch, J.M. Goust and H.H. Fudenberg, In preparation.

29. D.R. Webb and H.H. Fudenberg, Unpublished observations (1971).

30. J.M. Goust, E.H. Eylar and H.H. Fudenberg, In preparation.

31. M.S. Ascher, W.J. Schneider, F.T. Valentine and H.S. Lawrence, *In vitro* properties of leukocyte dialysates containing transfer factor. *Proc. Nat. Acad. Sci. (Wash.)* **71**, 1178 (1974).

32. J.M. Goust and H.H. Fudenberg, In preparation.

33. K.S. Zuckerman, J.A. Neidhart, S.P. Balcerzak and A.F. Lobuglio, Immunologic specificity of transfer factor. *J. Clin. Invest.* **54**, 997 (1974).
34. C. Henry and H.H. Fudenberg, Unpublished observations.
35. H.H. Fudenberg and T. Welch, Unpublished observations.
36. H.H. Fudenberg, T. Welch and J.M. Goust, Unpublished observations.

NEW FRONTIERS OF CANCER ACTIVE IMMUNOTHERAPY

G. MATHE

*Institut de Cancérologie et d'Immunogénétique (INSERM),
Hôpital Paul-Brousse* and Service d'Hématologie de l'Institut Gustave-Roussy†*

Active immunotherapy (AI) of cancer is a form of manipulation of the patient's immune machinery composed of T- and B-lymphocytes and of macrophages. It was introduced 11 years ago [1, 2] in an attempt to kill tumor cells left by chemotherapy, which is unable to kill "the last cell" because it obeys first-order kinetics [3–5]. This clinical use of AI for treatment of residual minimal disease still seems to be its most rational indication. This is what my initial experimental studies suggested.

1. EXPERIMENTAL STUDIES

As a matter of fact, my first work on L1210 leukemia treated after the tumor is established, this condition is the definition of active immunotherapy [6, 7], clearly showed that combining irradiated tumor cells and a systemic immunity adjuvant (living, fresh BCG) is able to cure mice, but only if the number of neoplastic cells is equal or inferior to 10^5 (Fig. 1) [1].

The superiority of the combination of the specific stimulus and BCG was confirmed by another experiment in which mice, inoculated with 10^3 living L1210 leukemia cells, were cured only by associated both agents and not by administering one of them alone (Fig. 2). The same is true of immunoprophylaxis of this leukemia, which is the application of immunomanipulation before the tumor is grafted or induced [7]. In this case, however, BCG applied alone is able to prolong survival significantly [8].

These two conclusions were confirmed by Parr in London [9].

The effect of AI can be obtained on mice inoculated with more than 10^5 cells, for example 5×10^6, and treated, 6 days before immunomanipulation, by a dose of 6-mercaptopurine able to reduce this population to 10^5 [6].

Interestingly, when mice are treated by chemotherapy, for example with cyclophosphamide before AI, BCG alone is able to induce cures [10] (Fig. 3).

* 14–16, avenue Paul-Vaillant Couturier, 94800-Villejuif, France.
† 16 bis, avenue Paul-Vaillant Couturier, 94800-Villejuif, France.

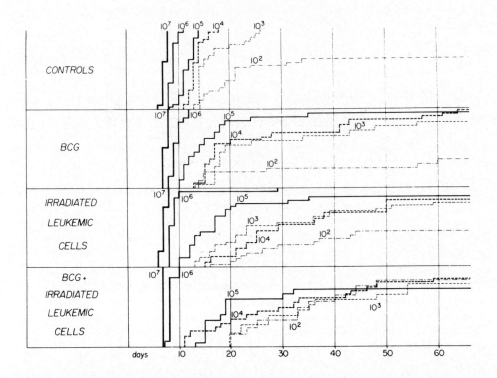

Fig. 1. Cumulative mortality of mice grafted with 10^2 to 10^7 L1210 leukemia cells, untreated or treated in the 24 hr following the graft by BCG (1 mg intravenously) (repeated injections) or irradiated leukemic cells (one injection) or a combination of BCG and leukemic cells.

The above conclusions are valid for other grafted leukemias such as Rauscher grafted leukemia [11], and E♂G2 leukemia [12] and also for spontaneous AkR leukemia treated when mice are 6 months old [13].

They are valid for the use of *Corynebacterium parvum* administered to mice carrying leukemia, which have received cyclophosphamide as cell reduction chemotherapy [14] (Fig. 4).

In all these experiments, the irradiated cells are injected i.d. and BCG i.v. All our experiments on tumors are conducted using a BCG dose of 1 mg i.v., which we showed to be the optimal dose in the hemolytic "plaque-forming" cell test. Increasing the dose eliminates the effect [7]. S. Orbach *et al.* [16], who works in our laboratory, showed that this is due to stimulation of T suppressor-lymphocytes.

BCG is also effective in mice when administered on scarifications, or with a heaf gun [17] (Fig. 5). It is not effective when introduced through a gastric catheter.

Unfortunately, immunoresistance does exist, as shown by an experiment in which BCG was given repeatedly, starting at day +1 after 10^3 L1210 leukemia cells inoculation: in some animals, after the initial increase in tumor volume, the latter decreases until the neoplasia disappears. In others, this volume does not stop increasing, which indicates primary resistance. In others again the curve of this volume, after increasing normally, is broken to form a plateau: the latter can persist for a long time, but finally the curve rises again and the animals die; this fact suggests the appearance of

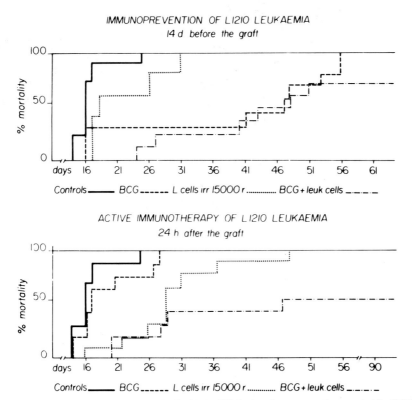

Fig. 2. Cumulative mortality of mice grafted with L1210 leukemia, untreated or treated by BCG (1 mg intravenously) (first injection 14 days before the graft and injections repeated each 4 days) or irradiated leukemic cells (one injection 14 days before the graft) or a combination of both. Cumulative mortality of mice grafted with L1210 leukemia and untreated by BCG (1 mg intravenously) (first injection 24 hr after the graft and injections repeated each 4 days) or irradiated leukemic cells (one injection 24 hr after the graft) or a combination of both.

secondary resistance [8]. We also studied toxicology, starting with mice. Histologically, after administration of 1 mg of BCG, manifestations of septicemia are seen, particularly granulomas and giant cells [19] (Fig. 6). They are more important after i.v. than after s.c. injection.

In monkeys, we observed the same manifestations in an experiment devoted to studying the toxicology of i.v. BCG administration. Five injections of 100 mg were little while one injection of 1 g was not [20].

2. CLINICAL STUDIES

2.1. In 1964 we started applying BCG on scarifications and irradiated allogeneic tumor cells i.d. to *acute lymphoid* leukemia (ALL) patients. This treatment was given after remission induction and complementary cell reduction chemotherapy [2]. The length of remission was compared to randomized controls and not submitted to immunomanipulation. A difference appeared so quickly that we had to stop introducing patients into the trial for obvious ethical reasons. When considering the curve of immunotherapy patients, three segments can be seen: the first characterizes subjects who

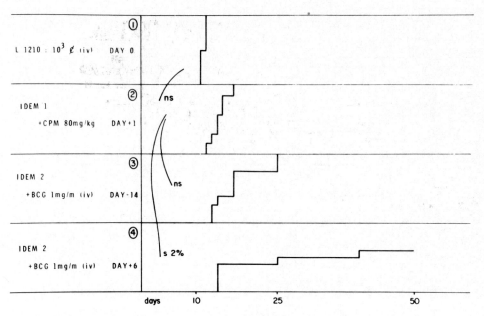

Fig. 3. Immunotherapeutic effect of BCG administered 5 days after injection of 80 mg/kg of cyclophosphamide.

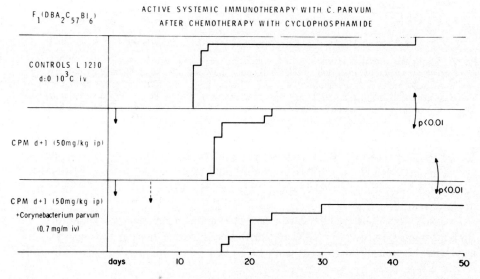

Fig. 4. Treatment of Lewis tumor by radiotherapy followed by active systemic immunotherapy with BCG.

relapsed like the controls, which suggests that more cells were left by complementary chemotherapy than AI is able to control. The second concerns patients who relapsed late, suggesting the possibility of immunoresistance which we had observed experimentally [1, 8]. The third, which concerns one-third of the patients, has been a plateau extending from the thousandth day to the tenth year (Fig. 7). This plateau is considered as the expression of cure expectancy in ALL [21].

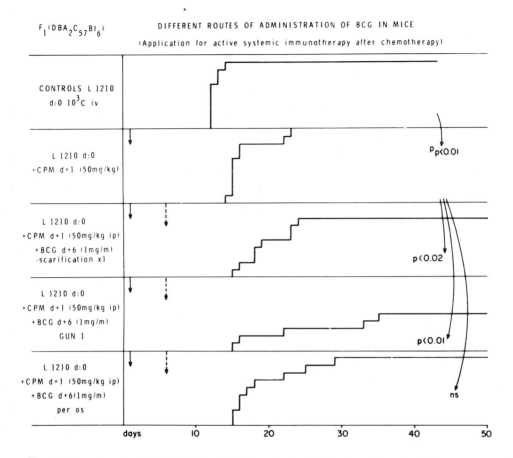

Fig. 5. Different routes of administration of BCG in mice (application for active systemic immunotherapy after chemotherapy).

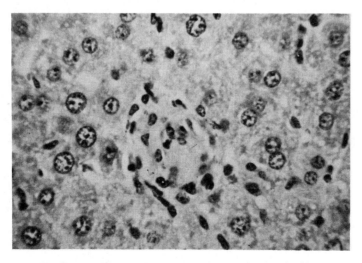

Fig. 6. A specific granuloma in the liver of BCG-treated mice.

Since 1964, we have applied AJ to 200 ALL patients. Such treatment induces BCG bacteriema as indicated by granulomas like the one shown in Fig. 8. However, it induces no major toxicity: no patient dies, which is very different from the results of so-called maintenance chemotherapy during which 10% to 20% [22, 23] or even more die during a complete remission of drug complications; the last publication of the Memphis group [24] mentioned "50% crippling or lethal leucoencephalopathy" in ALL patients in complete remission.

On the basis of the results for the first hundred patients, it may be observed [25] that: (a) the younger the patients, the better the results; (b) the smaller the volume of the leukemic mass, as judged by leukocytosis of spleen volume, the better the results; (c) prognosis differs according to the cytological types we described [26, 27] : some, such as

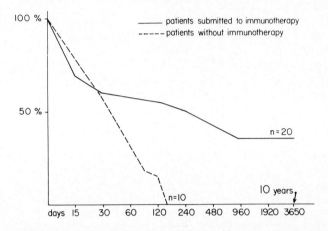

Fig. 7. Actuarial curves of duration of remission of patients treated by active immunotherapy after the end of chemotherapy (protocol 1) (note that time scale is geometrical).

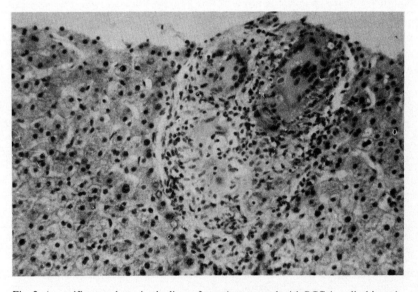

Fig. 8. A specific granuloma in the liver of a patient treated with BCG (needle biopsy).

the prolymphoblastic type, seem insensitive to AI; others, such as the microlymphoblastic type, seem AI sensitive [28]. It is interesting to note that more than 80% of the patients of all ages belonging to this latter type are included in the plateau expressing cure expectancy. It is also interesting to note that a computerized statistical analysis of the correlation between the different prognosis factors showed that they all depend on the cytological type (Figs. 10 and 11).

Immunological investigation was conducted by counting rosette-forming cells, membrane IgC carrying cells and peroxidase positive cells present in the peripheral blood. The results showed a significant increase of so-called "null cells" [29].

2.2. Other tumor cells which seem sensitive to AI are lymphosarcoma cells. *Terminal leukemic lymphosarcoma* patients were treated by chemoradiotherapy according to the above principle and were then submitted to AI using BCG and lymphosarcoma cells (Fig. 12). Figure 13 shows the results of eighteen out of forty patients who entered complete remission: five are in perfect clinical and hematological conditions after 13 to 70 months [30].

These results are significantly better than those of historical controls submitted only to maintenance chemotherapy.

2.3. *Acute myeloid leukemia* (AML) has been shown to be sensitive to AI by Powles *et al.* [31] and by Vogler *et al.* [32]. The latter's curves are very similar in shape to our ALL curves. Gutterman *et al.* [33] also published interesting results for this disease. In a phase II trial, the only ethical type of trial which can be authorized in the light of the preceding results, we submitted eighteen AML patients to AI with BCG and AML irradiated cells. Our remission and survival medians are significantly longer than those of our historical controls submitted to maintenance chemotherapy (Table 1). However we did not obtain a plateau, which suggests that cell reduction by chemotherapy may be insufficient [34].

Table 1

	MEDIANS		
	of first complete remissions (FCR)		of survival after FCR
Maintenance chemotherapy	EORCT first trial	32 weeks	55 weeks
	EORTC second trial	34 weeks	N.D.
	EORTC Villejuif patients in both trials	26 weeks	52 weeks
	Vogler *et al.*	26 weeks	
	Powles *et al.*	26 weeks	46 weeks
	Gutterman	60 weeks	
Chemotherapy interspersed with immunotherapy	Gutterman	72 weeks	77 weeks
	Powles	58 weeks	
Chemotherapy followed by immunotherapy	Powles	48 weeks	83 weeks
	Vogler	39.4 weeks	
	Mathé	60 weeks	104 weeks

N.D. = not determined.

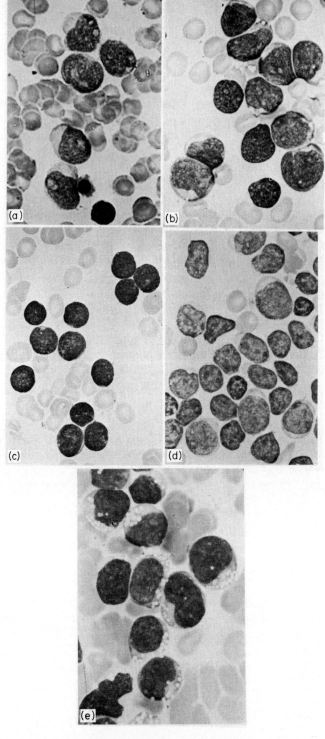

Fig. 9. The different subvarieties of acute lymphoid leukemias: (a) Acute lymphoid leukemia, prolymphoblastic (PLbAL). (b) Acute lymphoid leukemia, macrolymphoblastic (MLbAL). (c) Acute lymphoid leukemia, microlymphoblastic (mLbAL). (d) Acute lymphoid leukemia, prolymphocytic (PLcAL). (e) Acute lymphoid leukemia, immunoblastic.

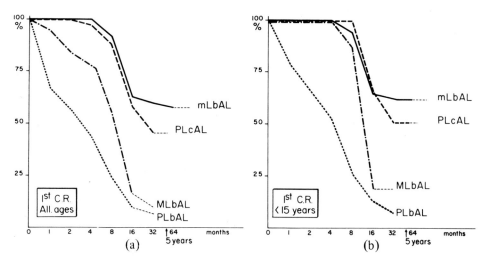

Fig. 10. (a) Comparative cumulative duration of first remission of the different cytological varieties of acute lymphoid leukemia (all ages) (actuarial curves). (b) Comparative cumulative duration of first remission of the different cytological varieties of acute lymphoid leukemia (patients younger than 15 years). (Note that time scales are geometrical.)

2.4. AI is being applied on a few *solid tumors* for residual imperceptible disease after surgery in cases for which prognosis was poor. The most recent results for melanoma patients published by Gutterman *et al.* [35] show that, as in AML patients, this treatment is significantly effective, but only of slight benefit to patients.

These results indicate that, in such disease, greater chemotherapy cell reduction and improved immunotherapy are essential to further detection progress. These are in fact the aims of our present research in the field of AI development.

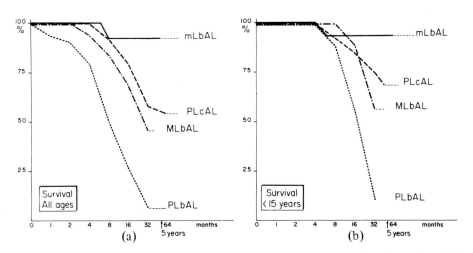

Fig. 11. (a) Comparative cumulative survival of the different cytological varieties of acute lymphoid leukemia (all ages) (actuarial curves). (b) Comparative cumulative survival of the different cytological varieties of acute lymphoid leukemia (patients younger than 15 years) (actuarial curves). (Note that time scales are geometrical.)

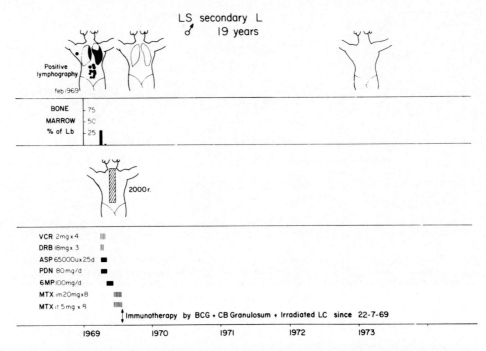

Fig. 12. Treatment with chemo-radiotherapy followed by active immunotherapy of a lymphosarcoma complicated by leukemia. CB = *Corynebacterium*; LC = leukemic cells.

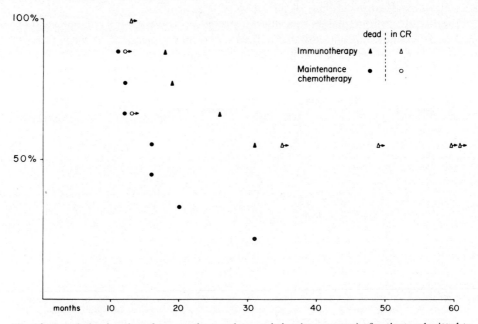

Fig. 13. Cumulative duration of apparently complete remission (upper curve) of patients submitted to active immunotherapy after cell-reduction chemoradiotherapy for terminal lymphosarcoma converted into leukemia. The second curve concerns patients with similar disease treated with maintenance chemoradiotherapy without immunotherapy.

3. DEVELOPMENT

3.1. Chemotherapy and AI interspersion

In view of the hypothesis of insufficient preimmunotherapy-chemotherapy-cell-reduction, and bearing in mind the tumor volume curve, which during AI may be a long plateau until resistances appear and growth resumes [6], one is tempted to intersperse AI with chemotherapy. This is precisely what Powles *et al.* [31] did in their first trial on AML patients in which they observed a difference between AI patients and controls. But the overall results of this trial are not better than those of another study by the same authors in which chemotherapy was completed before AI [36].

Moreover, a recent experiment conducted on L1210 leukemia in which we gave first BCG and then cyclophosphamide (CPM) suggests that chemotherapy and AI interspersion may be contra-indicated. As a matter of fact, BCG given before CPM reduces the effect of the latter [10] (Fig. 14). The mechanism of this deterioration is accounted for in an experiment in which BCG and then CPM were applied to mice carrying allogeneic skin grafts: the result was a considerable prolongation of transplant survival compared to that produced by CPM alone. This suggests that BCG administration before chemotherapy may potentiate the latter's immunosuppressive effect [37] (Fig. 15).

Thus even though there are grounds for interspersion, more research is needed on the kinetics of the reciprocal effects of chemotherapy and immunotherapy.

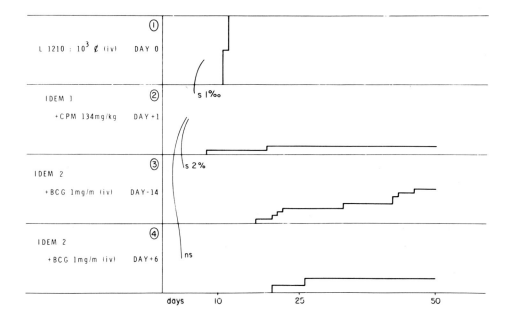

Fig. 14. Deterioration by BCG given before 134 mg/kg of cyclophosphamide on its antileukemic effect.

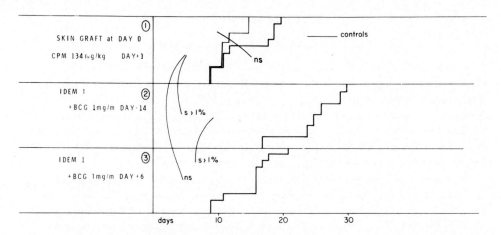

Fig. 15. Cumulative curve of skin-graft rejection: effect of the sequential combination of BCG and cyclophosphamide (134 mg/kg) on the survival of C_3H skin graft on $(DBA/2 \times C_{57}Bl/1)F1$ mice recipients.

3.2. Specific immunomanipulation

I have contrasted the need for combining irradiated tumor cells and BCG in animals not submitted to chemotherapy before AI, with the strong effect of BCG given alone in mice previously submitted to chemotherapy. It is possible that oncostatics cause specific stimulation by killing cells. Irradiated tumor cells are therefore not necessary under all conditions. As to whether an adjuvant is always necessary, the answer is no: in this connection, Bekesi and Holland [38], working on AkR leukemia, and others, especially Simmons *et al.* [39], working on solid tumors, obtained remarkable results with neuraminidase-treated cells as suggested by Currie and Bagshawe [40]. Submitting spontaneous leukemia AkR mice to BCG and cells treated or not treated with neuraminidase, we did not obtain any difference as a result of this cell manipulation [13].

An attempt by Doré *et al.* [41] at grafted leukemia prophylaxis, using cells treated with neuraminidase or papain enhanced tumor growth compared to the controls, whereas the use of non-manipulated irradiated cells produced a beneficial effect.

By preparing soluble tumor-associated-antigen (TAA) from Rauscher grafted leukemia, Martyre *et al.* [42], working in our laboratory, were able to cure animals in an immunotherapy experiment when the extract was injected sufficiently early. In an immunoprophylaxis experiment, the same preparation for which the cells were destroyed by a hypertonic 3M KCl solution produced a significant effect. When the cells were lysed by a hypotonic sodium chloride solution, tumor growth was enhanced [43] (Fig. 16).

Much work therefore remains to be done on TAA, more especially as it is suspected of being under certain conditions a circulatory blocking factor, as shown, among others, by Baldwin *et al.* [44].

3.3. Non-specific immunomanipulation

Although BCG was effective either when applied on scarifications [2] or with a heaf gun [31], it was considered as medieval by modern researchers and harsh by sensitive

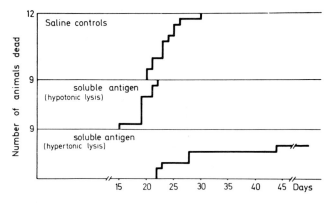

Fig. 16. Influence of soluble antigen on mortality prophylaxis from RC19 leukemia.

physicians. Thus we set up a battery of tests to detect adjuvant(s) which might be administered in a satisfactory quantitative manner. The tests included in this screening battery [45, 46] are listed in Table 2. They are: (a) a non-specific macrophage activation test [47]; (b) the hemolytic plaque-forming cell (HPFC) test; (c) prophylaxis of L1210 leukemia; and (d) prophylaxis of solid Lewis tumor.

Table 2. *Tests and Methods Used for the Screening of Immunity Systemic Adjuvants*

Technique	Day 0	Injection of the adjuvant Before [a]	Results
1 Macrophage activation	Sample taken of peritoneal macrophages	Days +3, +7 or +14	Tumor cell non-specific lysis (^{51}Cr release) [48]
2 HPFCT (Jerne)	10^9	Day +14 (BCG) Day +2.5 (others)	PFC at day +4
3 L1210	10^3 leukemic cells i.v.	Day +14 (BCG) Day +2.5 (others)	Mortality
4 Lewis tumor	2×10^6 tumor cells s.c.	Day +14 (BCG) Day +2.5 (others)	Mortality

[a] The administration of the antigen (Jerne test) [2]; or the inoculation of the tumors [3, 4].

Table 3. *Fresh Pasteur Institute BCG* in the Immunoprophylaxis of L1210 Leukemia and Lewis Tumor*

Leuk.	I[†]	Administration routes						
		i.v.		i.p.		i.d.		s.c.
		Significance	I	Significance	I	Significance	I	Significance
L1210 leukemia	1.6	S‡ at 5%	1	NS	1	NS	1	NS
Lewis tumor	2.6	S‡ at 1%	1	NS	1	NS	0.8	S at 2%

* BCG is injected at day −14.
† I − Median of survival of experimental animals/median of the controls.
‡ Statistics: non-parametric test of Wilcoxon. S, significant. NS, not significant.

First we compared several BCG preparations and observed that only the fresh living Pasteur Institute preparation is constantly active in all the tests [48].

We then screened several extracts of mycobacteria. Only MER is effective in all the tests, whereas the hydrosoluble extracts (Hui II and WSA) [49, 50] are only effective in the HPFC test.

Other agents have also been tested: some, such as *Corynebacteria* and polynucleotides, are active. This screening brings us back to the importance of the administration route. I should like to stress that, although i.v. injected BCG exerts a favorable effect on L1210 leukemia and solid Lewis tumor, the same agent injected s.c. has no effect on the leukemia and enhances Lewis tumor growth (Table 3) [45, 46].

Such enhancement has been seen in man by authors who practice local immunotherapy by intratumoral BCG injection [51–53].

We have also observed some cases of enhancement after i.v. injection of BCG in man (from 1 mg to 1.5 mg), in the course of an immunorestoration trial by different adjuvants in immunodepressed cancer patients [54]. Although BCG applied to one scarified area three times a week is the best means of inducing immunorestoration, this mycobacteria injected i.v. has never produced the same effect.

Hence, conditions of AI may not be identical in man and mice, and we must avoid being exclusive when extrapolating conclusions from experiments on mice to clinical protocols. We must not reject results obtained by Gutterman *et al.* [55] in man not based on experimental data, such as those of chemotherapy and immunotherapy combinations in the case of voluminous tumors. These results are also of interest even if they are due, at least partially, to an effect of BCG on hemopoietic stem cells [56, 57], which allows administration of stronger or more frequent doses of chemotherapy.

REFERENCES

1. G. Mathé, Immunothérapie active de la leucémie L1210 appliquée après la greffe tumorale. *Rev. Fr. Etud. Clin. Biol.* **13**, 881 (1968).
2. G. Mathé, J.L. Amiel, L. Schwarzenberg, M. Schneider, A. Cattan, J.R. Schlumberger, M. Hayat and F. de Vassal, Active immunotherapy for acute lymphoid leukaemia, *Lancet*, **1**, 697 (1967).
3. H.E. Skipper, F.M. Schabel and W.S. Wilcox, Experimental evaluation of potential anticancer agents. XIII. On the criteria and kinetics associated with "curability" of experimental leukemia. *Cancer Chemoth. Rep.* **35**, 1 (1964).
4. H.E. Skipper, F.M. Schabel and W.S. Wilcox, Experimental evaluation of potential anticancer agents. XIV. Further study of certain basic concepts underlying chemotherapy of leukemia. *Cancer Chemoth. Rep.* **45**, 5 (1965).
5. H.E. Skipper, F.M. Schabel and W.S. Wilcox, Experimental evaluation of potential anticancer agents. XXI. Scheduling of arabinosyl cytosine to take advantage of its S-phase specificity against leukemia cells. *Cancer Chemoth. Rep.* **51**, 125 (1967).
6. G. Mathé, Active immunotherapy. *Adv. Cancer Res.* **14**, 1 (1971).
7. G. Mathé, *Introduction to Active Immunotherapy of Cancer: Its Immunoprophylaxis and Immunoprevention.* 1 vol., Heidelberg, New York, Springer-Verlag, 1976 (in press).
8. G. Mathé, P. Pouillart and F. Lapeyraque, Active immunotherapy of L1210 leukaemia applied after the graft of tumor cells. *Br. J. Cancer,* **23**, 814 (1969).
9. I. Parr, Response of syngeneic murine lymphomata to immunotherapy in relation to the antigenicity of the tumour. *Br. J. Cancer,* **26**, 174 (1972).
10. G. Mathé, O. Halle-Pannenko and C. Bourut, Immune manipulation by BCG administered before or after cyclophosphamide for chemoimmunotherapy of L1210 leukemia. *Europ. J. Cancer,* **10**, 661 (1970).
11. G. Mathé, P. Pouillart and F. Lapeyraque, Active immunotherapy of mouse RC19 and E♀K1 leukemia applied after the intravenous transplantation of the tumour cells. *Experientia,* **27**, 446 (1971).
12. J.L. Amiel and M. Berardet, Essai de traitement de la leucémie E♂G2, association chimiothérapie et immunothérapie active non spécifique et spécifique. *Rev. Fr. Etud. Clin. Biol.* **14**, 685 (1969).

13. G. Mathé, O. Halle-Pannenko and C. Bourut, Active immunotherapy of AkR mice spontaneous leukemia. *Exp. Hematol.* **1**, 110 (1973).
14. M. Martin, Treatment of L1210 leukemia by cyclophosphamide followed by *C. parvum. Biomedicine* (in press, 1976).
15. M. Martin, Treatment of Lewis tumor by local therapy followed by BCG administration. *Biomedicine* (in press, 1976).
16. S. Orbach-Arbouys and M. Geffard, Induction of suppressor cells by BCG pretreatment of the donor as a possible way of control of a graft-versus-host reaction. *Exp. Hematol.* (in press, 1976).
17. M. Martin, Comparison of three modalities of administration (on scarification) with a heaf gun or through a gastric catheter to mice for L1210 leukaemia. *Biomedicine* (in preparation, 1976).
18. J. Lheritier. Unpublished data.
19. A Khalil, H. Rappaport, C. Bourut, O. Halle-Pennenko and G. Mathé, Histologic reactions of the thymus, spleen, liver, lymph nodes to i.v. and s.c. BSC injections. *Biomedicine*, **22**, 121 (1975).
20. M. Martin, S. Jurcyzk-Procyk, P. Dubouche, M. Gheorghiu and S. Orbach-Arbouys, Experimental toxicity studies in mice and monkeys of fresh live BCG. 17th Meeting of the European Society for Toxicology, Montpellier, June 1975 (in press).
21. G. Mathé, J.L. Amiel and L. Schwarzenberg, Acute lymphoid leukemias: clinical and cytological features. In: *Acute Childhood Leukemia*, edited by C. Pochedly, vol. 16, p. 1. Modern problems in paediatrics. Basel, Karger, 1975.
22. J.V. Simone, E. Holland and W. Johnson, Fatalities during remissions of childhood leukemia. *Blood* **39**, 759 (1972).
23. J. Bernard, M. Boiron, C. Jacquillat and M. Weil, Recent results in acute leukemias at the Hospital Saint-Louis. In: *Nomenclature, Methodology and Results of Clinical Trials in Acute Leukemias*, edited by G. Mathé, P. Pouillart and L. Schwarzenberg, vol. 43, p. 151. R.R.C.R. Heidelberg, Springer-Verlag, 1973.
24. R. Aur, M. Verzosa, O. Hustu, J. Simone and L. Barker, Leukoencephalopathy (LEP) during initial complete remission (CR) in children with acute lymphocytic leukemia (ALL) receiving methotrexat (MTX). *Proc. Am. Ass. Cancer Res.* **16**, 92 (1975) (abstract 365).
25. G. Mathé, P. Pouillart, L. Schwarzenberg, M. Hayat, F. de Vassal, and M. Lafleur, Prognostic factors in acute leukaemias. In: *Advances in the Biosciences*, p. 145, 1 vol., Oxford, Pergamon Press, 1975.
26. G. Mathé, P. Pouillart, M. Sterescu, J.L. Amiel, L. Schwarzenberg, M. Schneider, M. Hayat, F. de Vassal, C. Jasmin and M. Lafleur, Subdivision of classical varieties of acute leukemia: correlation with prognosis and cure expectancy. *Europ. J. Clin. Biol. Res.* **16**, 554 (1971).
27. G. Mathé, D. Belpomme, D. Dantchev, P. Pouillart, C. Jasmin, J.L. Misset, M. Musset, J.L. Amiel, J.R. Schlumberger, L. Schwarzenberg, M. Hayat, F. de Vassal and M. Lafleur,, Immunoblastic acute lymphoid leukaemia: an indescribed type. *Biomedicine*, **20**, 333 (1974).
28. G. Mathé, P. Pouillart, L. Schwarzenberg, J.L. Amiel, M. Schneider, M. Hayat, F. de Vassal, C. Jasmin, C. Rosenfeld, R. Weiner and H. Rappaport, Attempt at immunotherapy of 100 acute lymphoid leukemia patients. Some factors influencing results. *Nat. Cancer Inst. Monogr.* **35**, 361 (1972).
29. R. Joseph, Lymphocytes and macrophages in cancer patients. In: *BCG in Cancer Patients*, edited by G. Mathé, Heidelberg, Springer-Verlag (in preparation, 1976).
30. G. Mathé, Phase II trial of immunotherapy in leukaemic lymphosarcoma patients. *Biomedicine* (in press, 1976).
31. R. Powles, T.J. McElwain, P. Alexander, D. Crowther, G. Fairley and M. Pike, Immunotherapy of acute myeloblastic leukemia in man. In: *Investigation and Stimulation of Immunity in Cancer Patients,* edited by G. Mathé and R. Weiner, vol. 47, p. 499. R.R.C.R., Heidelberg, Springer-Verlag, 1974.
32. W.R. Vogler and Y.K. Chan, Effect of Bacillus Calmette-Guerin (BCG) in prolongation of remissions in acute myeloblastic leukemia (AML). *Proc. Am. Ass. Cancer Res.* **15**, 164 (1974) (abstract 723).
33. J.U. Gutterman, V. Rodriguez, G. Mavligit, M.A. Burgess, E. Gehan, E.M. Hersh, K.B. McCredie, R. Reed, T. Smith, J.P. Bodey,Jr. and E.J. Freireich, Chemo-immunotherapy of adult acute leukemia prolongation of remission in myeloblastic leukemia with BCG. *Lancet,* **2**, 1405 (1974).
34. G. Mathé, M. Musset, L. Schwarzenberg, M. Hayat, F. de Vassal, J.L. Amiel, P. Pouillart and J.L. Misset, Phase II trial of immunotherapy of acute myeloid leukemia. *Biomedicine*, **23**, 291 (1975).
35. J.U. Gutterman, M. McBride, E.J. Freireich, G. Mavligit, E. Frei III, and E.M. Hersh, Active Immunotherapy with BCG for recurrent malignant melanoma. *Lancet,* **1**, 208 (1973)
36. Powles, R. Immunotherapy for acute myelogenous leukemia using irradiated and unirradiated

cells. *Cancer*, **34**, 1558 (1974).
37. G. Mathé, O. Halle-Pannenko and C. Bourut, Potentiation of a cyclophosphamide-induced immunodepression by the administration of BCG. *Transplant. Proc.* **6**, 431 (1974).
38. J.G. Bekesi and J.F. Holland, Combined chemotherapy and immunotherapy of transplantable and spontaneous murine leukemia in DBA/2 and AkR mice. In: *Investigation and Stimulation of Immunity in Cancer Patients,* edited by G. Mathé and R. Weiner, vol. 47, p. 357. R.R.C.R., Heidelberg, Springer-Verlag, 1974.
39. R.L. Simmons and A. Rios, Immunotherapy of cancer: immunospecificity rejection of tumors in recipients of neuraminidase-treated tumor cells plus BCG. *Science,* **174**, 591 (1971).
40. G.A. Currie and K.D. Bagshawe, Tumour specific immunogenicity of methylcholanthrene-induced sarcoma cells after incubation in neuraminidase. *Br. J. Cancer,* **23**, 141 (1969).
41. J.F. Doré, M.J. Hadjiyannakis, A. Coudert, A. Guibout, L. Marholev and K. Imai, Use of enzyme-treated cells in immunotherapy of leukaemia. In: *Investigation and Stimulation of Immunity in Cancer Patients,* edited by G. Mathé and R. Weiner, vol. 47, p. 387. R.R.C.R., Heidelberg, Springer-Verlag, 1974.
42. M.C. Martyre, Immunotherapy of Rauscher grafted leukemia with soluble tumor associated antigen. *Biomedicine* (in press, 1976).
43. M.C. Martyre, R. Weiner and O. Halle-Pannenko, The *in vivo* activity of soluble extract obtained from RC19 leukemia: the effect of the method of extraction. In: *Investigation and Stimulation of Immunity in Cancer Patients*, edited by G. Mathé and R. Weiner, vol. 47, p. 405. R.R.C.R., Heidelberg, Springer-Verlag, 1974.
44. R.W. Baldwin, J.G. Bowen, M.J. Embleton, M.R. Price and R.A. Robins, Cellular and humoral immune interactions during neoplastic development. In: *The Role of Immunological Factors in Viral and Ancogenic Processes,* edited by R.F. Beers, R.C. Tilgham and E.G. Bassett, p. 393. Baltimore, Johns Hopkins Univ. Press, 1974.
45. G. Mathé, M. Kamel, M. Dezfulian, O. Halle-Pannenko and C. Bourut, An experimental screening for "systematic adjuvants of immunity" applicable in cancer immunotherapy. *Cancer Res.* **33**, 187 (1973).
46. G. Mathé, O. Halle-Pannenko, I. Florentin, M. Bruley-Rosset, M. Kamel, I.J. Hiu and C. Bourut, The second generation of EORTC-ICIG experimental screening for systemic immunity adjuvants. Its significance for cancer immunotherapy. A comparison of BCG and its hydrosoluble extract. *Europ. J. Cancer* **11**, 801 (1975).
47. M. Bruley-Rosset, I. Florentin, A.M. Khalil and G. Mathé, Non-specific macrophage activation by systemic adjuvants. Evaluation by lysosomal enzyme and *in vitro* tumoricidal activities. *Int. Arch. Allergy Applied Immunobiology* (in press, 1975).
48. G. Mathé, O. Halle-Pannenko and C. Bourut, BCG in cancer immunotherapy. II. Results obtained with various BCG preparations in a screening study for systemic adjuvants applicable to cancer immunoprophylaxis or immunotherapy. *Nat. Cancer Inst. Monogr.* **39**, 107 (1973).
49. I.J. Hiu, Water soluble and lipid free fraction from BCG with adjuvant and antitumor activity. *Nature (New Biol.)* **238**, 241 (1972).
50. A. Adam, R. Ciorbanu, J.F. Petit and E. Lederer, Isolation and properties of a macromolecular, water-soluble, immuno-adjuvant fraction from the cell wall of *Mycobacterium smegmatis. Proc. Nat. Acad. Sci. USA,* **69**, 851 (1972).
51. N.L. Levy, M.S. Mahaley Jr. and E.D. Day, Serum-mediated blocking of cell-mediated anti-tumor immunity in a melanoma patient: association with BCG immunotherapy and clinical deterioration. *Int. J. Cancer*, **10**, 244 (1972).
52. R.S. Bornstein, M.J. Mastrangelo, H. Sulit, D. Chee, J.W. Yarbo, L. Prehn and R.T. Prehn, Immunotherapy of melanoma with intralesional BCG. *Nat. Cancer Inst. Monogr.* **38**, 213 (1973).
53. N.L. Levy, Use of an *in vitro* microcytotoxicity test to assess human tumor specific cell-mediated immunity and its serum-mediated abrogation. *Nat. Cancer Inst. Monogr.* **37**, 85 (1973).
54. M.C. Simmler, L. Schwarzenberg and G. Mathé, Attempt at immunorestoration of BCG of immuno-depressed patients. In: *BCG in Cancer Patients,* edited by G. Mathé, Heidelberg, Springer-Verlag (in preparation, 1976).
55. J.U. Gutterman, G. Mavligit, J.A. Gottlieb, M.A. Burgess, C.E. McBride, L. Einhorn, E.J. Freireich and E.M. Hersh, Chemo-immunotherapy of disseminated malignant melanoma with dimethyl tri-azenoimidazole carboxamide and Bacillus Calmette-Guerin. *New England J. Med.* **291**, 592 (1974).
56. G. Mathé, Prevention of chemotherapy complications: time, toxicity, pharmacokinetic, pharmacodynamic and logistic factors. In: *Complications of Cancer Chemotherapy,* edited by G. Mathé and R.K. Oldham, vol. 49, p. 124. R.R.C.R., Heidelberg, Springer-Verlag, 1974.
57. P. Pouillart, T. Palangie, L. Schwarzenberg, H. Brugerie, J. Lheritier and G. Mathé, Effect of BCG on hematopoietic stem cells: experimental and clinical study. *Cancer Immunol. Immunoth.* (in press, 1976).

THE IMMUNOTHERAPY OF ACUTE MYELOBLASTIC LEUKAEMIA

J.M.A. WHITEHOUSE

*Imperial Cancer Research Fund, Department of Medical Oncology,
St Bartholomew's Hospital, West Smithfield, London EC1A 7BE*

In 1890 Behring and Kitasato [1] were able to prepare an antiserum to tetanus toxin-- the first description of an antibody. The significance of this discovery was readily appreciated and its potential amplified towards the management of human malignant disease. The last 80 years have seen every conceivable attempt to exploit the possibility that tumours may express antigens which are not normally found on cells of the tissue of origin. Early experiments mainly utilized attempts at passive immunization with sera raised to tumour extracts or homogenates [2].

Others tried to stimulate the host's "specific" immune response using "vaccines" [3] or by injecting tumour homogenates directly into the patient [4]. Although the results obtained were variable, many investigators tended to look upon their own results with a degree of uncritical optimism. Publications in this field accelerated towards 1929 when Woglom published a critical review of the situation [5]. His deflationary perspective so quelled both animal and human investigators alike that only sporadic publications appeared until syngeneic populations of animals allowed a genuine scientific approach to such studies in the 1940s.

Using such populations it became readily apparent that at least two types of tumour antigens could be demonstrated; an individual specific tumour antigen in carcinogen induced tumours, and group specific tumour antigens shared by all tumours produced by a particular virus. It was also found that by various immunological manipulations it was possible to protect animals against otherwise tumourigenic doses of tumour cells, providing evidence that such animals had been "immunized" [6]. This original work has been considerably amplified in animal studies to show that some tumours express more antigen than others and that some tumours are more immunogenic than others [7].

Unfortunately spontaneously arising tumours in animals, which more readily approximate to malignant tumours in man, do not obey such attractive principles, nor are they so easy to study. This fact may, in part, explain the difficulty which has existed in man in defining tumour specific antigens despite the clarity of the animal model data. Indeed, the identification of tumour specific antigens in man and the definition of their relevance to the course of the tumour has proved difficult.

Early studies in a solid tumour (malignant melanoma) suggested that some patients with this condition have circulating antibodies directed against tumour specific antigens present both on the membrane and within the cytoplasm of the tumour cells [8–12]. However, the technical problems associated with membrane immunofluorescent studies on cells isolated from solid tumours and the identification of antibodies to cytoplasmic components of proliferating cells in the sera of patients with a wide variety of different pathologies [13] underline the difficulties of interpreting these early data.

Serum cytotoxicity studies have also failed adequately to define the role of circulating antibody in human malignant disease. In contrast a considerable body of evidence has been presented that lymphocyte cytotoxicity is related to the expression of tumour antigens [14, 15] and that this cytotoxicity is influenced by the extent of the disease and by circulating factors presumed to be either antibody [16] or antigen–antibody complexes [17].

In the case of the acute leukaemias, early work by Fridman and Kourilsky [18] and Powles *et al.* [19], using the mixed lymphocyte reaction (MLR) with blast cells and autologous remission lymphocytes, suggested the leukaemic blast cells carried on their surface antigens which were not present on normal autologous bone marrow cells. Others [19–21] were able to show that immunization of patients with stored autologous acute leukaemia cells caused an increase in the *in vitro* recognition of leukaemic cells by autologous lymphocytes. Lymphocytes cytotoxic to stored autologous leukaemic blast cells have also been reported [22].

Attempts to define a specific cytotoxic antibody in the serum of patients with acute leukaemia have been disappointing. Using membrane immunofluorescence, Dore *et al.* [23] studied twenty-two patients with leukaemia (thirteen acute lymphoblastic leukaemia, nine acute myelogenous leukaemia) for circulating antibody. None was found but one patient's cells were found to have membrane-bound immunoglobulin. Similar techniques were used to examine leukaemic cells from twenty different patients with acute myeloblastic leukaemia. Immunoglobulin-bearing cells were found in half (Whitehouse and Ferguson, unpublished observation). Although the indirect immunofluorescence technique was used it was not possible to demonstrate circulating antibodies to the leukaemic cells.

More recently, Gutterman *et al.* [24] have demonstrated a much greater frequency of patients having immunoglobulin-bearing leukaemic cells. The significance of these observations has yet to be explained. More conclusive evidence suggesting the presence of tumour specific antigens on the surface of AML cells has come from the studies of Metzgar *et al.* [25] who used an antiserum to AML cells raised in primates to demonstrate antigens present on the surface of AML cells and chronic myeloid leukaemic (CML) cells which were not found on normal bone marrow cells.

Cumulatively, these studies suggest that there is on the surface of many AML cells some foreign protein which may distinguish them from the normal cells of the tissue of origin. While this protein may represent a true tumour specific antigen, such a definitive marker has proved elusive to many of the immunological techniques employed and the significance of the various findings remains as yet unestablished. Nonetheless, the MLR studies, plus the more recent work by Metzgar *et al.* [25], lend support to the existence of such tumour specific antigens, which if they are immunogenic in the host may play some part in influencing the resultant course of the disease. It seems likely that an immunological response to such antigens will be weak. Otherwise, it would be more readily demonstrable and the impact on the disease process more obviously significant.

Nevertheless, animal experiments suggest that under certain circumstances manipulation of immune mechanisms can influence the course of malignant disease.

ANTI-TUMOUR IMMUNIZATION STUDIES IN ANIMALS

The most logical way in which to immunize an animal against a tumour is to do so using the specific tumour antigen. Membrane extracts may be used for this purpose, but this method suffers from the disadvantage that fragile antigenic determinants may be damaged in the extraction procedure. Viable cell suspensions irradiated to prevent implantation offers an alternative means of presenting tumour antigen. This active specific immunization has been widely exploited in animal experiments. Non-specific stimulators of the immune mechanism with bacterial antigens such as BCG or *Corynebacterium parvum* have also been employed. Alternative methods of immune stimulation or immunization are summarized in Table 1.

Table 1. *Some of the Potential Methods of Immunotherapy of Human Tumours*

	Specific	Non-specific
ACTIVE	Sterilized tumour cell vaccines	BCG
		Zymosan
	Antigen extracts	Antireticular serum
	Helper determinants	Corynebacteria
	Heterogenization	Levamisole
PASSIVE	Anti-tumour antisera	Normal serum components
	"Deblocking" sera	Properdin
		Complement
ADOPTIVE	Sensitized allogeneic or xenogeneic lymphoid cells	Non-sensitized allogeneic lymphoid cells
		Graft-versus-tumour

Taken from Currie [41].

Conventional animal experiments have shown that active immunization with tumour cells can prevent implantation of a tumour by a dose of cells which would normally be sufficient to produce a tumour. Such immunization is considerably less successful when it follows the successful implantation of a tumour, a situation which resembles attempts to immunize the tumour-bearing host in man. Experiments in the L1210 leukaemia [26] showed that mice could be cured provided that the tumour load did not exceed 10^5 cells if they received BCG or irradiated leukaemia cells within 24 hr of challenge. Parr [27] reported similar findings using the L5178Y lymphoma, showing that if 10^3 living cells of the L5178Y lymphoma are given intraperitoneally and the animals receive no further treatment they all die within 28 days. However, when irradiated tumour cells are given 24 hr later some of the animals fail to develop lymphomas, if the cells are given 3 days later the effect is minimized, and if they are not given until 7 days later the effect is abolished.

BCG alone was also found to have a similar effect, but the combination of both BCG and irradiated lymphoma cells was superior to either alone, suggesting that the BCG fulfills a role as an adjuvant by amplifying the immune response non-specifically.

Table 2. *Non-specific Stimulation with Bacterial*
Antigens

1. Increased antibody production
2. Increased numbers of rosette-forming lymphocytes
3. Increased phagocytosis
4. Increased homograft rejection
5. Increased interferon production

Table 2 summarizes various phenomena attributed to the administration of BCG.
Various extracts of BCG have been shown to be similarly effective and other bacterial
antigens such as *Corynebacterium parvum* provoke similar reactions. These are particularly
interesting in the light of experiments carried out by Currie and Bagshawe [28]
suggesting that careful timing of the combination of immunotherapy and chemotherapy
may significantly increase the effectiveness of each, a feature which may be particularly
relevant to the management of acute leukaemia.

These workers showed that in a transplanted fibrosarcoma in mice, treatment with
cyclophosphamide followed by *C. parvum* was effective in preventing the growth of
the tumour but only when the *C. parvum* was given 12 days after treatment with
cyclophosphamide. When the *C. parvum* was given 0, 3, 6 or 16 days following the
cyclophosphamide none of the animals survived to 100 days, whereas when it was
given on the 12th day 70% of the animals survived in excess of 100 days. The results
of this study suggest that the timing of the immunotherapy is critical, for if it is given
too soon the immunosuppressant effect of the cyclophosphamide is still active and the
cell mediated immune response still suppressed, whereas if the *C. parvum* is given too
late regrowth has occurred among the tumour cells surviving the chemotherapy with
cyclophosphamide and the immune response is then insufficient to eliminate the
increasing number of sarcoma cells.

Such critical timing is obviously difficult to achieve in the human situation. Since
immunological cell kill is more likely to be effective when only few abnormal cells
remain, these experiments illustrate certain important principles if immunotherapy is to
be applied to AML in man; namely, that for immunotherapy to be effective, chemotherapy must be utilized to maximally reduce the leukaemic cell burden; that the host
must be capable of reacting to an immune stimulus; and lastly, that the timing of the
immunotherapy must be such that the response is not depressed by recent chemotherapy,
but not left so late that the leukaemic cell population is rapidly increasing.

ANTI-TUMOUR IMMUNIZATION (IMMUNOTHERAPY) IN HUMAN AML

In order to justify the term "immunotherapy", an observed therapeutic effect must
follow an immunological manipulation. The usage of this word has been widely coined
and applied to situations where immunological mechanisms are presumed to be operative
and in anticipation of therapeutic benefit. Effector mechanisms in this situation are,
however, still very much under critical study since it is possible that any therapeutic
advantage may result from non-immunological responses. Despite this, however, there is
a variety of data to suggest that the application of immunological principles to the

management of acute leukaemia in complete remission may have advantages in terms of prolonged survival and the ease of attainment of second remission.

Encouragement for the hypothetical advantages of immunotherapy came from the study of Mathé et al. [29] who selected a group of patients who were in complete remission from ALL following 2 years of intensive chemotherapy. Thirty patients were assigned to four groups. Ten patients received no further treatment; eight patients received 150 μg of fresh pellicle grown Pasteur BCG by scarification every 4 days for 1 month and then weekly until relapse; five patients received weekly subcutaneous injections of 4×10^7 allogeneic leukaemic cells either treated with dilute formalin or irradiated prior to injection and seven patients received both BCG and allogeneic cells. While all of the patients who received no further treatment had relapsed at 130 days, only 9/20 of those receiving BCG, cells, or both, had done so. There was no significant difference between these three groups, but seven patients remained in remission $4\frac{1}{2}$ to 7 years after treatment. Although animal experiments in the L1210 and L5178Y lymphomas in mice had suggested that BCG or irradiated malignant cells, or both, might be effective therapeutically, this study provided the first evidence that such treatment might prove effective in man.

Two subsequent major controlled trials, one by the British Medical Research Council (Report by Leukaemia Committee and Working Party on Leukaemia in Children) [30] and the other by the United States Cancer Study Group A [31], failed to demonstrate any benefit from BCG. In both studies children with ALL achieving their first complete remission were randomized to one of three groups — either no further treatment, standard maintenance chemotherapy, or BCG. In neither of the studies did BCG show any statistical advantage over the no-treatment groups, and both were inferior to maintenance chemotherapy.

Leventhal et al. [32] used BCG plus irradiated leukaemic cells in children with ALL, but found no benefit over methotrexate alone. Any benefit which these studies might have shown would have been overshadowed by the advances in remission maintenance achieved by Pinkel and his co-workers [33] who have so improved the prognosis of acute lymphoblastic leukaemia that potential benefits which might accrue from immunotherapy in ALL will now be extremely difficult to assess.

This contrasts with acute myeloblastic leukaemia in which a relatively poor prognosis and rapid relapse rate make the demonstration of therapeutic benefit more readily apparent. Since the results of chemotherapy alone in the maintenance of complete remission in acute myeloblastic leukaemia suggested that this form of maintenance offered little hope of dramatically improving survival, and since animal experimental data encouraged a trial of immunotherapy in man, a remission maintenance trial was started at St Bartholomew's Hospital. Patients with AML were randomized on admission to receive either chemotherapy alone or chemotherapy in combination with weekly BCG (Glaxo given by a multipuncture gun to a depth of 2 mm, delivering approximately 1×10^6 organisms), plus injections of irradiated allogeneic leukaemic cells once complete remission was achieved. These results have been published [34, 35] and are summarized in Table 3. The trial was planned so that each group received identical treatment including chemotherapy, the only difference being that one arm received, in addition, BCG plus irradiated leukaemic cells.

Several comments can be made about the results of this study. Firstly, the group receiving chemotherapy alone did not survive as long as some other groups who received

Table 3. *Results of All Patients with Acute Myelogenous Leukaemia Entering Complete Remission*

Group	No. of patients	Median duration first remission (days)	Median duration of survival from onset of first remission (days)
Chemotherapy only	21	191	295
Chemotherapy plus immunotherapy	32	313	520

These results represent a further follow-up on the study previously reported by Powles *et al.* [35].

chemotherapy alone (MRC unpublished results [36]) and also the deaths occurring in the Bart's group resulted from relapse of AML and were not chemotherapy induced deaths. These factors suggest that this form of chemotherapy was less efficient than others in maintaining remission. Secondly, the group receiving chemotherapy plus immunotherapy survive longer than any of the chemotherapy alone groups, and significantly longer than our own chemotherapy alone group, clearly demonstrating therapeutic benefit from the injections of BCG and allogeneic irradiated leukaemic cells.

On the basis of immunological arguments so far presented, the specific active element of the immunotherapy might be expected to be the major contributor to the effectiveness of the technique. However, the various effects of BCG include certain non-specific actions which may be as important as those specific immunological effects of irradiated cells. Since only a very weak immune response may occur, the non-specific effects elicited by the BCG may be more important.

Evidence is already accumulating that BCG without irradiated cells may prolong the complete remission duration in acute myeloblastic leukaemia [37]. Particularly impressive in the context are the results of Gutterman *et al.* [38]. Fourteen patients received the combination of chemotherapy plus immunotherapy and only four of these have relapsed, the median duration of remission being in excess of 72 weeks and thus likely to exceed that achieved using BCG and irradiated cells in the study reported by Powles *et al.* [34]. Twenty-one patients received chemotherapy alone and twelve have relapsed, the median duration of complete remission being 60 weeks. Other workers have reported similar results [39]. BCG from a variety of sources has been used in these studies so that they will be difficult to compare satisfactorily. Recently methanol extractable residues (MER) of BCG have been used to replace BCG in the maintenance of complete remission. Prolongation of remission and survival have been reported when this is used in place of BCG [40].

If BCG achieves its effect in prolonging survival through non-immunological mechanisms, then the hypothetical arguments suggesting that the immunotherapeutic effect would only be useful when the residual tumour population is small no longer applies. Indeed, an overall stimulus to host resistance might contain the disease equally well even when limited overt disease is apparent. Currie [41] has suggested that mixing viable non-irradiated cells with BCG might potentiate the effect of the specific active component of immune stimulation, thus achieving the optimum benefit from each. This form of immunotherapy has been given to eleven AML patients at St Bartholomew's

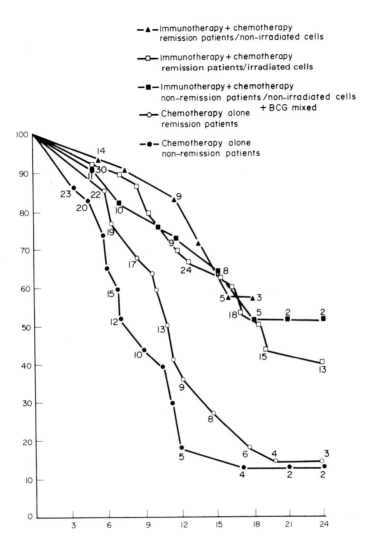

Fig. 1. Survival of AML patients alive after 4 months' treatment.

▲ Fourteen patients who achieved complete remission were treated
   with chemotherapy and BCG with non-irradiated cells.
□ Thirty patients who achieved complete remission were treated with
   chemotherapy and BCG with irradiated cells, as described by
   Powles *et al.* [35].
■ Eleven patients who failed to achieve complete remission were
   treated with chemotherapy and non-irradiated cells mixed with BCG.
○ Twenty-two patients who achieved complete remission were treated
   with chemotherapy alone.
● Twenty-three patients who failed to achieve remission were subsequently
   treated with chemotherapy alone.

Hospital who had achieved partial remission only. The survival curves of these patients
can be plotted with those of other patients who are in either complete or partial remission
3 months after starting chemotherapy. Five groups of patients can be examined (Fig. 1).

1. Twenty-three patients who failed to achieve complete remission maintained with chemotherapy alone.
2. Twenty-two patients maintained in complete remission with chemotherapy alone.
3. Thirty patients who were maintained in complete remission with conventional chemotherapy and BCG plus irradiated cells as described by Powles *et al.* [35].
4. Fourteen patients maintained in complete remission with chemotherapy and BCG plus non-irradiated allogeneic leukaemic cells.
5. Eleven patients maintained in partial remission with chemotherapy and a mixture of BCG plus allogeneic non-irradiated leukaemic cells.

It is apparent from these curves that those patients given immunotherapy as part of their maintenance survive significantly longer than those receiving only chemotherapy. The adage that patients in complete remission survive longer than those who are not can be questioned. Patients who are not in complete remission, but who had immunotherapy, fared better than those in complete remission who had chemotherapy alone. Eleven patients who were not in complete remission more than 4 months after the onset of treatment were given BCG mixed with allogeneic non-irradiated leukaemic cells without further chemotherapy. These patients were symptomatically and clinically well and had only small numbers (between 6% and 10%) of blast cells in the bone marrow, with the exception of one patient who had 25% infiltration. Five patients achieved complete remission from 2 to 6 months after the cessation of chemotherapy and beginning mixed BCG plus cells. The duration of these remissions has ranged from 6 weeks to $4\frac{1}{2}$ months. These results collectively encourage arguments in favour of a beneficial role for BCG and allogeneic irradiated cells in the maintenance of acute leukaemia without as yet identifying the active component.

Powles [34] reported a group of patients in complete remission maintained with BCG plus irradiated allogeneic leukaemic cells alone, given at separate sites, whose remission lengths and survival were identical to those in patients maintained with both chemotherapy and immunotherapy, and better than those patients who had maintenance with chemotherapy only. This evidence is supported by data from Freeman *et al.* [42] and throws doubts on the value of the maintenance chemotherapy as used in our studies.

There has been new speculation about the possible mechanism of action of BCG, namely that it stimulates the normal bone marrow and enables the balance between the normal cells and the leukaemic cells to be changed in favour of the former [34]. Experimental evidence supporting this comes from the work of Mathé *et al.* [43] which showed that BCG protected the normal bone marrow in animals from damage produced by cyclophosphamide. In the series reported by Clarkson [34] the duration of complete remission maintained by intensive chemotherapy is very similar to our own study achieved with immunotherapy, and since the quality of life for patients receiving intensive chemotherapy is undoubtedly diminished when compared with that of patients receiving immunotherapy, with or without moderate chemotherapy the vital question is to determine whether manipulations using combinations of BCG and allogeneic leukaemic cells, or one or other alone, can produce survivals equal to or better than those achieved by intensive chemotherapy.

REFERENCES

1. E. Behring and Kitasato: Ueber das Zustandekommen der Diphtherie-Immunität und der Tetanus-Immunität bei Thieren. *Dtsch. med. Wschr.* **49**, 1113 (1890).
2. E. Vidal: Sérothérapies des tumeurs malignes. *Conférence Internationale du Cancer (Paris, 1910),* p. 293 (1911).
3. A.F. Coca, G.M. Dorrance and M.G. Lebredo: Vaccination in cancer II. A report of the results of vaccination therapy as applied in 79 cases of human cancer. *Z. Immun. Forsch.* **13**, 543 (1912).
4. T.H. Kellock, H. Chambers and S. Russ: An attempt to procure immunity to malignant disease in man. *Lancet,* **1**, 217 (1922).
5. Woglom, W.H.: Immunity to transplantable tumours. *Cancer Rev.* IV, 3, 4, p. 9 (1929).
6. L. Gross: Intradermal immunization of C3H mice against a sarcoma that originated in an animal of the same line. *Cancer Res.* **3**, 326 (1943).
7. R.W. Baldwin: Membrane associated antigen in chemically induced tumours. *Ser. Haemat.* V, **4**, 67 (1972).
8. D.L. Morton, R.A. Malmgren, E.C. Holmes and A.S. Ketcham: Demonstration of antibodies against human malignant melanoma by immunofluorescence. *Surgery,* **64**, (1), 233 (1968).
9. M.G. Lewis, R.L. Ikonopisov, R.C. Nairn, T.M. Phillips, G. Hamilton-Fairley, D.C. Bodenham and P. Alexander: Tumour-specific antibodies in human malignant melanoma and their relationship to the extent of the disease. *Brit. Med. J.* **3**, 547 (1969).
10. M.M. Romsdahl and I.S. Cox: Human malignant melanoma antibodies demonstrated by immunofluorescence. *Arch. Surg. Chicago,* **100**, 491 (1970).
11. N.M. Muna, S. Marcus and C. Smart: Detection by immunofluorescence of antibodies specific for human malignant melanoma cells. *Cancer,* **23**, 88 (1969).
12. H.F. Oettgen, T. Aoki, L.J. Old, E.A. Boyse, and E. de Harven: Suspension culture of a pigment producing cell line derived from a human malignant melanoma. *J. Nat. Cancer Inst.* **41**, 827 (1968).
13. J.M.A. Whitehouse: Circulating antibodies in human malignant disease. *Brit. J. Cancer,* **28**, Suppl. I, 170 (1973).
14. I. Hellström, K.E. Hellström, G.E. Pierce and J.P.S. Yang: Cellular and humoral immunity to different types of human neoplasm. *Nature,* **220**, 1352 (1968).
15. J. Bubenik, P. Perlmann, K. Hemstein and G. Moberger: Immune response to urinary bladder tumours in man. *Int. J. Cancer,* **5**, 39 (1970).
16. I. Hellström and K.E. Hellström: Some aspects of the immune defense against cancer. II. *In vitro* studies on human tumours. *Cancer,* **28**, (5), 1269 (1971).
17. G.A. Currie and C. Basham: Serum mediated inhibition of the immunological reactions of the patient to his own tumour: a possible role for circulating antigen. *Brit. J. Cancer,* **26**, 427 (1972).
18. W.H. Fridman and F.M. Kourilsky: Stimulation of lymphocytes by autologous leukaemic cells in acute leukaemia. *Nature,* **224**, 227–279 (1969).
19. R.L. Powles, L.A. Balchin, G. Hamilton-Fairley and P. Alexander: Recognition of leukaemic cells as foreign before and after auto-immunisation. *Brit. Med. J.* **1**, 486 (1971).
20. D.C. Viza, O. Bernard-Degani, C. Bernard and R. Harris: Leukaemia antigens. *Lancet,* **2**, 493 (1969).
21. J.U. Gutterman, G. Mavligit, K.B. McCredie, E.J. Freireich and E.M. Hersh: Autoimmunisation with acute leukaemia cells: demonstration of increased lymphocyte responsiveness. *Int. J. Cancer,* **11**, 521 (1973).
22. B.G. Leventhal, R.H. Halterman, E.B. Rosenberg and R.B. Herberman: Immune reactivity of leukaemia patients to autologous blast cells. *Cancer Res.* **32**, 1820 (1972).
23. J.F. Dore, L. Marholev, D.E. Colas, H. La Noue, F. de Vassal, R. Motta, I. Harsak, G. Seman, and G. Mathé: New antigens in human leukaemic cells, and antibody in the serum of leukaemic patients. *Lancet,* **2**, 1396 (1967).
24. J.U. Gutterman, R.D. Rossen, W.T. Butler, K.B. McCredie, G.P. Bodey, E.J. Freireich and E.M. Hersh: Immunoglobulins in tumour cells and tumour-induced lymphocytes. Blastogenesis in human acute leukaemia. *New Engl. J. Med.* **4**, 169 (1973).
25. R.S. Metzgar, T. Mohanakumar, R.W. Green, D.S. Miller and D.P. Bolognesi: Human leukaemia antigens: partial isolation and characterization. *J. Nat. Cancer Inst.* **52**, (5), 1445 (1974).
26. G. Mathé, P. Pouillart and F. Lapeyraque: Active immunotherapy of L1210 leukaemia applied after the graft of tumour cells. *Br. J. Cancer,* **23**, 814 (1969).
27. I. Parr: Response of syngeneic murine lymphomata to immunotherapy in relation to the antigenicity of the tumour. *Br. J. Cancer,* **26**, 174 (1972).
28. G.A. Currie and K.D. Bagshawe: Active immunotherapy with *Corynebacterium parvum* and chemotherapy in murine fibrosarcomas. *Brit. Med. J.* **1**, 541 (1970).

29. G. Mathé, J.L. Amiel, L. Schwarzenberg et al.: Active immunotherapy for acute lymphoblastic leukaemia. *Lancet*, **1**, 697 (1969).
30. Report to the medical research council by the leukaemia committee and the working party on leukaemia in childhood: Treatment of acute lymphoblastic leukaemia: comparison of immunotherapy (BCG), intermittent methotrexate, and no therapy after a five-month intensive cytotoxic regimen (Concord trial). *Brit. Med. J.* **4**, 189 (1971).
31. R. Heyn, W. Borges and P. Joo et al.: BCG in the treatment of acute lymphocytic leukaemia (ALL). *Proc. Am. Ass. Cancer Res.* **14**, 45 (1975).
32. B.G. Leventhal, A. Le Pourheit, R.H. Halterman et al.: Immunotherapy in previously treated acute lymphatic leukaemia. *Nat. Cancer Inst. Monogr.* **39**, 177 (1973).
33. J. Simone: Acute lymphocytic leukaemia in childhood. *Seminars in Hematology*, **11**, 25 (1974).
34. R.L. Powles: Immunotherapy for acute myelogenous leukaemia using irradiated and unirradiated leukaemia cells. *Cancer*, **34**, 1558 (1974).
35. R.L. Powles, D. Crowther, C.J.T. Bateman et al.: Immunotherapy for acute myelogenous leukaemia. *Brit. J. Cancer*, **28**, 365 (1973).
36. B.D. Clarkson: Acute myelocytic leukaemia in adults. *Cancer*, **30**, 1572 (1972).
37. W.R. Vogler and Y-K. Chan: Prolonging remission in myeloblastic leukaemia by tice-strain Bacillus Calmette-Guerin. *Lancet*, **2**, 128 (1974).
38. J.U. Gutterman, E.M. Hersh, V. Rodriguez, K.B. McCredie, G. Mavligit, R. Reed, M.A. Burgess, T. Smith, E. Gehan, G.P. Bodey Sr., and E.J. Freireich: Chemoimmunotherapy of adult acute leukaemia. Prolongation of remission in myeloblastic leukaemia with BCG. *Lancet*, **4**, 1405 (1974).
39. M.G. Whiteside, M.N. Gauchi, C.M. Paton, A. Foy and J.M. Stone: Immunotherapy in the maintenance period of acute non-lymphatic leukaemia. *Proceedings of the XV Congress of the International Society of Haematology, Jerusalem*, Abstract, Part II, p. 295 (1974).
40. D.W. Weiss, Y. Stupp and G. Izak: Treatment of acute myelocytic leukaemia patients with the MER tubercle bacillus fraction. *Proceedings of the 5th Congress of the Transplantation Society, Jerusalem*, p. 74 (1974).
41. G.A. Currie: Cancer and the immune response. *Current Topics in Immunology Series*, **2**, Edward Arnold, London, 1974.
42. C.B. Freeman, R. Harris, C.G. Geary, M.J. Leyland, J.E. MacIver, I.W. Delamore: Active immunotherapy used alone for maintenance of patients with acute myeloid leukaemia. *Brit. Med. J.* **4**, 571 (1973).
43. G. Mathé, O. Halle-Pannenko and C. Bourut: Immune manipulation by BCG administered before or after cyclophosphamide for chemo-immunotherapy of L1210 leukaemia. *Eur. J. Cancer*, **10**, 661 (1974).

IMMUNOTHERAPY OF HUMAN SOLID TUMORS: PROLONGATION OF DISEASE-FREE INTERVAL AND SURVIVAL IN MALIGNANT MELANOMA, BREAST AND COLORECTAL CANCER*

JORDAN U. GUTTERMAN, GIORA M. MAVLIGIT, MICHAEL A. BURGESS,
JUAN O. CARDENAS, RICHARD C. REED, GEORGE R. BLUMENSCHEIN,
JEFFREY A. GOTTLIEB, CHARLES M. McBRIDE and EVAN M. HERSH

*Departments of Developmental Therapeutics and Surgery[†],
The University of Texas System Cancer Center, M.D. Anderson Hospital
and Tumor Institute, 6723 Bertner Avenue, Houston, Texas 77025*

SUMMARY

Results of immunotherapy with BCG in patients with malignant melanoma, colorectal carcinoma, and breast cancer are described. The first study demonstrated that high doses of living BCG organisms (6×10^8) viable units delivered by scarification in the upper arms and legs prolonged the disease-free interval and survival of 52 malignant melanoma patients with regional lymph node metastases compared to 218 surgical control patients. Patients with trunk and extremity, but not head and neck melanoma, benefited from BCG, suggesting the importance of the delivery of BCG into the tumor involved lymphatics. The second study demonstrated that lyophilized Pasteur BCG given by scarification or 5-FU plus BCG prolonged the post-operative disease-free interval and survival of 73 patients with colorectal carcinoma of the Duke's C classification (positive mesenteric lymph nodes) compared to 58 surgical control patients.

The principles of intermittent chemotherapy combined with BCG immunotherapy first developed in patients with disseminated melanoma and acute myelogenous leukemia have been confirmed in a series of patients with disseminated breast cancer: 45 patients treated with a combination of 5-FU, Adriamycin, and Cyclophosphamide (FAC) plus BCG by scarification showed prolongation of remission, as well as overall survival compared to a group of 44 consecutive patients treated with FAC chemotherapy without immunotherapy. The limitations of BCG immunotherapy as well as speculations for future developments of immunotherapy are discussed.

* This work was supported by Contract NO1-CB-33888 and PHS Grant 1R 26 CA 15458-01 from the National Institutes of Health, Public Health Service, Bethesda, Maryland 20014. Drs. Gutterman and Mavligit are the recipients of Career Development Awards (CA 71007-02 and CA 00130-01, respectively) from the National Institutes of Health, Education, and Welfare, Bethesda, Maryland 20014.

† Reprint requests should be mailed to: Jordan U. Gutterman, M.D., Associate Professor of Medicine, M.D. Anderson Hospital and Tumor Institute, 6723 Bertner Avenue, Houston, Texas 77025.

INTRODUCTION

Immunotherapy of human cancer is not a new medical discipline. Since early in the twentieth century there was evidence suggesting that immunological manipulation of the tumor cancer patient can favorably modify tumor growth [1–3].

The systematic treatment of human cancer, however, received a major impetus in the late 1960s with publication of papers by (a) Mathé and co-workers showing that BCG could prolong the disease-free interval and survival of children with acute lymphoblastic leukemia after major cytoreduction with chemotherapy [4], (b) E. Klein showing that induction of delayed hypersensitivity could control skin cancers (reviewed in ref. 5) and (c) Morton, showing that intratumoral inoculation of BCG caused regression of melanoma skin nodules [6].

The benefit of immunotherapy in prolonging disease free interval and survival has been confirmed in adult acute myeloblastic leukemia by several investigators with the use of BCG plus chemotherapy or BCG and tumor cells plus chemotherapy [7–11].

The use of systemic active "non-specific" immunotherapy with immunopotentiating agents in human solid tumors presented a dilemma in 1971. Would acceleration or enhancement of tumor growth occur because of the induction of so-called blocking antibodies or other enhancing factors? This was a theoretical possibility because of the demonstration that in animal model solid tumors, but rarely in leukemia, tumor enhancement by immunological adjuvants had been reported [12].

Our program of immunotherapy for human solid tumors was initiated in the Department of Developmental Therapeutics at M.D. Anderson Hospital and Tumor Institute in the fall of 1971. Following the principles outlined by Mathé that immunotherapy would work best in the minimal residual disease situation [12], we initiated a trial of BCG immunotherapy following the surgical resection of recurrent melanoma in regional lymph nodes [13]. Malignant melanoma was selected because several investigators had published data suggesting the existence of tumor-associated antigens in this disease [14–17]. In addition, Morton had shown that intra-tumor inoculation of BCG in melanoma nodules induced significant regression of tumor in immunocompetent patients [6]. Our initial phase 1 trial comparing different doses and strains of BCG was published in 1973 [13]. In that report, we suggested that the use of high doses of BCG by scarification (that is 6×10^8 viable units) on a weekly basis for 3 months and then every other week prolonged the disease-free interval and survival of patients with stage III melanoma (regional lymph node metastases removed by surgery). A lower dose of BCG (that is 6×10^7 viable units) was less effective. The stable variety of BCG, the Tice lyophilized strain, appeared to be more beneficial than the liquid Pasteur BCG.

This paper will summarize an up-dated analysis of that study. Although BCG has clearly proved to be beneficial in patients with melanoma, several critical factors are necessary to achieve a positive clinical effect including the dose of BCG, the anatomical location of the tumor referable to the site of BCG application, the amount of residual disease, and the immunological competence of the host.

Following the demonstration that BCG could prolong the disease-free interval and survival of patients with recurrent melanoma [13], we initiated a similar study in patients with Duke's C classification of colorectal cancer. The preliminary report of this study has been published [18, 19].

The second major application of immunotherapy in human solid tumors that was initiated in April 1972 was the use of BCG immunotherapy in combination with chemo-therapy for patients with disseminated metastases. The major questions asked were: (1) could immunotherapy combined with chemotherapy increase remission rates? (2) could immunotherapy prolong chemotherapy induced remissions? and (3) could immunochemotherapy prolong the overall survival of solid tumor patients compared to chemotherapy alone?

The first study of immunochemotherapy of disseminated melanoma with BCG was published in 1974 [2]. The chemotherapeutic drug Imidazole Carboxamide (DTIC) was combined with fresh Pasteur BCG in patients with disseminated melanoma. The major results were: (1) remission rates regional to sites of BCG administration were increased, (2) remissions were prolonged with chemoimmunotherapy compared to chemotherapy alone, and (3) the overall survival of patients on chemoimmunotherapy was significantly prolonged compared to chemotherapy alone [20].

The principles learned from this initial chemoimmunotherapy study in melanomas were then extended to patients with metastatic breast cancer. These results are summar-ized below. The principles of chemoimmunotherapy were successfully applied to breast cancer patients.

Therefore, this paper will describe the results of adjuvant BCG in melanoma and colorectal carcinoma and the results of chemoimmunotherapy in disseminated breast cancer.

PATIENTS AND METHODS

Following the surgical removal of recurrent melanoma in regional lymph nodes BCG was given by scarification weekly for 3 months and then every other week in the upper arms and legs as previously described [13]. Two dose levels of lyophilized Tice and liquid Pasteur were compared, 6×10^7 and 6×10^8 viable units. The disease-free interval and survival of fifty-two patients with regional lymph node metastases (stage III) entered on study from November 1971 through July 1973 were evaluated. The data were compared to similar data for 218 stage III patients treated by surgery alone at M.D. Anderson Hospital from 1965 to 1971. Further details of the patient groups are described in reference 13.

The second adjuvant study evaluated a total of fifty-eight patients with colorectal cancer of the Duke's C classification. These patients had their primary and definitive surgery for colorectal cancer either at M.D. Anderson Hospital or elsewhere. Patients were randomized to receive BCG either alone or in combination with oral doses of 5-FU. The lyophilized Pasteur BCG was administered by scarification in a dose of 6×10^7 viable organisms weekly for 3 months and then every other week thereafter. 5-FU was originally given in a dose of $100 \, mg/m^2$ four times a day for 5 days and repeated every 4 weeks. More recently, the dose of 5-FU has been increased to $150 \, mg/m^2$ in a similar schedule. Patients were randomized to receive BCG on days 7, 14 and 21 of each course during the first three courses, and on days 7 and 21 thereafter [18, 19].

The historical control group included a large-scale natural history group of patients with colorectal cancer who were consecutively operated on at M.D. Anderson Hospital during the period of 10 years prior to the initiation of the immunotherapeutic trial. An historical control group with seventy-three patients of the Duke's C classification is shown.

Forty-seven patients with disseminated breast cancer were entered on study between March 1 through 15 August 1974. Before chemoimmunotherapy, the patients were evaluated for metastatic disease with the following tests: physical examination, complete blood counts, urinalysis, test of liver and renal functions, chest X-ray, liver scan, electroencephalogram, metastatic bone survey and bone marrow biopsy. Two patients died within the first 2 weeks of treatment. Forty-five patients were considered evaluable with an adequate trial of one or more courses of treatment.

The experimental design of the chemoimmunotherapy was as follows: 5-Fluorouracil (5-FU) 500 mg/m^2 intravenously on days 1 and 8 of each chemoimmunotherapy course, Adriamycin–50 mg/m^2 intravenously on day 1, and Cyclophosphamide–500 mg/m^2 intravenously on day 1. Lyophilized Tice strain BCG in a dose of 6×10^8 viable units was given by scarification in a rotating fashion on the upper arms and upper legs as previously described [4, 20] on days 9, 13 and 17 of each course. Courses were repeated every 21 days if blood counts permitted.

If, during the previous course, the lowest absolute granulocyte count did not fall below 2000 and the lowest platelet count did not fall below 100,000 all three chemotherapeutic agents were increased by an amount of 20%. If the blood counts fell to less than 1000 granulocyte count and/or less than 50,000 platelet count, all agents were decreased by 20%. No drug change was required for patients whose blood counts fell between these levels. However, if the patient had morbidity (i.e. documented infection and/or hemorrhage), all agents were decreased 25–40% regardless of change in blood counts.

The total dose of Adriamycin was limited to 500 mg/m^2 because of the known increase in the incidence of cardiotoxicity above this dose level [21]. Adriamycin was discontinued if any evidence of cardiac toxicity developed. Severe diarrhea or cerebellar ataxia, attributable to 5-FU, required withholding of this agent until resolution of these symptoms. Subsequently, 5-FU was reintroduced at a 20% reduced level. The development of severe stomatitis was an indication to lower the dose of both 5-FU and Adriamycin by 20%.

The following definitions were used: complete remission, complete disappearance of all objective and subjective disease manifestations; partial remission, 50% of greater reduction in the areas of all measurable tumor; stabilization, less than 50% reduction or less than 25% increase in tumor size for at least 2 months; progression, 50% of greater increase in tumor masses or appearance of any new masses; relapse, reappearance of the tumor mass.

Survival was measured from onset of treatment to death or date of last follow-up examination. FAC-BCG was continued for a minimum of two courses. Then therapy was stopped only with evidence of unequivocal progression.

The responses to therapy with FAC-BCG were compared to the response of a consecutive series of forty-four patients treated in an identical fashion with FAC chemotherapy alone just prior to this study from 15 August 1973 until 1 March 1974 [22].

The criteria for admission to these studies were identical. All patients with clinical evidence of disseminated breast cancer were admitted for therapy.

Table 1 shows that the FAC and FAC-BCG were comparable in the major features known to be associated with prognosis in breast cancer [23]. The distribution of visceral and non-visceral metastases was similar. The frequency of hormonal manipulation, the proportion of pre- and post-menopausal patients and the median time to dissemination,

Table 1. *Clinical Features of 45 Patients treated with FAC-BCG and 44 treated with FAC*

	FAC-BCG	FAC
Clinical Feature		
Median age	56	51
(range)	(29–72)	(29–67)
Median disease-free interval	16	15
	(0–140)	(0–104)
Pre-menopausal (at diagnosis)	40%	44%
Prior hormone therapy	69%	79%
Prior chemotherapy	7%	7%
Site of Metastases		
Lymph node	44%	52%
Soft tissue	50%	84%
Lung	44%	55%
Pleura	11%	16%
Liver	27%	20%
Bone	49%	66%

were nearly identical (Table 1).

The statistical methods used included the chi square test for testing difference in remission rate, a generalized Wilcoxon test with a one-tailed analysis [24] for testing differences between remission and survival curves, and a method of Kaplan and Meier for calculating and plotting remission and survival curves [25].

RESULTS

A. Adjuvant BCG in Malignant Melanoma

Figure 1 shows the disease-free interval for patients with stage III disease compared to the control series. Although the total number of relapses in both the high and the low BCG groups was identical, the time to relapse was prolonged for those patients treated with the high dose compared to the control series. There was no benefit for patients treated with low dose BCG. The difference in the disease-free interval for the high dose BCG compared to the surgical control group is significant at the 0.03 level.

Figure 2 shows the overall survival for the preceding group of patients. There was no benefit for those patients who were treated with low doses of BCG. In contrast, there was a significant prolongation of survival time for patients who were treated with the high dose of BCG. The difference in survival compared to the surgical control series is highly significant at 0.002.

We next examined the efficacy of BCG correlated with the site of the original primary lesion. Patients with trunk melanoma, metastatic to regional lymph nodes of the axilla or inguinal region benefited most strikingly compared to the surgical control group. As shown on Figure 3, patients who received the high dose of BCG had a significant prolongation of the disease-free interval ($p = 0.05$). Although the patients treated with low dose BCG also had prolongation of disease-free interval, this as yet has not reached statistical significance.

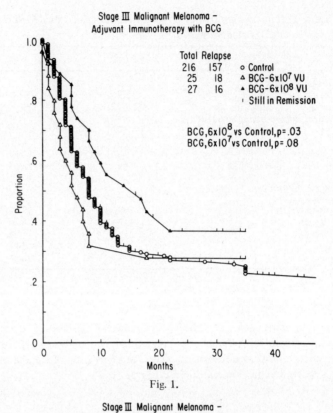

Fig. 1.

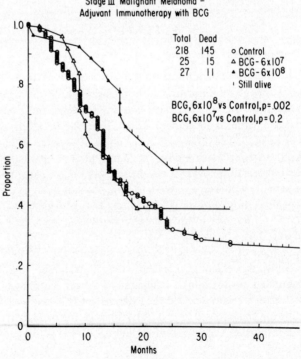

Fig. 2.

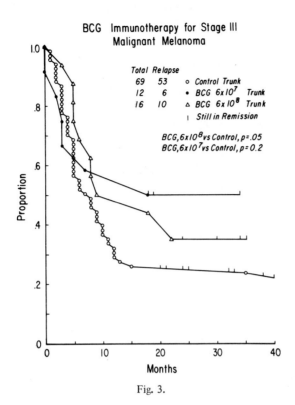

Fig. 3.

On Fig. 4 is shown the survival of these patients. Survival has been prolonged for both groups of patients with trunk melanomas. However, the group who received the high dose has already had a statistical significance prolonged survival ($p = 0.006$). The low dose has not reached stastical significance ($p = 0.1$).

In sharp contrast with the encouraging results for trunk melanoma patients, those with head and neck melanoma have not benefited from BCG. Figure 5 shows the disease-free interval for patients who received BCG compared to the controls. Both groups of patients had recurrences as rapidly as the surgical controls. One should note that the six patients who received low dose BCG had an accelerated and statistically shorter time to recurrence compared to the surgical controls.

Figure 6 shows survival for the preceding group of patients. There was no significant difference in survival for either BCG group compared to the surgical group.

Because of limited space we will not present data with extremity melanoma. However, those treated with high dose, but not low dose, had significant prolongation of disease-free interval and survival. Thus, the data would suggest the importance of administering BCG into the tumor involved lymphatics since patients with trunk and extremity, but not head and neck melanoma, benefited from BCG.

Figure 7 shows the importance of immunological evaluation prior to immunotherapy in the prediction of prognosis with non-specific immunotherapy. The most useful immunological test to predict survival has been delayed hypersensitivity reaction after primary immunization with keyhole limpet hemocyanin (KLH). These data include

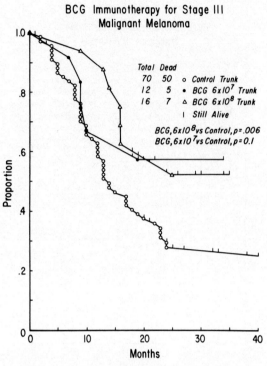

Fig. 4.

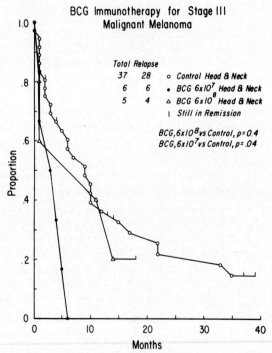

Fig. 5.

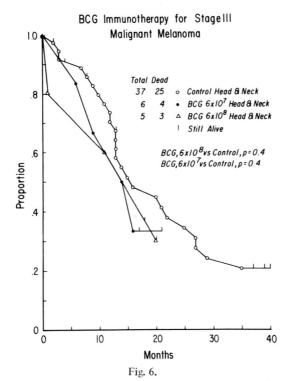

Fig. 6.

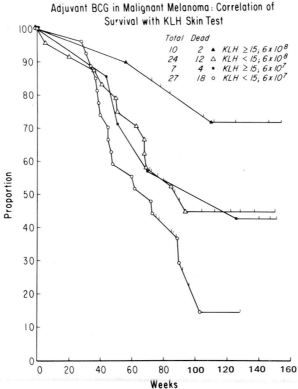

Fig. 7.

patients with stages III and IVA (distant metastases removed by surgery) Gutterman, submitted for publication). Of the ten patients who had a vigorous primary immune response
to KLH and who were treated with high doses of BCG, only two have died to date. In
contrast, the poorest survival was noted in those patients who had a KLH skin test of less
than 15 mm and who were treated with low dose BCG. Intermediate and equivalent survivals were noted for those patients with a KLH less than 15 mm who received high dose
BCG and those with a vigorous KLH response ($\geqslant$ 15 mm) who received the low dose BCG.
The data strongly suggest that preimmunotherapy immunocompetence as well as dose of
immunopotentiating agent play an important role in the eventual outcome of immunotherapy. A combination of vigorous immunity with the high dose of BCG results in the
best prognosis; a combination of relatively weak immunity with a low dose of BCG results
in the worst prognosis.

B. Adjuvant Therapy in Duke's C Colorectal Carcinoma

Twenty-six of fifty-eight patients received BCG alone. The disease-free interval of
this group is shown in Fig. 8. Five of twenty-six patients have relapsed and the 75
percentile is 15.1 months compared to 10.1 months in the controls ($p = 0.12$). The two
deaths in the whole study occurred in the BCG alone group (Fig. 9). The 75 percentile of
surviving patients has not been reached yet, but since these two deaths occurred relatively
early (6 and 13 months) the p value is estimated at 0.18.

Further analysis with break-down according to the number of involved mesenteric
lymph nodes, among both the treated patients and the controls, revealed that at the
time of analysis, BCG alone appeared to confer statistically significant protection in
terms of the disease-free interval and survival among patients who had six or more

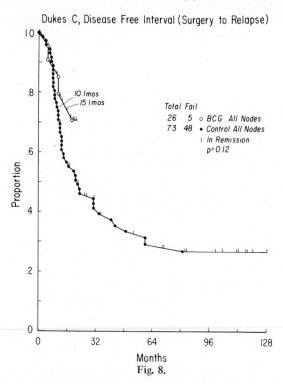

Fig. 8.

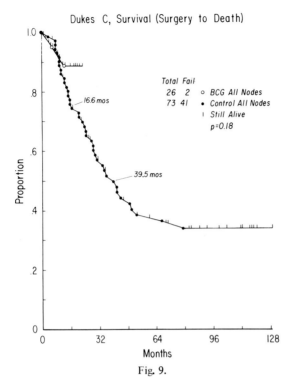

Fig. 9.

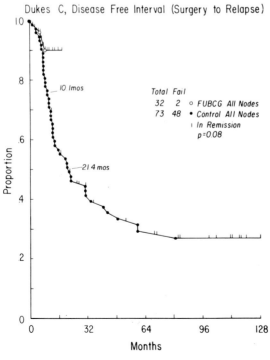

Fig. 10.

involved lymph nodes, and only marginal protection among patients with five or less involved lymph nodes. However, the sub-groups are too small and more cases are needed before a more conclusive statement can be made.

   Thirty-two of fifty-eight patients received the combination of 5-FU plus BCG. The disease-free interval of this group is shown in Fig. 10. Only two of thirty-two patients have relapsed and the 75 percentile has not been reached yet with an estimated *p* value of 0.08 compared to the controls. More striking is the total survival of patients who have received 5-FU plus BCG (Fig. 11). No death has occurred among the thirty-two patients. The two patients who had a relapse went into a complete and a partial remission respectively by using more intensive chemotherapy. In the one who achieved the complete remission, disease was detected in the liver (positive liver scan, elevation of LDH, persistent elevation of CEA). After three courses of combination chemotherapy with Methyl CCNU, Methotrexate, and Ftorafur plus weekly vaccinations with BCG, the liver scan, LDH, and plasma CEA levels all returned to normal.

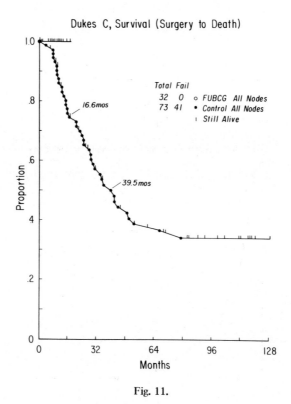

Fig. 11.

   Further break-down according to the number of involved lymph nodes among treated (5-FU plus BCG) patients and controls revealed that the combination of 5-FU plus BCG conferred statistically significant protection in terms of disease-free interval and survival regardless of the number of lymph nodes involved. Again, the numbers are still too small and more follow-up time is needed before a definitive conclusion can be drawn.

C. Chemoimmunotherapy of Metastatic Breast Cancer

Forty-five patients received an adequate trial of one or more courses of therapy (see ref. 33 for details). Thirty-four (75.5%) patients achieved a partial or complete remission. Fourteen patients (30%) had a complete remission and twenty (43%) achieved a partial remission. The disease was stable for two or more months in nine of forty-five patients (20%); only two patients (4.5%) had a progression of their disease. These results are essentially the same reported previously for the FAC without BCG regimen.

The duration of remission for patients achieving a partial remission with FAC-BCG compared to FAC alone is shown in Fig. 12. Seventeen of twenty-six patients on chemotherapy alone have relapsed with a median time to relapse with a projected media to $10\frac{1}{2}$ months. The differences are significant at the 0.009 level.

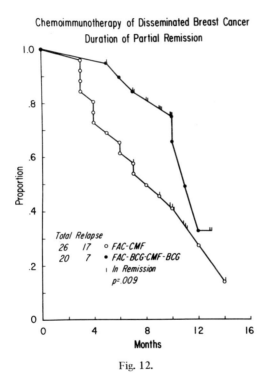

Fig. 12.

Only two of six chemotherapy patients achieving complete remission and five of fourteen chemoimmunotherapy patients have relapsed. The durations of complete remission are identical at this time.

The survival of the FAC and FAC-BCG treated patients who achieved partial remission is shown in Fig. 13. Only one of twenty partial remission patients on FAC-BCG has died, compared to eleven of twenty who have achieved partial remission with chemotherapy alone. These differences are statistically significant at the $p = 0.02$ level. None of the fourteen FAC-BCG patients achieving complete remissions have died, compared to two of six on FAC alone.

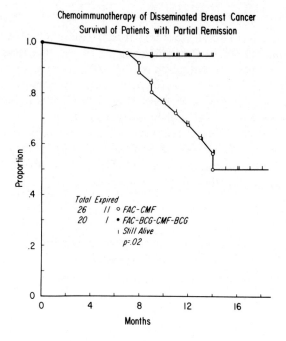

Fig. 13.

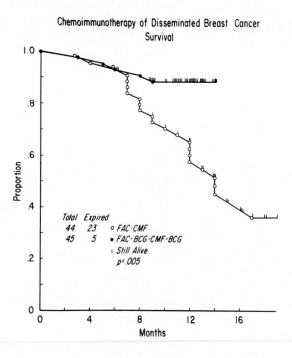

Fig. 14.

The survival of all treated patients on FAC-BCG and FAC alone is shown on Fig. 14. The median survival for FAC was 14 months which is superior to previously described combination chemotherapy programs for disseminated breast cancer. Only five of forty-five patients on chemoimmunotherapy have died. The median follow-up time is already 12+ months. The survival of the latter group is significantly longer than the former group ($p = 0.005$).

Chemoimmunotherapy was well tolerated. Although the requirement quality of supportive care was similar for both groups of patients, thrombocytopenia appeared to be less for patients on FAC-BCG compared to FAC alone.

DISCUSSION

Based on the principles first outlined by Mathé [4, 12] immunotherapy appears to be effective in the minimal residual disease situation. Specifically, patients whose solid tumor (melanoma) has spread to regional lymph nodes appear to have a delayed onset of recurrent metastases and a prolonged survival when treated with adequate trials of BCG. Although early, it appears that patients with Duke's C classification of colorectal cancer will also have a delayed recurrence time and prolonged survival.

From the detailed analysis of the melanoma study, however, many clinical as well as therapeutic variables are necessary to achieve a positive effect. In the first place, the dose of immunoadjuvant appears to be critically important in melanoma patients. Patients treated with high dose have benefited more than patients treated with a 1-log lower dose of BCG. Secondly, the principles outlined in a variety of animal model studies showing the importance of contact between BCG and tumor cells appear to be important in man [26–28]. BCG was administered to the regional lymphatics of the trunk and extremities. Patients with trunk and extremity melanoma benefited from BCG. BCG was not administered into the regional lymphatics of the head and neck region. We speculate that this regional difference may explain the lack of benefit noted in the head and neck of melanoma patients. In contrast, Morton, who achieved positive results in all regional areas, administered BCG into the head and neck lymphatics [29]. There are now at least four published studies demonstrating the efficacy of BCG in patients with regional node metastases [13, 30–32].

It is reassuring that the principles first learned from the combination of chemo-immunotherapy for disseminated melanoma have been confirmed and extended to metastatic breast cancer.

This study indicates that the prognosis of patients with disseminated breast cancer has been significantly improved by the addition of immunotherapy with living BCG organisms to combination chemotherapy. The duration of remission as well as survival of remission patients, and the overall survival of all patients on chemoimmunotherapy, are superior to results carried out immediately prior to this study with chemotherapy alone [33], as well as compared to results with combination chemotherapy or single-agent chemotherapy programs reported in the literature [34, 35].

The results, therefore, confirm and extend the principles learned from the initial combination of chemoimmunotherapy trials reported by us for malignant melanoma [20] and acute myelogenous leukemia [9]. In these studies, remission rates were not significantly increased (except for tumor sites regional to BCG scarification), but remission durations and overall survival were significantly increased with chemoimmuno-

248
CLINICAL TUMOR IMMUNOLOGYCLINICAL TUMOR IMMUNOLOGY

therapy compared to chemotherapy alone. Thus, this is the first disseminated malignant disease of high incidence wherein immunotherapy combined with chemotherapy has been shown to significantly improve prognosis.

Despite the encouraging and positive results with BCG, improved modalities of immunotherapy and combination chemotherapy are needed to increase the remission rates in visceral regions as well as shift the balance of partial remissions to complete remissions. Recently, Currie and co-workers reported that a combination of active specific (tumor cells) combined with non-specific BCG immunization improved the remission rates in melanoma compared to the use of chemotherapy alone [36]. We have confirmed these results in a small series of melanoma patients [37] and will begin to test this combination in metastatic breast cancer. In addition, we have speculated that the delivery of an intravenous adjuvant into the visceral areas, such as liver and lungs, may improve response rates compared to the use of BCG by scarification. This hypothesis has been tested in metastatic melanoma and has confirmed that response rates for patients with liver metastases may be improved by this modality of therapy [37]. Thus, the use of intravenous *C. parvum* or intravenous BCG may be a logical next step in the management of disseminated breast cancer.

Since the maximal benefit of immunotherapy with living BCG organisms may be limited by the wide range of viable/non-viable counts in various lots of BCG as well as by the differences in anti-tumor activity of various strains, the use of more standardized non-viable preparations of mycobacterial and other bacterial organisms or synthetic immunopotentiating agents should be evaluated in breast cancer. MER, a non-viable extract of BCG, has prolonged survival in acute myelogenous leukemia [38]. Levamisole, a synthetic immunopotentiating agent, prolonged disease-free interval and survival in resectable breast cancer [39]. *Corynebacterium parvum* plus chemotherapy has prolonged survival in patients with metastatic breast cancer compared to chemotherapy alone [40].

Finally, since adjuvant chemotherapy alone has been shown to prolong disease-free interval and survival in patients with histologic evidence of spread of regional lymph nodes [42, 42], programs of combination chemotherapy and active immunotherapy are now indicated early in the disease.

Additional immunotherapeutic approaches with possible different mechanisms of action and toxicity that should be combined with BCG include a transfer factor which has shown activity in breast cancer [43]. Additionally, since there is increasing evidence that tumor viruses are related to the pathogenesis and/or etiology of breast cancer the use of anti-viral and anti-tumor substances such an Interferon which has prolonged the disease-free interval in operable osteogenic sarcoma patients [44] needs to be investigated.

In conclusion, further trials of immunotherapy and immunochemotherapy of early and disseminated solid tumors are clearly warranted. With increased understanding of the host—tumor relationships [45], the application of scientifically sound programs of cellular engineering [46] should lead to improved prognosis of cancer patients over the next decade.

REFERENCESREFERENCES

1. H.C. Nauts: *The Apparently Beneficial Effects of Bacterial Infection on Host Resistance to Cancer.* New York Cancer Research Institute (Monograph 8), 1969.
2. E.M. Hersh, J.U. Gutterman and G.M. Mavligit: *Immunotherapy of Cancer in Man—Scientific*1. H.C. Nauts: *The Apparently Beneficial Effects of Bacterial Infection on Host Resistance to Cancer.* New York Cancer Research Institute (Monograph 8), 1969.
2. E.M. Hersh, J.U. Gutterman and G.M. Mavligit: *Immunotherapy of Cancer in Man—Scientific*

Basis and Current Status. Monograph, Springfield, Illinois, Charles C. Thomas, Publishers, 1973, 141 pp

3. J.U. Gutterman, G.M. Mavligit, R.C. Reed and E.M. Hersh: Immunochemotherapy of human cancer. *Seminars in Oncology,* **1,** 409–423 (1974).

4. G. Mathé, J.L. Amiel, L. Schwarzenberg *et al.*: Active immunotherapy for acute lymphoblastic leukemia. *Lancet,* **1,** 697–699 (1969).

5. E. Klein and O.A. Holtermann: Immunotherapeutic approaches to the management of neoplasms. *Nat. Cancer Inst. Monogr.* **35,** 379–402 (1972).

6. D.L. Morton, F.R. Eilber, R.A. Malmgren *et al.*: Immunological factors which influence response to immunotherapy in malignant melanoma. *Surgery,* **68,** 158–164 (1970).

7. R.L. Powles, D. Crowther, C.J.T. Bateman *et al.*: Immunotherapy for acute myelogeneous leukemia. *Br. J. Cancer,* **28,** 365–376 (1973).

8. W.R. Vogler and Y-K. Chan: Prolonging remission in myeloblastic leukemia by Tice-strain Bacillus Calmette-Guerin. *Lancet,* **2,** 128–131.

9. J.U. Gutterman, E.M. Hersh, V. Rodriguez, K.B. McCredie, G. Mavligit, R. Reed, M.A. Burgess, T. Smith, E. Gehan, G.P. Bodey, Sr. and E.J. Freireich: Chemoimmunotherapy of adult acute leukemia: prolongation of remission in myeloblastic leukemia with BCG. *Lancet,* **2,** 1405–1409 (1974).

10. M. Whiteside, *Immunotherapy of Acute Myeloblastic Leukemia, Cancer* (in press).

11. J. Whitaker, Personal communication.

12. G. Mathé: Active immunotherapy. *Adv. Cancer Res.* **14,** 1–36 (1971).

13. J.U. Gutterman, G. Mavligit, C. McBride, E. Frei, III, E.J. Freireich and E.M. Hersh: Active immunotherapy of recurrent malignant melanoma with systemic BCG. *Lancet,* **1,** 1208–1212 (1973).

14. D.L. Morton, R.A. Malmgren, E.C. Holmes and A.S. Ketcham: Demonstration of antibodies against human malignant melanoma by immunofluorescence. *Surgery,* **64,** 233–240 (1968).

15. M.G. Lewis, R.L. Ikonopisov, R.C. Nairn *et al.*: Tumour-specific antibodies in human malignant melanoma and their relationship to the extent of the disease. *Br. Med. J.* **3,** 517–522 (1969).

16. G. Mavligit, J.U. Gutterman, C.M. McBride and E.M. Hersh: Tumor-directed immune reactivity and immunotherapy in malignant melanoma. Current status. *Prog. Exp. Tumor Res.* **19,** 222–252 (1974).

17. J.U. Gutterman, G. Mavligit, R. Reed, S.P. Richman, C.M. McBride and E.M. Hersh: Immunology and immunotherapy of human malignant melanoma: historical review and perspectives for the future. *Seminars in Oncology,* **2,** 155–174 (1975).

18. G.M. Mavligit, J.U. Gutterman, M.A. Burgess, J.F. Speer, R.C. Reed, R.C. Martin, C.M. McBride, E.M. Copeland, E.A. Gehan and E.M. Hersh: Immunotherapy: its possible application in the management of large bowel cancer. *Amer. J. Digest. Dis.* **19,** 1047–1053 (1974).

19. G.M. Mavligit, J.U. Gutterman, M.A. Burgess, N. Khankhanian, G.B. Seibert, J.F. Speer, R.C. Reed, A.V. Jubert, R.C. Martin, C.M. McBride, E.M. Copeland, E.A. Gehan and E.M. Hersh: Adjuvant immunotherapy and chemoimmunotherapy in colorectal cancer of the Duke's C Classification. Preliminary results. *Cancer,* **36,** 2421–2427 (1975).

20. J.U. Gutterman, G.M. Mavligit, J.A. Gottlieb, M.A. Burgess, C.M. McBride, L. Einhorn, E.J. Freireich and E.M. Hersh: Chemoimmunotherapy of disseminated malignant melanoma with dimethyl trizeno imidazole carboxamide and Bacillus Calmette-Guerin. *New Eng. J. Med.* **291,** 592–597 (1974).

21. R.A. Minow, R.S. Benjamin and J.A. Gottlieb: Adriamycin cardiomyopathy, an overview with determination of risk factors. *Cancer Chemotherapy Reports* (in press).

22. J.O. Cardenas, J.U. Gutterman, J.A. Gottlieb *et al.* (submitted for publication).

23. S.J. Cutler: The prognosis of treated breast cancer. In: *Prognostic Factors in Breast Cancer* A.P. Forrest, P.B. Kunkler, Edinburgh and London, E. & S. Livingston Ltd., 1968. pp. 20–31.

24. E.A. Gehan: A generalized Wilcoxon test for comparing arbitrarily singly-censored samples. *Biometrika,* **52,** 203–223 (1965).

25. E.L. Kaplan and P. Meier: Non-parametric estimation from incomplete observations. *J. Amer. Stat. Ass.* **53,** 457–481 (1958).

26. B. Zbar, I.D. Bernstein and H.J. Rapp: Suppression of tumor growth at the site of infection with living Bacillus Calmette-Guerin. *J. Nat. Cancer Inst.* **46,** 831–839 (1971).

27. R.W. Baldwin and M.V. Pimm: BCG immunotherapy of rat tumors of defined immunogenicity. *Nat. Cancer Inst. Monogr.* **39,** 11–17 (1973).

28. L. Milas, J.U. Gutterman, I. Basic, N. Hunter, G. Mavligit, E.M. Hersh and H.R. Withers: Immunoprophylaxis and immunotherapy for a murine fibrosarcoma with *C. granulosum* and *C. parvum. Int. J. Cancer,* **14,** 493–503 (1974).

29. F.R. Eilber, D.L. Morton, E.C. Holmes, F.C. Sparks and K.P. Ramming: Immunotherapy with BCG for lymph node metastases from malignant melanoma. *New Engl. J. Med.* **294,** 237–240 (1976).

30. A.Z. Bluming, C.L. Vogel, J.L. Ziegler *et al.*: Immunological effects of BCG in malignant melanoma: two modes of administration compared. *Ann. Int. Med.* **76**, 405–411 (1972).
31. D.L. Morton, F.R. Eilber, E.C. Holmes, J.S. Hunt, A.S. Ketcham, M.J. Silverstein and F.C. Sparks: BCG immunotherapy of malignant melanoma. A seven year experience. *Ann. Surgery,* **180**, 635–643 (1974).
32. R.L. Ikonopisov: The use of BCG in the combined treatment of malignant melanoma. *Behring Inst. Mitt.* **56**, 206–214 (1975).
33. J.U. Gutterman, G.M. Mavligit, M.A. Burgess, J.O. Cardenas, G.R. Blumenschein, J.A. Gottlieb, C.M. McBride, K.B. McCredie, G.P. Bodey, V. Rodriguez, E.J. Freireich and E.M. Hersh: Immuno-therapy of human solid tumors and acute leukemia with BCG: Prolongation of disease free interval and survival. *Cancer Immunol. Immunoth.* (in press, 1976).
34. R. Cooper: Combination chemotherapy in hormone resistant breast cancer. *Proc. Am. Ass. Cancer Res.* 10–15 (1969).
35. S.K. Carter: The chemical therapy of breast cancer. *Seminars in Oncology,* **1**, 131–141 (1974).
36. G.A. Currie and T.J. McElwain: Active immunotherapy as an adjunct to chemotherapy in the treatment of disseminated malignant melanoma. A pilot study. *Br. J. Cancer,* **31**, 143–156 (1975).
37. J.U. Gutterman: unpublished data.
38. D.W. Weiss, Y. Stupp, N. Many and C. Izak: Treatment of acute myelocytic leukemia (AML) patients with the MER tubercle bacillus fraction: a preliminary report. *Transplant Proc.* **7**, 545–552 (1975).
39. A.F. Rojas, E. Mickiewicz, J.N. Feierstein, H. Glait and A.J. Olivari: Levamisble in advanced human breast cancer. *Lancet,* **1**, 211–215 (1976).
40. L. Israel and B. Halpern: Le *Corynebacterium parvum* dans les cancers advancés. Première évaluation de l'activité thérapeutique de cette immunostimuline. *Nouv. Press. Med.* **1**, 19–23 (1972).
41. B. Fisher, P. Carbone, S.G. Economour, R. Frelick, A. Glass, H. Lerner, C. Redmond, M. Zelen, P. Band, D.L. Katrych, N. Wolmark, and E.R. Fisher: 1-Phenylalanine mustard (L-Pam) in the management of primary breast cancer. A report of early findings. *New England J. Med.* **292**, 117–122 (1975).
42. G. Bonadonna, A. Lattuada, F. Rilke and A. Banfi: Controlled study with local radiotherapy (RT) versus RT plus CTX-VCR-PRED (CVP) in non-Hodgkin's lymphoma. *Proc. Am. Ass. Cancer Res.* **16**, 188 (# 752) (1975).
43. H.F. Oettgen, L.J. Old, J.H. Farrow *et al.*: Effects of dialyzable transfer factor in patients with breast cancer. *Proc. Nat. Acad. Sci.* **71**, 2319–2323 (1974).
44. N. Strander: *J. Nat. Cancer Inst.* (in press, 1976).
45. *Immunobiology of the Tumor–Host Relationship,* edited by Richard T. Smith and Maurice Landy. Academic Press, New York, 1975. pp. 360.
46. R.A. Good: Immunodeficiencies of man and the new immunobiology. In: *Immunodeficiency in Man and Animals,* edited by D. Bergama. Sinauer Ass., Inc., Sunderland, Mass., 1975.

ABSTRACTS

ACTIVE ROSETTES IN BCG-TREATED MELANOMA PATIENTS AND UNTREATED LEUKAEMIC CHILDREN

J. Bertoglio, Annie Bourgoin, K. Gronneberg and J.F. Dore

Centre Léon Bérard, 28, rue Laënnec, 69373 Lyon Cedex 2, France

Active E-rosettes were repeatedly measured in nine melanoma patients submitted to BCG treatment, and studied in nine children with untreated acute lymphoblastic leukaemia.

Each melanoma patient in this study was tested on three to six occasions over a period of time extending from 2 to 5 months. Four of them were under BCG treatment for at least 7 months at the time of the first determination and showed stable values within the normal range (27.9 ± 4.9%, as determined in twenty normal healthy donors). The five other patients were tested first at the beginning of the treatment and showed values increasing steadily from the lower normal limit to the upper one. In these patients, no significant variation in membrane immunoglobulin bearing-lymphocytes (B-cells) was seen over the same period of time, whereas T (E-rosettes forming) lymphocytes remained stable or showed a tendency to decrease. Active E-rosettes being considered as reflecting a subpopulation of differentiated T-cells, these results would indicate that BCG treatment could eventually act through differentiation of T-cells.

In two of the leukaemia patients, more than 90% of the blast cells were found to form E-rosettes and active rosette formation could be demonstrated in 10% and 20% of the blast cells respectively. In two other patients 10% and 37% of the blast cells were respectively shown to form E-rosettes but no active rosettes. These results seem to indicate that leukaemic lymphoblasts may form active rosettes.

LONG-TERM IMMUNOLOGICAL STUDIES IN PATIENTS WITH ADVANCED COLORECTAL CANCER

B.R. Bullen, G.R. Giles, T.G. Brennan

St James's Hospital, Leeds, Great Britain

It is generally stated that patients with advanced malignant disease are immunosuppressed, thus allowing their tumour to progress. We have examined some immune reactions in patients with advanced colorectal cancer over a period of from 5 to 14 months. Our aim was to obtain an assessment of the changes of the immune status of patients with metastatic cancer with time, and relate these studies to the course of the malignant process.

Nine patients were studied and their immune status assessed monthly by means of a dose response of lymphocyte transformation to phytohacmagglutinin (PHA), leucocyte migration in the presence of colonic tumour antigen, plasma protein electrophoresis, immunoglobulin and carcinoembryonic antigen (CEA) levels. All patients received intermittent chemotherapy throughout the study.

Results

Mean CEA levels increased with time but were only markedly elevated in four patients. PHA responses showed a tendency to improve towards normality, four of the six patients who died during the study having normal PHA transformation studies at their last investigation. Evidence of blocking in autologous serum was only found in two patients.

At the beginning of the study only one-third of the patients exhibited sensitization to tumour antigen in the leucocyte migration assay. With time this proportion improved to more than 75% exhibiting sensitization. The only patient failing to show any sensitization in autologous or homologous sera at any time had the poorest prognosis. Plasma protein electrophoresis appeared normal apart from the α_2 globulins which were elevated in those patients having the shortest survival times. IgC, IgM and IgA levels remained largely within normal limits throughout the study.

Conclusions

The immunologically suppressed state of patients with advanced colorectal cancer may be improved by simple symptomatic treatment and intermittent chemotherapy. However, a return of normal immunological parameters is not necessarily associated with control of the malignant process.

IMMUNOLOGICAL STUDIES DURING IMMUNOTHERAPY IN CHRONIC MYELOCYTIC LEUKEMIA

Nicole Carpentier-Bricteux and Gerard Degiovanni

Institut de Médecine, département d'Hématologie (Pr. J. Hugues) et département de Chirurgie expérimentale (Pr. G. Lejeune), Université de Liège, Belgique

In an attempt to prevent blastic crisis, twenty patients with chronic myelocytic (CML), controlled by chemotherapy, were given immune stimulation: thirteen with BCG plus allogeneic blast cells, seven with BCG alone. Immunizing cells were derived from three lymphoid tissue culture cell lines established from the peripheral blood of a patient with acute myelogenous leukemia (RPMI 6410) and two patients with blastic crisis of CML (RPMB 7642 and 7481). These cells have been shown to carry antigens specifically associated with leukemic myeloblasts (Metzgar and Sokal, 1975). During immunotherapy, all patients increased their skin test reactivity versus antigens unrelated to the immune stimulation (Varidase, Candida and Trichophyton extracts) as well as to components of the vaccine mixture (PPD, fetal calf serum, cell homogenates). The K-cell cytotoxic activity of circulating lymphocytes was assessed *in vitro* against antibody-coated normal human and heterologous cultured target cells. This non-specific cytotoxicity varied greatly from patient to patient but remained unchanged during vaccination. Nineteen of the twenty patients failed to develop an *in vitro* direct cell-mediated immune response against the immunizing blast cells. In contrast to those stimulated by BCG alone, all patients receiving blasts developed highly efficient antibodies cytotoxic for these cells either in presence of complement or of normal lymphoid cells. This humoral immune response increased continuously, reaching a plateau after the sixth vaccination. Part of the antibodies seemed to be directed against transplantation antigens; after their absorption with normal lymphocytes, a significant cytotoxicity of the antisera against normal PHA-stimulated lymphocytes was lost while no substantial decrease of the humoral cytotoxicity to immunizing cells was recorded. These results suggest the development of a specific antibody activity against leukemia associated antigens during immunotherapy of CML with allogeneic blast cells.

PROGNOSTIC CORRELATIONS IN MALIGNANT MELANOMA

A.L. Claudy, J. Viac, N. Pelletier, N. Fouad-Wassef, A. Alario and J. Thivolet

Laboratoire d'Immunopathologie, Clinique Dermatologique, Hôpital Edouard Herriot, 69374, Lyon Cedex 2, France

Fifty-two patients with malignant malanoma were studied histologically and by various assays to determine cell mediated immune responses. Delayed cutaneous reactivity to tuberculin, candidin and DNCB, PHA and PWM induced lymphocyte blastogenesis and total E-rosette count are not statistically impaired compared to normal individuals. The active E-rosette count drops significantly below 15% among patients whose tumour is growing rapidly, and return to normal quickly after starting chemotherapy (BCG therapy was ineffective to modify the counts). The fall of active E-rosette count occurred on average 1.52 months before the clinical appearance of metastasis. No hypothesis can be advanced for the reason why a fall in the percentage of active E-rosette count below 15% in melanoma patients means a poor prognosis. A direct correlation between histological data, active E-rosette count and evolution can be demonstrated. Two-thirds of patients with superficial spreading melanomas have both normal active E-rosette counts and a long survival, while only half of patients with nodular melanomas have normal active E-rosette count and a shorter survival. According to these data, melanoma patients can be subdivided into five groups in terms of prognosis:

1. nodular melanomas with a deep level of invasion and a low active E-rosette count: poor prognosis;
2. nodular melanomas with a high active E-rosette count: careful follow up, uncertain prognosis;
3. superficial spreading melanomas with a high active E-rosette count: good prognosis;
4. superficial spreading melanomas with a low active E-rosette count: uncertain prognosis;
5. lentigo maligna melanomas with a constant high active E-rosette count: excellent prognosis.

The results suggest that both the histopathological findings and the active E-rosette count may be valuable tests to help assess the prognosis in malignant melanoma patients.

FAILURE OF ALLOGENEIC LEUKEMIC CELLS TO STIMULATE IN MIXED LYMPHOCYTE CULTURE

D. Collavo, G. Biasi, A. Colombatti and L. Chieco-Bianchi

Laboratory of Experimental Oncology, Institute of Pathological Anatomy, University of Padova

Studies on mixed lymphocyte reaction (MLR) in humans suggest that lymphoblastoid cell lines, which have the characteristics of thymus-derived (T) lymphocytes, fail to activate normal allogeneic lymphocytes. In contrast, leukemic cell lines, which have bone-marrow-derived (B) lymphocytes characteristics, are potent stimulators.

We have observed that both primary virus-induced murine leukemias and murine leukemic cell lines induced by virus, chemical or physical agents do not stimulate normal spleen cells differing at the H-2 complex or at M-locus. Repeated attempts to detect inhibitory factors possibly secreted in the culture medium by a transplantable Moloney virus-induced leukemia (YC8) gave negative results. Similarly, no important variations were observed when YC8 cells were pretreated with neuraminidase, to enhance their antigenicity, or preincubated to shed potentially masking immunoglobulins bound to the cell surface. Using a "three-party" system, an adherent fraction of the leukemic cells interfered with the MLR of normal allogeneic cells. Nevertheless, even after removal of this cell fraction non-adherent leukemic cells did not stimulate normal allogeneic lymphocytes.

The characterization of the leukemic cell populations used, as to their T- or B-cell origin, revealed that in all cases T-cell markers are present. Since evidence exists that I-region associated antigens (Ia) (which may be related to MLR activating determinants) and M-locus stimulatory products are absent or weakly expressed on T-cells, the T-cell origin of tumors is a possible explanation of their lack of stimulating capacity.

In a ^{51}Cr release assay, leukemic cells were able to generate *in vitro* cytotoxic T-lymphocytes (CTL). The tumor cells could sensitize allogeneic normal lymphocytes to kill specifically normal as well as leukemic targets, even when no stimulation was detected in parallel mixed lymphocyte cultures.

These results indicate that killer cell generation does not depend on the stimulatory capacity of the sensitizing cells.

INTERACTION OF ANTIMICROCOCCUS ANTIBODIES WITH THE LYMPHOID SYSTEM

P. de Baetselier, R. Hooghe, J. Grooten, C. Hamers-Casterman and R. Hamers

Different bacterial vaccines have been used in cancer immunotherapy with some success. However, the mode of action of these vaccines is still not fully understood. Some of these vaccines can elicit very high levels of homogeneous antibody populations to the bacterial cell wall components. These produced anti-carbohydrates share the same specificity as plants lectins (*N*-acetylglucose-amine, fucose, glucose) and like the latter would interfere with the immune system.

The following observations support this idea:

1. Rabbit antimicrococcus antibodies exert a significant immuno-suppressive-like action when injected in new-born mice. Half of the litter population was injected with antimicrococcus antibodies, the other half with pool rabbit immunoglobulins. After the treatment an amplification of IgM synthesis (between 10 and 57%) and a depletion of IgG level (between 0 and 45%) was observed in the experimental mice.

2. Fluorescent rabbit anticarbohydrates (prepared from antimicrococcal antisera) bind on rabbit lymphocytes with typical spot and cap formation. The percentage of labelled cells (between 2 and 10%) depends on the anticarbohydrate used and rabbit lymphocytes tested.

3. These fluorescent anticarbohydrates also bind on certain well-established cell lines. They appear to be more selective than fluorescent ConA which binds all the cell lines tested. The antitumor immunoprotection with bacterial vaccines may be conferred by an immune response to the bacterial cell wall carbohydrates. These antibodies elicited in the response would cross-react with tumor polysaccharide and this might inhibit tumor growth. On the other hand, our results suggest that the produced anticarbohydrates bind on their own lymphocytes. This would indicate a breakdown of tolerance against the host membrane components, and would lead to detrimental auto-immune effects.

CYTOTOXIC EFFECTS OF LYMPHOCYTES FROM MELANOMA PATIENTS AND HEALTHY DONORS TESTED IN PARALLEL ON MELANOMA CELLS FROM SHORT-TERM CULTURES, A CELL LINE (NKI-4) AND T24 BLADDER CARCINOMA CELLS. PRESENCE OF TAA ON NKI-4 CELLS?

Jan E. de Vries and Philip Rümke

The Netherlands Cancer Institute Dept. of Immunology, Sarphatistraat 108, Amsterdam

By means of a microcytotoxicity test, using target cells from melanoma cell lines, we found that lymphocytes from healthy donors showed cytotoxic effects to the same extent as did lymphocytes from melanoma patients. To see whether in addition to these "spontaneous" cytotoxic effects, melanoma specific reactions were still detectable (demonstrating the presence of TAA on melanoma cells after prolonged culture) lymphocytes from fourteen stage I, six stage II, thirty-two stage III melanoma patients and thirty-nine healthy donors were as far as possible tested in parallel on target cells from eighteen different short-term cultures, a melanoma cell line (NKI-4) and a bladder-carcinoma cell line (T24).

Compared to a medium control, lymphocytes from healthy donors and melanoma patients showed more frequent and stronger cytotoxic effects on NKI-4 than on T24 cells. Within the different lymphocyte donor groups enormous variations in cytoxic effects were found. However, stage I and II melanoma patients showed significant stronger mean cytotoxic effects on NKI-4 cells than did lymphocytes from the healthy donor group, whereas the mean cytotoxic effects on NKI-4 cells were also significantly stronger than on T24 cells. This may indicate that in addition to "spontaneous" cytotoxic effects, specific reactions towards NKI-4 cells might be present.

Lymphocytes from healthy donors showed in general no or weak cytotoxic effects on melanoma cells from short-term cultures, whereas lymphocytes from melanoma patients showed in about 40% of the cases tested significant cytotoxic effects. This implies that the use of melanoma cells from short-term cultures in a standardized way may enable us to monitor individual patients during the course of the disease. So more attention has to be focused on the use of target cells from short-term cultures, particularly since these cells also reflect much more than the *in vivo* situation.

LYMPHOCYTE POPULATIONS IN CHRONIC LYMPHOCYTIC LEUKEMIA (CLL)

H.-D. Flad,[*] C. Huber,[†] K. Bremer,[‡] U. Fink [§] and H. Huber[†]

Lymphocytes of the peripheral blood and thoracic duct lymph were studied in patients with CLL and patients with non-hematological diseases. When stimulated *in vitro* with PHA lymph lymphocytes of CLL patients responded markedly as determined by ^{14}C-thymidine incorporation, whereas blood lymphocytes showed a delayed or diminished response. The response of blood and lymph lymphocytes of control patients was equal. Using purified[125] I-labelled antisera against K-, λ-, μ-

and γ-chains and radioautography it was found that the percentage of lymphocytes bearing K and μ determinants was higher in the blood than in the lymph. Control patients showed a much lower percentage of lymphocytes with immunoglobulins, which was equal in blood and lymph. Preliminary experiments suggest that the antibody-dependent lymphocyte mediated cytotoxicity is diminished in the blood of CLL patients compared to the cytotoxic activity found in the blood of normal individuals. Furthermore, the membrane dynamics of HL-A-anti-HL-A complexes on the surface of blood and lymph lymphocytes were studied by means of membrane fluorescence. In CLL, the percentage of lymph lymphocytes showing "cap formation" within 2 hr was higher in the lymph than in the blood. Using autotransfused ^{3}H-cytidine labeled blood lymphocytes, it is shown that the recovery of labeled cells in the lymph of CLL patients within 48 hr is diminished compared to controls.

It is concluded that in CLL the leukemic cells are B-cells whose capacity to recirculate from blood to lymph is impaired. Only a minor population of PHA-responsive T-cells appears to recirculate normally. Consequently, the concentration of T-cells is higher in the lymph than in the blood, and the leukemic B-lymphocytes accumulate in the vascular pool. The impaired ability for recirculation and "cap formation" suggests a membrane abnormality of the CLL cell. (Supported by Deutsche Forschungsgemeinschaft and Oesterreichische Forschungsfond).

* Department of Clinical Physiology, University of Ulm, Ulm, Germany.
† Department of Medicine, University of Innsbruck, Innsbruck, Austria.
‡ Department of Medicine, Division of Haematology, University of Essen, Essen, Germany.
§ Division of Haematology, Department of Medicine, Technical University of Munich, Munich, Germany.

ACTIVE IMMUNOTHERAPY IN ACUTE MYELOID LEUKAEMIA

C.B. Freeman, G.M. Taylor and R. Harris

Department of Medical Genetics, St. Mary's Hospital, Manchester M13 0JH

C.G. Geary, J. E. MacIver, I.W. Delamore

University Department of Clinical Haematology, Manchester Royal Infirmary, Manchester M13

The duration of first remission (23 weeks) in a small group (7) of acute myeloid leukaemia (AML) patients maintained with irradiated allogeneic leukaemic cells and BCG, after initial induction and consolidation chemotherapy, was similar to that achieved in comparable trials using conventional chemotherapy [1]. In a second series of twenty patients in the MRC 6th AML trial, to whom the same immunotherapy was given but without prior consolidation chemotherapy, the median duration of first remission was considerably shorter (11 weeks).

Compared with patients receiving other therapeutic protocols, there was a remarkably high reinduction rate following relapse in both series of patients maintained with immunotherapy alone. In the first trial five out of six (83%) have achieved a second remission, one patient has achieved a total of six and another three remissions. In the second trial fourteen out of twenty have achieved second remissions, five have had three remissions and two patients are now in their 4th remission. The overall survival figures for both groups are encouraging, in group 1 four out of seven patients are alive with a current mean survival of 120 weeks and in group 2, ten out of twenty are alive with a current mean survival of 65 weeks.

The high reinduction rate may result from (1) a beneficial effect of immunotherapy, (2) the avoidance of drug resistance subsequent upon the use of less chemotherapy, (3) the avoidance of drug-induced immunosuppression, (4) early diagnosis of relapse or a combination of these factors. Preliminary data from all centres involved in the MRC 6th AML trial would indicate that patients receiving immunotherapy have a higher second remission rate than those patients maintained on the same chemotherapy alone (immunotherapy plus chemotherapy 11/20 second remissions (55%), chemotherapy alone 2/8 second remissions (25%)). Although the numbers are small these figures could be most readily explained if it is postulated that immunotherapy is exerting some beneficial effect.

1. Freeman *et al.*, *Brit. Med. J.* 4, 571–573 (1973).

CIRCULATING CARCINOEMBRYONIC ANTIGEN (CEA) LEVELS IN AUSTRALIAN NORMAL AND HOSPITAL POPULATIONS

M.A. Frost and A.S. Coates

*The Walter and Eliza Hall Institute of Medical Research,
and the Royal Melbourne Hospital, Victoria, Australia*

In a study designed to assess the value of current available methods for immunodiagnosis of human cancer, circulating carcinoembryonic antigen (CEA), levels were measured in 124 healthy control subjects not selected by smoking history, and in 425 hospital patients, by the zirconyl phosphate gel radioimmunoassay method using materials supplied by Hoffman-La Roche Inc.

The mean value obtained for normal persons was 2.2 ng/ml (± 1.2 ng/ml S.D.) giving a range of 0–4.6 ng/ml. No effect of age, sex or ABO blood group on CEA levels was found. Of 124 normal persons, two (1.6%) gave values exceeding 5 ng/ml. Among hospital patients highly elevated CEA levels exceeding 20 ng/ml were obtained in forty-six patients: forty-five of these (98%) had a diagnosis of cancer. Moderately elevated levels, 10–20 ng/ml, were obtained in nineteen patients; eleven of these (58%) had a diagnosis of cancer. Mildly elevated levels, 5–10 ng/ml, were obtained in sixty-seven patients; only twenty-three of these (34%) had cancer.

Conversely of the 110 cancer patients studied, 65% had CEA levels exceeding 5 ng/ml, 46% exceeded 10 ng/ml and 38% exceeded 20 ng/ml. Values exceeding 20 ng/ml were more frequent in patients with metastatic cancer (42%) than localized cancer (27%).

Cigarette smoking was found to be significantly associated with elevated CEA levels among the 257 patients with non-malignant diseases; 32% of those patients smoking more than 15 cigarettes daily had elevated CEA levels, compared with (8%) of other patients with similar diseases. The prevalence of elevated CEA levels among patients with non-malignant diseases increased progressively according to the number of cigarettes smoked daily; 8% of non- and ex-smokers, 22% of light smokers (1–14 cigarettes daily), 31% of moderate smokers (15–29 cigarettes daily) and 39% of heavy smokers (30 or more cigarettes daily) had CEA levels exceeding 5 ng/ml.

A similar relationship between the prevalence of elevated CEA levels and number of cigarettes smoked daily was also found among the normal population of the town of Busselton in Western Australia.

Thus highly elevated levels were virtually specific for cancer, while moderately and mildly elevated levels were correspondingly less specific, occurring also in patients with non-malignant diseases, particularly those who smoked.

INCREASED EXPRESSION OF A NORMAL LYMPHOCYTE MEMBRANE ANTIGEN ON CHRONIC LYMPHATIC LEUKEMIA CELLS

A. Hekman

The Netherlands Cancer Institute, Amsterdam, Holland

Rabbit antisera against 3 M KCl extracts from tonsil lymphocytes were found to show a consistently stronger reaction with CLL cells than with normal peripheral lymphocytes, without absorption. The degree of difference between the two cell types was not the same with different methods. In complement-dependent methods the antisera reacted with CLL cells to high titers (*ca.* 1/40 in cytotoxicity, 1/128 in immunoadherence, 1/32 in immunofluorescence with an anti-C_3' conjugate), whereas reactions with normal lymphocytes were often negative, with occasional titers up to 1/4. Nevertheless the antisera could be completely absorbed with normal lymphocytes, for which approximately twice as many normal cells as CLL cells were needed. In immunofluorescence with an anti-Ig conjugate and in immunoferritin labeling experiments normal lymphocytes always gave a positive reaction. Reactions with CLL cells were again about twice as strong. From these data it may be concluded that these antisera detect an antigen of the normal lymphocyte membrane that on CLL cells is increased to approximately twice the normal amount. For reasons as yet unknown the reaction of normal lymphocytes in C'-dependent methods is much weaker than would be expected from the amount of antigen present as detected by other methods.

The increase in antigen expression seems to be specific for CLL cells. Control cells included lymphocytes from cord blood and from patients with infectious mononucleosis, and two lymphoid cell lines, Raji and EB-3. The few cases of other leukemias (2 ALL, 1 AML, 1 CML) also reacted as normal cells. Tonsil lymphocytes could not be tested because of poor viability. Separation of normal lymphocytes into T- and B-cells did not increase the cytotoxic reaction. Together with the lack of increased reactivity of B-cell lines this seems to exclude a correlation between the increased antigen expression and the B-cell character of CLL cells.

STUDIES ON THE BIOLOGICAL AND CHEMICAL NATURE OF A COMPONENT IN TRANSFER FACTOR WITH IMMUNOLOGICALLY NONSPECIFIC ACTIVITY

Kai Krohn, Arja Uotila, Pentti Gröhn, Jugani Väisänen and Kari-Matti Hiltunen

The Institute of Biomedical Sciences, University of Tampere, Tampere 52, Finland

Fractionation of human leucocyte dialysates on Sephadex G-10 yielded nine fractions, of which fractions I, III and VI could transfer Oidiomycin sensitivity: fraction VI could further induce skin sensitivity to PPD in uremic subjects. Further analysis of fraction VI on thin-layer chromatography revealed three components. Two of these were identified as tyrosine and a ribose containing nucleotide: these components were clearly contaminants from adjacent, biologically inactive fraction V. The remaining spot adsorbed u.v. light strongly at 254 nm and had a slight fluorescence at 366 nm. This spot was isolated preparately from TLC plate and analysed further for its biological and chemical character. In generalized sarcoidosis, skin reactions to six different antigens could be induced in patients who before the transfer were skin test negative but had a positive *in vitro* reaction as measured by blast transformation test. This component also increased the number of E-rosette-forming cells in cases of sarcoidosis and malignant melanoma. Chemical studies revealed no phosphorus, d-ribose and d-deoxyribose, thus definitely ruling out the possibility of the compound being a nucleotide. The nitrogen content was 14%. Ninhydrin test was negative but the spot could be stained by the *N*-halogenation—ortho—Tolidine method, a reaction specific for secondary amines. The component resisted treatment with pronase and could not be hydrolysed with 6 N HCl for 20 hr at $120°C$. We must therefore conclude that there is no proof for this active component of TF being a polynucleotide or a peptide. The component probably contains a heterocyclic ring. Our results indicate that part of TF's activity is due to the action of an immunologically nonspecific component.

CYTOTOXICITY OF HUMAN PERIPHERAL BLOOD LYMPHOCYTES FOR BLADDER CARCINOMA CELLS AND UNRELATED SHORT-TERM CULTURES

M. Moore and Nicola Robinson

Khristie Hospital and Holt Radium Institute, Patterson Laboratories, Manchester M20 9BX

In an analysis of the specificity of the cell-mediated immune reaction to carcinoma of the human urinary bladder, experiments were performed to determine the cytotoxicity of peripheral blood lymphocytes from patients with bladder carcinoma for bladder cancer (T24)- and normal bladder (HCV)-derived cell lines and as well as several unrelated human tissue-derived cells in short-term culture originating from a variety of other cancers, normal and foetal tissues. In parallel, the cytotoxicity of lymphocytes from patients with a variety of untreated malignant diseases and non-malignant genitourinary conditions was simultaneously assessed against the same targets.

Effector cells prepared from bladder cancer patients by Ficoll-Triosil sedimentation of peripheral blood were toxic for both T24 cells and several unrelated short-term cultures while under comparable conditions HCV cells and cells originating from a squamous carcinoma of skin were resistant. Greater selectivity of reactivity of bladder cancer patients' lymphocytes for T24 cells was achieved by alternative methods of lymphocyte purification, viz. defibrination of venous blood, gelatin sedimentation, nylon column incubation and Tris-NH$_4$Cl lysis of red cells. However, under these conditions of separation, effector cells from patients with unrelated cancers, not appreciably cytotoxic for targets derived from tissues other than the bladder, also frequently reduced the survival of T24 cells. The pattern of reactivity was thus one of target cell sensitivity rather than tumour- or organ-specificity. The importance of using several target cells in tests of tumour specificity and purified lymphocyte populations is emphasized in this study.

SPONTANEOUS CELL-MEDIATED CYTOTOXICITY (SCMC) OF NORMAL HUMAN LYMPHOCYTES AGAINST ^{51}Cr-LABELED HUMAN MELANOMA CELLS: A PHENOMENON MEDIATED BY LYMPHOTOXIN

H.H. Peter,[*] R.F. Eife[†] and J.R. Kalden[†]

In previous studies it was demonstrated that peripheral blood lymphocytes from healthy donors exhibit considerable SCMC when tested *in vitro* against ^{51}Cr-labeled IGR3 melanoma target cells. The lymphocytes were isolated by Ficoll density gradient centrifugation (*fraction F*), followed by removal of phagocytic and adherent cells (*fraction FFF*) and subsequent removal of cells adhering to IgG–anti-IgG columns (*fraction FFF-C*). The highest SCMC activity was found in the lymphocyte fraction depleted of mononuclear phagocytes (*fraction FFF*); activity in fraction F was slightly but not significantly lower, whereas the B-cell free fraction FFF-C showed strongly reduced SCMC although it contained the highest percentage of T-cells. Since SCMC paralleled very closely antibody-dependent cellular cytotoxicity (ADCC) at a lower level of sensitivity, it was suggested that in both assays the same non-phagocytic non-adherent, non-T-lymphocytes were operating as effector cells.

To gain further insight into the mechanism by which normal lymphocytes react against IGR3 target cells, the cell-free culture media from mixed lymphocyte tumor cell cultures (MLTC) were harvested after 6, 12 and 53 hr of incubation and tested for lymphotoxin activity (LTA) by measuring their inhibitory effect on DNA synthesis of growing target cell cultures. IGR3 and Hela monolayers served as target cells and against both cell types significant LTA was detectable already in cell-free culture media from 6-hr MLTCs with F and FFF effector lymphocytes, while only weak LTA was found in supernatants of MLTCs with FF-C lymphocytes.

The same cell-free media exhibiting LTA caused a strong increase in SCMC when added to mixtures of ^{51}Cr-labeled IGR3 target cells and freshly prepared normal lymphocytes of fractions FFF and FFF-C. This effect could not be removed by absorption of the supernatants with a solid phase rabbit–anti-human-Ig immunadsorbent, suggesting that it was not related to antibody. FFF-C lymphocytes which were unable to produce significant LTA in MLTCs with IGR3 melanoma cells induced nevertheless increased target cell lysis when reacted in SCMC assays with IGR3 target cells in the presence of LTA containing supernatants from MLTCs with FFF lymphocytes. Results from preliminary experiments indicate that the cell type in lymphocyte fraction FFF-C which cooperates with LTA belongs predominantly to the "Null" cell compartment.

In summary our data show that (a) the IGR3 melanoma cell line provides sensitive indicator cells for the estimation of LTA in both ^{51}Cr release assays and in assays measuring inhibition of DNA synthesis. (b) The production of non-specific LTA occurs in short-term MLTCs involving normal human peripheral blood lymphocytes and IGR3 melanoma cells. (c) High LTA is generated by lymphocytes of fractions F and FFF incubated with IGR3 stimulator cells, while very little LTA is generated by lymphocytes of the B-cell fraction FFF-C. (d) SCMC against IGR3 melanoma cells can be explained on the basis of a cooperation between a non-specific cytotoxic mediator produced by lymphocytes which are retained on IgG–anti-IgG columns (most likely B-cells) and an amplifying effect promoted by lymphocytes which are not retained on IgG–anti-IgG columns (most likely "Null" cells).

[*] Abteilung für Klinische Immunologie und Transfusionsmedizin, Medizinische Hochschule, Hannover, West Germany.
[†] Universitätskinderklinik, München, West Germany.

THE IMMUNE REACTION TO HUMAN BREAST CANCER TISSUE

M. Maureen Roberts

Department of Clinical Surgery, University of Edinburgh

The aim of this study was to determine the incidence of cellular and humoral immune reactions to autologous tumour in patients undergoing mastectomy for primary breast cancer. A group of patients who had benign tumours of the breast were similarly tested.

Methods

An extract of tumour tissue was prepared by high-speed centrifugation and dialysis, and the protein concentration standardized. Both supernatant and deposit fractions were tested.

The tests employed were (a) skin reactions to tumour extract and leucocyte migration using buffy coat cells in pooled human and autologous serum. Both tests were performed 21 days after mastectomy or biopsy; (b) Ouchterlony analysis and complement fixation by a micro-titre method using pre- and post-mastectomy serum samples.

Results

Cellular immunity. Only the deposit fraction of the extract gave positive reactions on either *in vivo* or *in vitro* tests. On electron microscopy this fraction was shown to contain the cell membranes. Strong positive reactions to tumour were observed in seven and moderate reactions in six of thirty-seven patients with breast cancer on skin testing. Eleven of forty patients were positive by the leucocyte migration test. Serum "blocking factors" were detected in only three patients. Identical results were found in the group of twenty-nine women with benign tumours of the breast, also tested with autologous tissue extracts. Fifteen were positive on skin testing, ten on leucocyte migration and blocking factors were detected in the serum of two patients.

Humoral immunity. Serum antibodies to breast cancer tissue were found in four of sixty patients by Ouchterlony analysis, and in two of forty tested by complement fixation. Tissue extracts of cancer were highly anti-complementary. No positive reactions were observed in a total of sixty patients with benign tumours tested by one or both methods.

Conclusion. The clinical relevance of these findings can only be determined when the prognosis of the patients is known. The incidence of cellular immune reactions at the time of mastectomy is 35% but this is also true in benign breast disease. The specificity of the reaction is therefore in doubt. On the other hand, humoral immune reactions, though infrequent, were found only in cancer, and this may be related to the abnormalities in serum and tissue immunoglobulins levels which are also present.

THE EFFECT OF RADIOTHERAPY, AND CHEMOTHERAPY AND METHANOL EXTRACTION RESIDUE OF AN ANTI-TUBERCULOSIS VACCINE ON PATIENTS WITH LUNG CANCER*

E. Robinson,[†] A. Bartal, Y. Cohen and R. Haasz

Rambam Government Hospital, The Aba Khoushy School of Medicine, Department of Oncology and Nuclear Medicine, Haifa, Israel

MER is a methanol extraction residue of BCG. It is a non-viable material which has been found to be an immunostimulant. We have previously reported that the combination of radiotherapy or chemotherapy with MER was more effective in retarding tumor growth and in prolonging the survival of tumor-bearing mice as compared to radiotherapy or chemotherapy alone. In man, phase I studies with MER have shown that it can be administered safely to patients, and that it stimulates their immune response. In the present study twenty-one patients with locally advanced or metastatic lung cancer were treated by radiotherapy and/or chemotherapy. Eleven of the patients received in addition to the conventional treatment immunotherapy by MER, and the other ten patients served as controls. MER was given on the back of the patients by ten injections each containing 0.1 mg for a total of 1.0 mg per treatment. The immunotherapy was repeated every month. Two to nine courses were given to each patient. The immune status of the patients was determined before and after each treatment by skin tests (PPD, Streptokinase–streptodornase, and candidine) and by lymphocyte culture stimulated by the same antigens and PHA.

There was no difference in the survival between the MER treated and control patients. But after MER treatment the skin reactivity to PPD became stronger (0.05 level) and the lymphocyte stimulation index to PPD and candidine becomes higher (0.02 for PPD and 0.01 for candidine).

Reports in the literature indicate a direct relationship between immunocompetence and survival in lung cancer. It seems that it is worthwhile to try the combination of conventional and MER treatment in patients with a smaller tumor load in the aim to achieve a better survival.

* This work was supported in part by a donation in memory of the late Luise Güterman, administered by the Office of the Administrator General and the Medical Research Fund.

† Associate Professor and Established Investigator of the Chief Scientist's Bureau, Ministry of Health.

ADJUVANT IMMUNOTHERAPY IN CARCINOMA OF THE PROSTATE

M.R.G. Robinson,* C.C. Rigby,† R.B.C. Pugh,† R.J. Shearer,† D.C. Dumonde‡ and L.C. Vaughan§

The prostate is a suitable organ for the direct injection of BCG (Bacille Calmette-Guerin) into tumours. A preliminary study with nine sensitized dogs has shown that intraprostatic injection of PPD (Purified Protein Derivative) produces a localized cell-mediated hypersensitivity reaction within the prostate without harming the normal tissues of the genito-urinary tract, and without producing a major constitutional disturbance.

Subsequently the prostates of six patients with advanced metastatic prostatic cancer have been injected with BCG (Glaxo Freeze-dried Vaccine) to see if adjuvant immunotherapy causes tumour destruction in this disease. The BCG has been given at weekly intervals, in increasing doses of 1 to 6 cm³, by multiple injections into the gland. Histological changes have been studied in Tru-cut needle biopsies.

The patients have not suffered a major constitutional disturbance following BCG prostatic injections, although most of them have had a mild pyrexial reaction for 48 hr. There has been no clinical evidence of damage to the urogenital tract. Two patients at post-mortem had granulomatous lesions in the lungs and liver, but none of the patients had evidence of hepatic dysfunction.

Histologically small focal granulomas have been found in the prostate after patients have received more than two injections of BCG. There has been destruction of tumour in these small areas, although adjacent tumour cells have not been affected. Four cases have shown an improvement in micturition and general condition. Two patients remained well 8 and 4 months after BCG injection respectively. One died 4 months later with carcinomatosis but no difficulty in micturition. The fourth patient died from a pulmonary embolus. Two patients have shown no subjective or objective clinical response.

Adjuvant immunotherapy with BCG should now be tried in patients with less advanced prostatic cancer, who have had the bulk of their tumour destroyed by transurethral resection and oestrogen therapy or orchidectomy.

* Pontefract General Infirmary, Yorkshire.

† Institute of Urology, London.

‡ Kennedy Institute of Rheumatology, London.

§ Royal Veterinary College, London.

ALKYLATING DRUG-CARRIER-IMMUNOGLOBULIN CONJUGATES FOR EXPERIMENTAL AND CLINICAL ANTI-CANCER THERAPY

G.F. Rowland, G.J. O'Neill and D.A.L. Davies

Searle Research Laboratories, High Wycombe, England

Drug-antibody conjugate (DRAC), designed to localize anti-cancer drugs at the tumour site, can show progressive loss of antibody activity and water-solubility with increasing levels of drug substitution. In the present work, conjugates were prepared by a technique which helps to overcome these problems. The alkylating agent phenylenediamine mustard is first linked to a carrier molecule (polyglutamic acid) using a water-soluble carbodiimide. The drug-carrier is then linked to immunoglobulin prepared from rabbit anti-mouse lymphoma serum to form a carrier linked drug-antibody conjugate ("Carrier-DRAC"). The conjugate contained 90 moles of drug per mole immunoglobulin, was water soluble and retained two-thirds of the original antibody activity. On injection into lymphoma bearing mice the conjugate was highly effective in suppressing tumour growth.

Phenylalanine mustard (Melphalan) was also linked to immunoglobulin by the carrier method. A conjugate with goat anti-human melanoma antibody was prepared containing 98 moles Melphalan per mole immunoglobulin. This preparation retained specific anti-tumour antibody activity, cross-reacting with melanoma of two patients.

EFFECT OF CHEMOTHERAPEUTIC DRUGS ON THE SENSITIVITY OF TUMOR CELLS TO KILLING BY ANTIBODY AND COMPLEMENT

M. Segerling,[*] S.H. Ohanian[†] and T. Borsos[†]

Antibody sensitized guinea-pig hepatoma cells, L-1 and L-10, are normally of higher resistance to killing by guinea-pig complement (GPC) than by human complement. This could not be ascribed to antigen expression, class of antibody, activation and fixation of the GPC components C4 and C3 to the cell surface. The high resistance to killing by GPC could be due to the lack of activation and fixation of the later acting complement components and/or repair mechanisms of cell surface sites damaged by antibody and GPC.

Seventeen hours pretreatment of the tumor cells with actinomycin D (25 μg/ml), hydroxy-urea (500 μg/ml), puromycin (20 μg/ml), mitomycin C (20 μg/ml), adriamycin (40 μg/ml) or azacytidine (20 μg/ml) render them susceptible to killing by antibody and GPC. Some preparations of tumor cells treated with cyclophosphamide (500 μg/ml), vincristine sulfate (20 μg/ml) or methotrexate (500 μg/ml) were rendered susceptible while other preparations were not rendered susceptible. Cytosine arabinoside (100 μg/ml) and 6-Mercaptopurine (500 μg/ml) and 5-Fluor-Uracile (500 μg/ml) were not effective.

The increased sensitivity to antibody-GPC mediated killing of the tumor cells was dependent of the concentration of the active drugs of the concentration of the antibody and of time and temperature. The effect of active drugs can be reversed in 7 hr and is dose and temperature dependent. The increased susceptibility of tumor cells is not due to increased expression of antigen or to increased binding of GP C4 and C3.

The studies indicate that intracellular events under metabolic and/or synthetic control modulate the susceptibility of tumor cells killing by complement. The results suggest that at least some part of the *in vivo* effectiveness of chemotherapeutic drugs may be due to their ability to increase the susceptibility of the tumor cells to immune attack by complement.

[*] Ruhr University, Bochum, Germany.

[†] National Institute of Health, Bethesda, U.S.A.

SUPPRESSION OF *IN VITRO* LYMPHOCYTE STIMULATION IN CANCER PATIENTS TREATED WITH RADIOTHERAPY

B. Serrou,[*] J.B. Dubois,[†] and C. Thierry[*]

Lymphoblastic transformation tests in sixty cancer patients have been performed before, during and after treatment with physical agents and the lymphocyte uptake of tritiated thymidine under the influence of mitogens such as phytohemagglutinin, pokeweed mitogen and concanavalin A has been evaluated. The results showed a marked depression in cellular immunity in patients treated in this manner. This depression can persist after irradiation which is a criterion for poor short-term prognosis. It might also repair to normal values with occasionally an increase over initial values, i.e. immunological rebound phenomenon which is a criterion for favorable short-term prognosis. The passage on fiberglass columns of lymphocytes from these patients demonstrated a non-adherent population (25% of the total population). In a large number of cases, the response of the non-adherent population to the same mitogens returned either to or above pre-treatment level, this being on a per-cell basis. This would suggest that the mitogen-responsive lymphocyte population may diminish under the effect of radiotherapy, in such a way that it could be masked by a non-responsive lymphocyte population. The possible existence of a depressor cell population, eliminated by passage on a fiberglass column, should also be considered.

[*] Department of Chemotherapy and Immunology, Centre Paul Lamarque, Hôpital St-Eloi, 34059, Montpellier, France.

[†] Department of Radiotherapy, Centre Paul Lamarque, Hôpital St-Eloi, 34059, Montpellier, France.

IMMUNO- VERSUS CHEMOTHERAPY DURING COMPLETE REMISSION (CR) OF ACUTE
LYMPHOBLASTIC LEUKEMIA (ALL)

EORTC Hemopathies Working Party*

Eighty-six ALL patients (<21 y.o.) in their first CR were randomized to receive for 1 year as
consolidation either polychemotherapy (P): successively (L-asparaginase + 6 MP), (6 MP +
prednisolone), (BCNU + cyclophosphamide) and (methotrexate + vincristine), or monochemotherapy
(M): methotrexate (MTX) interspersed by reinductions (Predn. + vincristine). The patients still in CR
after the year were again randomized, for maintenance by chemotherapy (C): (6 MP + MTX) interspersed by reinductions, or by immunotherapy (I): BCG + non-irradiated allogeneic ALL blasts.
During consolidation, no difference in relapses nor in death rate was seen between (P) and (M).
During maintenance, 3 deaths in CR occurred in (C): (3/17) in contrast to (I): (0/21). The % of
patients in CR after 2 years of maintenance was 62 in (I) and 55 or 85 in (C) depending on whether
death in CR was interpreted as relapse or withdrawal. The difference between (I) and (C) is not
significant. In conclusion, hitherto, (I) and (C) appear to be equal value for maintenance of ALL.

* Presented by P. Stryckmans, Secretary for the Group.

CELL-MEDIATED CYTOTOXICITY (CMC) IN PATIENTS WITH ACUTE MYELOID
LEUKAEMIA RECEIVING IMMUNOTHERAPY

G.M. Taylor, R. Harris and C.B. Freeman

Department of Medical Genetics, St. Mary's Hospital, Manchester M13 0JH

We are treating a number of acute myeloid leukaemia (AML) patients during remission with active
immunotherapy and without maintenance chemotherapy (see ref. 1) as part of the MRC 6th AML trial.
The treatment protocol is based on immunotherapy trials carried out at the Royal Marsden and St.
Bartholomew's Hospitals [2] and entails the weekly subcutaneous injection of X-irradiated
allogeneic AML blasts and BCG. If immunotherapy is to become an acceptable form of treatment
in AML, and cancer in general, objective measurement of its effects are necessary. To our knowledge
no evidence has been presented showing that lymphocytes from patients treated with active
immunotherapy using allogeneic AML blasts are capable of killing either allogeneic (donor) or
autochthonous blasts. Using the fact that allogeneic lymphocytes stimulate the differentiation of
killer cells in mixed lymphocyte culture we took lymphocytes from healthy controls and from AML
patients receiving immunotherapy and cultured them *in vitro* for 6 days, either alone or with AML
immunotherapy blasts (AML-I) or with cell lines. The lymphocytes were then harvested and tested
for cytotoxicity against ^{51}Cr-labeled AML-I test blasts and cell lines as target cells. Unstimulated
normal and patient lymphocytes were usually not cytotoxic to any of the target cells, whilst AML-I
stimulated normal lymphocytes were cytotoxic to AML-I targets only in 1/8 tests compared with
6/8 positive cytotoxic tests on AML patients. Control cultures consisting of normal or patient
lymphocytes stimulated with Raji (Burkitt's lymphoma) or MICH (lymphoblastoid) cells showed
similar cytotoxic effects on AML-I, Raji and MICH cells indicating that the response to AML-I
blasts in patients reflected their treatment with immunotherapy. Since normal individuals did not
develop cytotoxicity to AML-I blasts we conclude that patients possess a pool of memory
lymphocytes, resulting from immunotherapy, capable of restimulation *in vitro* by the AML-I blasts, and
to a lesser extent by cell-lines. We feel that this assay should be a useful method of evaluating the
response of patients to immunotherapy and in the search for tumour-associated antigens on the
patients' own leukaemia cells.

References

1. C.B. Freeman, R. Harris, C.G. Geary, M.J. Leyland, J.E. MacIver, and I.W. Delamore, *Br. Med. J.*,
   4, 571–573 (1973).
2. R, Powles, D. Crowther, C.J.T. Bateman, M.F.J. Beard, T.J. McElwain, J. Russel, T.A. Lister,
   J.M.A. Whitehouse, P.F.M. Wrigley, M. Pike, P. Alexander and G. Fairley-Hamilton,
   Br. J. Cancer, **28**, 365–376 (1973).

4

REMOVAL OF SUPPRESSION OF T-LYMPHOCYTES BY PROTEOLYTIC ENZYMES IN PATIENTS WITH CANCER

R.D. Thornes

Royal College of Surgeons in Ireland, Dublin 2

It was discovered by accident that the induction of fibrinolysis by the proteolytic enzymes, Brinase or Streptokinase, removes suppression of the cellular immune mechanism.

Enhanced proteolysis restores skin tests for delayed hypersensitivity, enhances PHA response, lymphocyte migration and rosetting of lymphocytes. The rate of resuppression of lymphocyte activity appears to be related to tumour load.

Our experience with fifty patients will be presented.

CLINICAL USE OF SIMULTANEOUS TWO-WAVELENGTH FLUORESCENCE MICROSCOPY IN PARAPROTEINAEMIA

B. Van Camp

Internal Medicine, Prof. P.P. Lambert, University Hospital Brugmann, V.U.B.

Using the immediate filter exchange system for FITC and TRITC [1], two antigenic determinants can be recognized simultaneously in one cell. The method for studying intracytoplasmic immunoglobulins in bone marrow by fluorescence microscopy has been extensively reported by Hijmans *et al.* [2].

By these means we studied thirty-five bone marrows of patients with monoclonal gammopathies (m.g.). They are presented on a clinical basis.

1. Nine patients with non-myelomatous m.g. showed "reactive plasmocytosis". Intracytoplasmicly a clone of plasma cells secreting only the paraprotein was found. They never exceeded 90% of immunocytes. The morphological appearance in fluorescence varied from normal plasma cells to rather lymphoid cells. The monoclonal proliferation perhaps started already at the level of the young lymphocyte. Therefore it could be interesting to study its surface immunoglobulins.
2. Twenty myeloma patients (13 IgG, 3 IgA, 1 IgM and 3 lambda) showed a clearcut malignant proliferation (more than 99% of immunocytes), with a definite suppression of the other Ig-secreting plasma cells. Some cases had less than 6% normal looking plasma cells, but were all secreting the paraprotein. The monoclonal reaction started thus already intracellular at the normal looking sites of the bone marrow. In addition in those patients showing more than 30 m.g. % Bence-Jones proteinuria, only light chain secreting cells were found.
3. Five treated myelomas and one macroglobulinaemia were also examined. Some of them were treated for over more than 6 years. Preliminary results show that the intracytoplasmic distribution followed quite closely the clinical picture. In one case reticulo-sarcomatous cells were seen secreting only light chains. Our first results suggest that a clinical remission can be detected and followed.

In conclusion, this fluorescence method can give a lot of information in patients with m.g.:
as a supportive diagnosis,
in cell morphology,
in the course of therapy.

This study was supported by a grant of the N.F.W.G.O., Belgium Nr. F.G.O.

References

1. W. Hijmans, H.R.E. Schuit and E. Hulsing-Hessellnk, *Ann N.Y. Acad. Sci.*, **177**, 290 (1971).
2. W. Hijmans, H.R.E. Schuit and F. Klein, *Clin. Exp. Immunol.* **4**, 457 (1969).

SPECIFICITY OF AN ANTISERUM FROM A MONKEY IMMUNIZED WITH HUMAN MELANOMA CELLS

C. Vennegoor

Dept. of Immunology, Antoni van Leeuwenhoekhuis, Sarphatistraat 108, The Netherlands

The aim of the study is the preparation of a strong and specific antiserum against malignant melanoma cells to enable screening of patients for reappearance of tumor in an early stage. Initial results with antisera from rabbits were unsatisfactory. Therefore, it was decided to immunize an animal more closely related to man (compare the work of Metzgar *et al., J. Nat. Cancer Inst.* **50**, 1065 (1975)). A *Macaca speciosa* was immunized with 1-month cultured melanoma cells (Dr. Balner and co-workers, REP/TNO, Rijswijk, The Netherlands). Antibodies were measured with the complement-dependent serum cytotoxicity test.

The pre-immunization serum was negative on all cells tested. The antiserum absorbed with pooled peripheral lymphocytes from twenty healthy donors was positive on 3/7 melanoma cell line cells tested, weakly positive on the melanoma cells used for immunization, and positive on brain cells. Negative reactions were found with normal peripheral lymphocytes, normal bladder, embryonal kidney, embryonal lung, bladder carcinoma, mammary carcinoma, and cervix carcinoma cell line cells. Cells from an originally negatively reacting melanoma cell line reacted strongly positive when they had become murine leukemia virus (MuLV)-producing after artificial infection. A 2 M KI extract prepared from membranes of melanoma cells showed a considerably higher inhibition of the complement-dependent serum cytotoxicity than an extract similarly prepared from normal peripheral lymphocytes. After absorption with melanoma or brain cells the antiserum became negative on melanoma cells, whereas it remained positive on melanoma cells after absorption with embryonal kidney cells. On brain cells the antiserum became negative after absorption with each of the three cell types mentioned.

These results indicate that it is possible to prepare specific antisera against malignant melanoma cells, although brain cells possess antigens which cross-react with those on the tumor cells.

ANTI-TUMOUR IMMUNOPROTECTION BY AN IMMUNOBACTERIAL–LECTIN APPROACH

R. Verloes,* G. Atassi and L. Kanarek

*Laboratory of Experimental Chemotherapy, Service de Médecine et d'Investigation Clinique, Institut Jules Bordet, Bruxelles, Belgium
Laboratorium voor chemie der proteinen, Instituut voor Moleculaire Biologie, Vrije Universiteit Brussel, St. Genesius Rode*

Our approach deals with a common feature of all tumours: the difference in viscosity of the tumour cell membrane.

Lectine, such as concanavalin A (ConA) and wheat germ agglutinin (WGA), bind to tumour cells and in a smaller degree to normal cells, but agglutinate only tumour cells or transformed cells [1].

Those plant proteins have a carbohydrate binding capacity, ConA binds to glucose and mannose residues, while WGA binds *N*-acetylglucosamine (NAG); they inhibit tumour growth *in vivo* but they have no therapeutical value because of their haemagglutinating capacity and toxic effect on normal cells [2].

Micrococcus lysodeikticus is a nonpathologic gram-positive bacterium that stimulates production of high titre antibodies and homogeneous structure as shown by electrophoresis and sequence [3].

Anti-micrococcus antibodies are directed either against the bacterium specific carbohydrate, mainly anti-glucose, or against the peptide of the peptidoglycan moiety of the cell wall.

As anti-micrococci have an anti-glucose specificity we used this immunobacterial system as an equivalent of ConA.

Further preparation of an antigen (CWC) consisted in coupling of a polymer of NAG on the peptide moiety of the cell wall of *M. lysodeikticus* in order to break down tolerance to the NAG polysaccharide.

By *in vivo* screening against leukemia L1210 in BDF mice and Ehrlich ascites tumour in BALB/C mice, we found that prior vaccinations with the antigen CWC protect mice against L1210 challenge and Ehrlich tumour, with cures of 14–28% of the animals and a mean survival time of 170–200% for 10^5 tumour cells.

Vaccinations with *M. lysodeikticus* enhance tumour growth while passive transfer of rabbit anti-microccocus antibodies cures mice of 10³ L1210 challenge, sometimes in 80% of the mice, depending on the antibody dose and specificity. Some anti-microccocus antibodies agglutinate lymphocytes, however they do not agglutinate RB cells of any species and vaccinations for years in rabbits did not reveal any toxicity or pathogenicity.

References

1. M.M. Burger, A difference in the architecture of the surface membrane of normal and virally transformed cells. *Proc. Nat. Acad. Sci. U.S.A.* **62**, 994 (1969).
2. M. Inbar, H. Ben-Bassat and L. Sachs, Inhibition of ascites tumor development by ConA. *Int. J. Cancer,* **9**, 143 (1972).
3. M. Van Hoegaerden, M. Wikler, R. Janssens and L. Kanarek, Antibodies to *Micrococcus lysodeikticus. Eur. J. Biochem.* **53**, 19 (1975).

* Predoctoral Fellow of the IWONL.

LYMPHOCYTE FUNCTIONS IN MYELOMA PATIENTS

O. Wetter and K.H. Linder

D-43 Essen, Hufelandstr. 55, Klinikum

Peripheral blood lymphocytes (PBL) and bone marrow lymphocytes (BML) of patients with multiple myeloma have been studied by mitogenic stimulation, spontaneous rosette formation (SRF) and surface-Ig. Eight out of eleven patients showed a reduced response to PHA when compared to PBL of normal individuals. Using ConA and PWM fifteen out of twenty patients showed an impaired reactivity. Considering PHA as a T-cell stimulant and PWM as a B-cell stimulant these results indicate an unspecific impairment of lymphocyte functions in myeloma patients.

Seven out of sixteen patients showed reduced SRF. We tried if inhibition of SRF by ALG would provide a more sensitive assay for lymphocyte function in myeloma. All nine patients treated so far showed a significantly reduced inhibition of SRF by ALG. Three out of these nine patients exhibited normal SRF. So, in these cases by ALG a previously undetected peculiarity in myeloma lymphocytes has been revealed.

BML of normals have been tested for rosette inhibition. Our preliminary results indicate a stronger resistance to inhibition by ALG in normal BML compared to normal PBL. Differences of the ability to form E-rosettes also have been found between PBL and BML of normals by other authors (Vogel, J.E., *et al., Proc. Nat. Acad. Sci. USA,* **72**, 1175 (1975)) and have been ascribed to lymphocyte maturation processes.

By immunofluorescence experiments no differences of surface-Ig have been found between normals and patients.

Summary

It has been found that PBL in myeloma patients often show an impaired mitogenic response. In addition and more specifically, inhibition of SRF by ALG reveals differences to normals. As rosette inhibition of PBL and BML has been found different in normals the results in myeloma patients could be explained by altered compartmentalization in such patients due to heavy bone marrow infiltration. Other explanations are possible. Lymphocytotoxins are present in sera of 70% of myeloma patients and may block ALG binding sites.

As myelomatosis is characterized by the accumulation of plasma cells generally considered of exclusive B-cell origin, the involvement of T-cells as shown by our results deserves further interest.

AUTHOR INDEX

Abelev, G.I. 97, 102
Adam, A. 222
Adkinson, N. F. 39
Adler, F. L. 189
Afanasyeva, A. C. 101
Aisenberg, A. C. 130, 143
Aitui, F. 204
Alario, A. 39, 252
Albert, S. 86
Alexander, E. L. 38
Alexander, P. 17, 26, 28, 170, 189, 221, 231, 262
Alford, T. C. 76, 86, 102
Almgard, L.E. 76
Alter, B. J. 17
Ambus, U. 76
Amery, W. 159, 168,
Amiel, J. L. 142, 220, 221, 232, 249
Andersen, V. 68, 76, 86
Anderson, J. M. 76
Anderson, L. L. 68
Andersson, B. 28
Anzai, T. 103
Aoki, T. 231
Arala-Chaves, M. P. 198
Ascher, M. S. 202, 204
Astarita, R. W. 102
Atassi, G. 264
Aur, R. 221
Aynsley-Green, A. 53

Bach, F. H. 17
Bach, J. F. 3, 4, 7
Bach, M. A. 7
Bagshawe, K. D. 218, 222, 226, 231
Baird, L. G. 157
Baker, M. 121
Baker, M. A. 121
Balcerzak, S. P. 205
Balchin, L. A. 231
Baldwin, R. W. 156, 218, 222, 231, 249
Balner 264
Balzarini, G. P. 86
Band, P. 250
Banfi, A. 250
Bansal, S. C. 68
Banzer, P. 53

Barker, C. R. 156
Barker, L. 221
Barnett, E. V. 39
Bartal, A. 259
Basham, C. 67, 231
Basic, I. 249
Bast, R. C., Jr. 157
Bateman, C. J. T. 232, 249, 262
Baumann, P. 53
Baxley, G. 39
Bean, M. A. 42, 45
Beard, M. E. J. 262
Behring, E. 223, 231
Bekesi, J. G. 218, 222
Belanger, L. 100, 103
Belanger, M. 103
Belohradsky, B. 38
Belpomme, D. 131, 142, 143, 144, 221
Ben-Bassat, H. 265
Bendixen, G. 74, 75, 76, 86
Benjamin, R. S. 249
Benjamini, E. 204
Bennett, S. I. 102
Bentwich, Z. 130, 142
Berardet, M. 220
Beraud, C. W. 130, 143
Bernard, C. 231
Bernard, J. 110, 221
Bernard-Degani, O. 231
Bernstein, L. D. 249
Bertoglio, J. 39, 251
Betuel, H. 39
Betz, E. H. 19, 28
Bhutani, L. K. 39
Biasi, G. 253
Bierensaadehaan, B. 102
Bini, A. 157
Biniaminov, M. 168
Bishop, G. 39
Bishop, G. B. 39
Bjerrum, O. 76, 86
Black, M. M. 85, 86
Bloom, B. 53
Bloomfield, C. D. 143
Blumenschein, G. R. 233, 250
Bluming, A. Z. 250
Bodenham, D. C. 231
Bodey, G. P. 231, 250

267

Bodey, G. P., Sr.   232, 249
Bodey, J. P., Jr.   221
Bodmer, J. G.   111
Bodmer, W. F.   110, 111
Boiron, M.   221
Bolognesi, D. P.   231
Bomford, R.   17
Bona, C.   17
Bonadonna, G.   250
Bondevik, H.   189
Bonmassar, A.   156, 157
Bonmassar, E.   153, 154, 156, 157
Bonnar, A. D.   52
Bonnard, G. D.   46
Bonner, W. A.   121
Booth, S. N.   95, 96, 102
Borella, L.   121, 143
Borges, W.   232
Bornstein, R. S.   222
Borsos, T.   86, 157, 261
Botto, H. G.   142
Botto, I.   143
Bourgoin, A.   39, 251
Bouroncle, B. A.   143
Bourut, C.   220, 221, 222, 232
Bowen, J. G.   222
Bowles, C.   39
Boyle, B. J.   156
Boyle, M. D.   18
Boyse, E. A.   4, 7, 231
Boyum, A.   189
Braylan, R. C.   143
Breenan, T. G.   251
Bremer, K.   254
Brennan, M.   86
Brenner, H. J.   68
Brouet, J. C.   121, 123, 130, 142, 143
Brower, P.   190
Brown, G.   115, 118, 121
Brugerie, H.   222
Brugmans, J.   168
Bruley-Rosset, M.   222
Brunner, K. T.   28, 41, 45, 46, 76, 194, 204
Bubenik, J.   231
Buffe, D.   99, 100, 101, 103
Bullen, B. R.   251
Burdick, J. R.   189
Burg, C.   28
Burger, M. M.   265
Burgess, M. A.   221, 222, 232, 233, 249, 250
Burtin, P.   97, 101, 102, 103
Butcher, D.   38
Butler, W. T.   231
Butterworth, A. E.   53
Byers, V.   39, 204
Byers, V. S.   39, 204

Cailleau, R.   86
Calderon, J.   18
Cameron, P.   17
Cameron-Mowat, D. E.   76
Campanile, F.   157

Campbell, A. C.   53
Campbell, C. B.   76
Canavari, S.   86
Cannon, G. B.   76, 77, 86
Capellaro, D.   115, 121
Carbone, P.   250
Cardenas, J. O.   233, 249, 250
Carnaud, C.   68
Carpentier-Bricteux, N.   252
Carr, M. C.   39, 142
Carter, S. K.   250
Caspary, E. A.   76
Catovsky, D.   121, 143
Cattan, A.   220
Ceppellini, R.   52
Cerottini, J.-C.   28, 41, 45, 46, 76, 194, 204
Cesarini, J. P.   xiv
Chambers, H.   231
Chan, Y-K.   221, 232, 249
Chantler, S.   39
Chapman, G. O.   156
Charlionnet, R.   103
Charreire, J.   7
Chavanel, G.   102
Chayvialle, J. A. P.   103
Chedid, L.   17
Chee, D.   222
Chelloul, N.   143
Chermann, J. C.   157
Chervenick, P.   17
Chess, L.   52
Chevalier, A.   143
Chieco-Bianchi, L.   253
Chin, A. H.   143
Chirigos, M. A.   156, 157, 168
Chu, T. M.   102
Ciorbanu, R.   222
Clarkson, B. D.   142, 230, 232
Claudy, A. L.   39, 252
Clausen, J. E.   75, 76
Clauvel, J. P.   130, 143
Clements, P. J.   39
Cleveland, R. P.   68
Clifford, P.   68
Coates, A. S.   256
Coca, A. F.   231
Cochran, A. J.   69, 75, 76, 85, 86
Cohen, A. M.   172, 189
Cohen, Y.   259
Cohn, Z. A.   11, 17
Colas, D. E.   231
Coligan, J. E.   101
Collatz, E.   102
Collavo, D.   253
Collins, R. D.   121, 130
Colombani, J.   111
Colombatti, A.   253
Connell, D. I.   28
Connolly, J. M.   52
Connor, R. J.   86
Coombs, R. R. A.   204
Cooper, A. G.   39
Cooper, G. H.   39

Cooper, M.   204
Cooper, R.   250
Copeland, E. M.   249
Coudert, A.   222
Cox, I. S.   231
Crowther, D.   221, 232, 249, 262
Crozier, C.   103
Cullen, P.   53
Currie, G. A.   45, 67, 156, 218, 222, 225, 226, 231, 232, 248, 250
Curtis, J.   39
Cutler, S. J.   249

Daniel, M. T.   121, 130, 143
Dantchev, D.   131, 142, 143, 144, 221
Darcy, D. A.   97
Dardenne, M.   7
Dausset, J.   68, 109, 110, 111
Davies, A. J. S.   6, 7
Davies, D. A. L.   68, 260
Day, E. D.   222
Dean, J. H.   76, 77, 86
de Baetselier, P.   253
Debois, J. M.   168
De Clerck, E.   10
De Cock, W.   168
De Cree, J.   168
Degani, O.   68
Degiovanni, G.   252
Degos, L.   110, 111
de Harven, E.   142, 231
De Hoff, R. T.   21, 28
deKernion, J. B.   190
Delamore, I. W.   232, 255, 262
Della Porta, G.   86
Delmas-Marsalet, Y.   109, 111
Delorme, E. J.   28, 189
de Marchi, M.   52, 53
de Nechaud, B.   103
Denk, H.   91, 101
Den Otter, W.   28
Deonhoff, M. J.   7
Desplaces, A.   143
de Vassal, F.   142, 220, 221, 231
de Vries, J. E.   44, 254
Dezfulian, M.   222
Dhar, P.   102
Dick, H. M.   111
Dickler, H. B.   204
Dickler, H. B., Jr.   39
Dissing, I.   76, 86
Djeu, J.   39
Doan, C. A.   143
Doering, T.   76, 86
Donnelly, F. C.   46
Donner, M.   28
Dore, J. F.   39, 218, 222, 224, 231, 251
Dorrance, G. M.   231
Douglas, S. D.   130
Dray, S.   171, 189
Drinker, C. K.   203
Drogemuller, C. R.   189

Dubois, J. B.   261
Dubouche, P.   221
Dumonde, D. C.   260
Dupuy, J. M.   110
du Rusquec, E.   142
Duval, D.   5
Dykes, P. W.   102
Dylsi, M.   102

Eckestorfer, R.   101
Economour, S. G.   250
Edginton, T. S.   97, 102
Edsymyr, F.   76
Edynak, E. M.   90, 101
Egan, M. L.   101
Egdahl, R. H.   170, 189
Eggleston, J. C.   143
Eife, R. F.   258
Eilber, F. R.   249, 250
Einborn, L.   222, 249
El Yafi, G.   130
Embleton, M. J.   222
Endo, Y.   103
Engers, H. D.   46
Epstein, W.   39
Evans, R.   17, 28
Eylar, E. H.   204
Ezer, G.   39

Fairley, G.   221
Fairley-Hamilton, G.   231, 262
Falk, J.   121
Farber, P. A.   68
Farrow, J. H.   250
Fefer, A.   156
Feierstein, J.N.   250
Feingold, N.   110
Feizi, T.   130
Ferguson   224
Festenstein, H.   51, 53
Feuilhade de Chauvin, F.   131, 142
Field, E. J.   76
Fink, U.   254
Fischer, R. E.   17
Fisher, B.   250
Fisher, E. R.   250
Fisher, J. C.   157
Fisher, P.   86
Fishman, M.   169, 189
Flad, H.-D.   254
Flandrin, G.   121, 130, 143
Flexner, J. M.   130
Florentin, I.   222
Foley, E. J.   27
Forrest, A. P.   249
Fossati, G.   86
Fouad-Wassef, N.   39, 252
Fourcade, M.   143
Fournier, C.   7
Foy, A.   232
Franchi, G.   168
Franco, P.   157

Frank, M.　130
Frank, M. M.　143
Frankson, C.　53
Franzén, S.　76
Fredriksen, G.　101
Freedman, S.　89, 101
Freedman, S. O.　89, 96, 102
Freeman, C.　53
Freeman, C. B.　230, 232, 255, 262
Frei, E., III　221, 249
Freireich, E. J.　221, 222, 231, 232, 249, 250
Frelick, R.　250
Freshney, R. I.　76
Fridman, W. H.　224, 231
Frisch, B.　121, 143
Fritze, D.　169, 190
Frizzera, G.　130
Froland, S.　142, 204
Fröland, S. S.　124, 130
Frost, M. A.　256
Fu, S. M.　130
Fudenberg, H. H.　31, 38, 39, 40, 142, 191, 198, 200, 203, 204, 205
Fudifin, D. J.　53

Gajl-Peczalska, K. J.　143
Gale, D. G.　53
Galetto, J.　143
Galton, D. A. G.　121, 143
Gaston, M.　157
Gauchi, M. N.　232
Geary, C. G.　232, 255, 262
Geffard, M.　221
Gehan, E.　221, 232, 249
Gehan, E. A.　249
Genin, J.　76, 86
George, M.　76
Gerard-Marchant, R.　143
Gery, I.　17
Gheorghiu, M.　221
Gibson, W. T.　157
Giese, J.　68
Giger, H.　21, 28
Giles, G. R.　251
Glait, H.　250
Glaser, M.　46
Glass, A.　250
Glew, D. H.　102
Glick, A. D.　130
Glynn, J. P.　151, 152, 156
Gold, J. M.　92, 102
Gold, Ph.　89, 93, 101, 102
Goldin, A.　147, 156, 157
Goldman, J. M.　121, 143
Goldstein, A.　3, 7
Goldstein, A. L.　39
Golub, E.　86
Gomard, E.　6, 45
Good, R. A.　203, 250
Gordon, S.　17
Gotch, F.　53
Gothoskar, B. P.　75
Gottlieb, A. A.　17

Gottlieb, J. A.　222, 233, 249, 250
Gottlieb, L. S.　103
Goust, J. M.　198, 202, 204, 205
Govaerts, A.　39, 107
Grace, W. R.　157
Granatek, C. H.　76
Grandjon, D.　131, 142, 143
Granger, G. A.　28
Grant, R. M.　76, 86
Greaves, M. F.　115, 118, 121
Green, I.　130, 143
Green, R. W.　231
Green, S. S.　46
Gren, I.　53
Grey, H. M.　142, 143
Griscelli, C.　39
Grob, P.　102
Gröhn, P.　257
Gronneberg, K.　39, 251
Grooten, J.　253
Gross, L.　231
Gross, R. L.　39
Gruca, S.　17
Guha, A.　7
Guibout, A.　222
Gutterman, J. U.　68, 76, 86, 213, 214, 220, 221, 222, 224, 228, 231, 232, 233, 248, 249, 250

Haasz, R.　259
Hackett, A. J.　39, 204
Hadgett, J.　28
Hadjiyannaki, M. J.　222
Hainz, H.　142
Häkkinen, J. P.　90, 101
Hakkinen, J. T.　97
Hakomori, S.　121
Hall, J. G.　28, 189
Halle-Pannenko, O.　220, 221, 222, 232
Hallgren, H. M.　143
Halliday, J. W.　76
Halliday, W. J.　67, 76
Halloran, P.　51, 53
Halper, J.　17
Halpern, B.　250
Halpern, B. L.　156
Halterman, R. H.　231, 232
Hamers, R.　253
Hamers-Casterman, C.　253
Hamilton, L. D.　189
Harding, B.　53
Hardisty, R. M.　111
Harris, R.　231, 232, 255, 262
Harsak, I.　231
Hayat, M.　xiv, 142, 221
Hayry, P.　4
Hayward, A.　121
Hayward, A. W.　39
Hekman, A.　256
Hellström, I.　39, 41, 45, 68, 76, 86, 231
Hellström, K. E.　28, 39, 41, 45, 68, 76, 86, 231

Hemstein, K. 231
Hendart, P. A. 101
Henderson, E. S. 111
Henry, C. 205
Herberman, R. B. 39, 44, 45, 46, 76, 77, 86, 102, 231
Hersh, E. M. 68, 76, 86, 221, 222, 231, 232, 233, 248, 249, 250
Hersy, P. 53
Herter, F. P. 102
Herzenberg, L. A. 121
Herzog, C. 39
Heyn, R. 232
Hibbs, J. B. 17, 18, 28
Hijmans, W. 263
Hiltunen, K-M. 257
Hirai, H. 102
Hirata, A. A. 102
Hirshaut, Y. 168
Hitzig, W. H. 203
Hiu, I. J. 222
Hoebeke, J. 168
Holden, H. T. 46
Holland, E. 53, 221
Holland, J. F. 218, 222
Hollinshead, A. C. 86, 93, 102
Holm, G. 39, 52, 53
Holmes, E. C. 231, 249, 250
Holtermann, O. A. 249
Holyner, H. 86
Holyoke, D. 95, 96, 102
Holyoke, E. D. 102
Holzner, J. H. 101
Hong, R. 39
Hooghe, R. 253
Hooper, J. A. 39
Horn, R. G. 130
Horowitz, S. 39
Hors, J. 109, 111
Houba, V. 53
Houchens, D. P. 147, 157
Howard, A. 52
Hoyle, D. E. 76
Hoyle, D. H. 86
Hsu, M. 204
Huber, C. 254
Huber, H. 197, 204, 254
Huchet, R. 142, 143
Hughes, L. E. 86
Hui, I. J. 220
Hulett, H. R. 121
Hulsing-Hesselink, E. 263
Humphreys, S. R. 156
Hunt, J. S. 250
Hunter, N. 249
Hustu, O. 221
Hutchison, D. J. 157
Hyat, M. 220

Iino, S. 103
Ikonopisov, R. L. 231, 249, 250
Imai, K. 222

Inbar, M. 265
Irlin, I. S. 102
Isbister, W. H. 67
Isliker, H. 102
Israel, L. xiv, 250
Izak, C. 250
Izak, G. 232
Izsak, F. C. 66, 68

Jackson, A. M. 69
Jacques, M. 168
Jacquillat, C. 221
Jaffe, E. S. 130, 143
Jamieson, G. C. 102
Janis, M. 17
Janossy, G. 115
Janssens, R. 265
Jasmin, C. 142, 221
Jeejeebhoy, H. F. 28
Jehn, U. W. 75, 76
Jerome, L. F. 76, 86
Jersild, C. 110
Jewell, D. P. 53
Johansson, B. 76
Johnson, R. K. 156, 157
Johnson, W. 53, 221
Johnston, J. O. 39, 204
Jondal, M. 39
Joo, P. 232
Jose, D. G. 68
Joseph, R. 131, 142, 143, 144, 221
Jubert, A. V. 249
Jurcyzk-Procyk, S. 221
Juy, D. 17

Kahan, B. D. 86
Kaizer, H. 143
Kalden, J. R. 258
Kamel, M. 222
Kanai, K. 103
Kanarek, L. 264, 265
Kaplan, A. M. 157, 237
Kaplan, E. L. 249
Kapp, F. 102
Karlsson, M. 46
Katrych, D. L. 250
Kay, M. M. 38
Kearny, G. 17
Keller, R. 17
Kellock, T. H. 231
Kelly, F. 76
Kern, D. H. 169, 171, 189, 190
Kersey, J. H. 143
Ketcham, A. S. 189, 231, 249, 250
Khalil, A. 221
Khalil, A. M. 222
Khankhanian, N. 249
Kiessling, R. 46
King, J. P. 102
Kirchner, H. 46
Kistler, G. S. 28

Kitasato   223, 231
Klein, E.   28, 41, 45, 46, 55, 68, 76, 249
Klein, F.   263
Klein, G.   28, 68, 86
Klockars, M.   17
Klouda, P. T.   109, 111
Komuro, K.   4, 7
Korhonen, L. K.   101
Kourilsky, F. M.   53, 109, 110, 224, 231
Kramkova, N. I.   102
Krohn, K.   257
Krupey, J.   102
Kubo, P. T.   143
Kunkel, H. G.   130, 142
Kunkler, P. B.   249
Kunze-Muhl, E.   86
Kupchik, H. Z.   102

Labaume, S.   130
Lacour, F.   76, 86
Lacour, J.   76, 86
Lafleur, M.   142, 143, 221
Lambert, L. H.   17
Lambert, L. M.   28
Lambert, R.   103
Lamon, E. W.   28
Lampen, N.   142
Landes, E.   68
La Noue, H.   231
Lapeyraque, F.   220, 231
Lardis, M. P.   101
Larochelle, J.   103
Larsen, O.   68
Lasfargues, E.   171
Lattes, R. G.   28
Lattuada, A.   250
Latty, A.   39
Laurence, D. J. R.   102
Lautenschleger, J. T.   101
Lavrin, D.   46
Law, L. W.   156
Lawler, S. D.   109, 111
Lawrence, H. S.   194, 202, 204
Lebredo, M. G.   231
Leclerc, J. C.   6, 45
Lederer, E.   222
Leech, J.   143
Leech, J. H.   130
Legrand, L.   111
Lehmann, F. G.   103
Leis, H. P., Jr.   86
Lejeune, F.   17
Lejeune, F. J.   9, 10, 18
Lejtenyi, M. C.   93, 102
Lelarge, N.   131
Lemerle, J.   103
Leonard, C. M.   86
Leonard, E.   86
Leonard, J.   102
Le Pourheit, A.   232
Lerner, C.   250
Leventhal, B. G.   227, 231, 232

Levin, A. S.   39, 204
Levine, P. H.   46
Levo, Y.   7
Levy, J.   39
Levy, J.-P.   45
Levy, N. L.   222
Lewis, M. G.   231, 249
Leyland, M. J.   232, 262
Lheritier, J.   221, 222
Liavac, I.   101
Lieberman, R.   39
Lille, I.   143
Lindberg, L.   68
Linder, K. H.   265
Lindop, G.   76
Lister, A.   121
Lister, T. A.   262
Littman, B. H.   68
Lobuglio, A. F.   17, 205
Loewi, G.   52
Logerfo, P.   102
Long, A.   86
Long, J. C.   130, 143
Loosli, R. M.   102
Lucas, D.   39
Luckasen, H. R.   143
Lukes, R. J.   121, 130
Lynch, H.   53
Lytton, B.   86

McBride, C.   76, 249
McBride, C. E.   222
McBride, C. M.   68, 86, 233, 250
McBride, M.   221
McCoy, J. L.   39, 46, 76, 77, 86
McCredie, K. B.   68, 221, 231, 232, 249, 250
McDermott, R. P.   52
Macdonald, H. R.   46, 52
McElwain, T. J.   221, 250, 262
Mach, J. P.   93, 94, 97, 102
MacIver, J. E.   232, 255, 262
McIvor, K.   17
Mackenzie, M. R.   143
Mackie, R. M.   69, 75, 76, 86
MacLennan, I.   51
MacLennan, I. C. M.   47, 52, 53
Macwright, C. G.   102
Mahaley, M. S., Jr.   222
Main, J. M.   27
Malmgren, R. A.   231, 249
Maluish, A.   67
Maluish, A. E.   76
Mann, R. B.   143
Mannick, J. A.   157, 170, 189
Mann-Whitney   70
Mantel, N.   156
Mantovani, A.   168
Many, N.   250
Marcus, S.   231
Marholev, L.   222, 231
Marquardt, H.   168
Marshal, E. K., Jr.   156

Martin, E. 101
Martin, F. 91, 102
Martin, G. R. 17
Martin, J. P. 103
Martin, M. 144, 221
Martin, M. S. 91, 102
Martin, R. C. 249
Martin-Chandon, M. R. 68
Martyre, M. C. 218, 222
Masseyeff, R. F. 103
Mastrangelo, M. J. 222
Mathé, G. 131, 142, 143, 144, 207, 213, 220,
221, 222, 227, 230, 231, 232, 234, 247, 249
Maurer, B. A. 77
Mavligit, G. 221, 222, 231, 232
Mavligit, G. M. 68, 76, 86, 233, 248, 249, 250
Mawas, C. 99, 103
May, W. 52
Meeus, L. 143
Meier, P. 237, 249
Melson, H. 11, 17
Meltzer, M. 86
Meltzer, M. S. 68
Mergen-Hagen, S. E. 17
Metchnikoff, E. 10, 17
Metzgar, R. S. 121, 224, 231, 252, 264
Michaelson, T. E. 130
Mickey, M. R. 108, 110
Mickiewicz, E 250
Middleton, M. 86
Mihich, E. 156, 157
Mikulska, Z. B. 28
Milas, L. 249
Miller, D. S. 121, 231
Miller, F. A. P. 7
Minow, R. A. 249
Misset, J. L. 142, 221
Moberger, G. 76, 231
Mohanakumar, T. 121, 231
Moore, M. 44, 257
Moore, T. L. 102
Morahan, P. S. 157
Moran, E. M. 130
Morris, B. 28
Morton, D. L. 231, 234, 249, 250
Motta, R. 231
Muna, N. M. 231
Munson, J. A. 157
Murphy, G. P. 102
Musset, M. 142, 221

Nairn, R. C. 231, 249
Nath, I. 39
Nathanson, L. 76
Natvig, J. B. 124, 130, 142
Nauts, H. C. 248
Navares, L. 143
Neidhart, J. A. 205
Nelson, D. S. 17
Nesbit, M. 143
Nesbit, M. E. 143

Neville, M. A. 102
Newberne, P. M. 39
Newman, E. S. 97
Nicolin, A. 154, 156, 157
Nilsonne, U. 68, 86
Nishi, S. 102
Noerjasin 43
Nossal, G. J. V. 142
Notkins, A. L. 68

Oates, G. D. 102
Oda, T. 103
Oettgen, H. F. 45, 168, 204, 231, 250
Ogata, Y. 68
Ogg, L. 69
Ohanian, S. H. 261
Okos, A. 121, 143
Old, L. J. 231, 250
Oldham, R. B. 86
Oldham, R. K. 77, 222
Olivari, A. J. 250
Olive, M. 86
Olivotto, M. 17
O'Neill, G. J. 260
Orbach, S. 208
Orbach-Arbouys, S. 221
Oren, M. E. 86
Orjasaeter, H. 91, 101
Ormerod, M. G. 18
Osoba, D. 7
Osserman, E. F. 17
O'Toole, C. 39, 43, 76
O'Toole, C. O. 46

Padarathsingh, M. 156
Palangie, T. 222
Papamichael, M. 121
Paque, R. E. 171, 189
Parie-Fisher, J. 53
Parks, L. C. 168
Parr, I. 207, 220, 231
Paton, C. M. 232
Paul, W. E. 53
Paulus, H. E. 39
Pearl, J. S. 28
Pearson, G. R. 157
Pearson, J. W. 155, 157, 168
Pees, H. 45
Pellegrino, M. A. 86
Pelletier, N. 39, 252
Perlmann, H. 52
Perlmann, P. 39, 46, 52, 76, 231
Pernis, B. 130
Perova, S. D. 102
Peter, C. R. 143
Peter, H. H. 44, 258
Peter, J. B. 39
Petit, J. E. 143
Petit, J. F. 222
Phillips, T. M. 231
Picard, F. 53

Pickbourne, P.   111
Pierce, G. E.   231
Pike, M.   221, 262
Pilch, Y. H.   169, 170, 171, 189, 190
Pimm, M. V.   249
Pinkel   227
Pinon, F.   142
Pinsky, C.   168
Pirofsky, B.   143
Pizzaia, L. M.   101
Plata, F.   42, 43, 45, 46
Platz, P.   111
Pleau, J. M.   7
Plow, E. F.   97, 102
Polley, M. J.   142
Polliack, A.   142
Pontvert, D.   131, 142
Postnikova, Z. A.   102
Pouillart, P.   142, 143, 144, 220, 221, 222,
    231
Powell, L. W.   76
Powles, R.   213, 217, 221, 262
Powles, R. L.   224, 228–232, 249
Prehn, L.   222
Prehn, R. T.   27, 222
Prendergast, R. A.   28
Preud'homme, J. L.   121, 123, 129, 130, 142,
    143
Price, M. R.   222
Prieur, A. M.   130
Pross, H.   46
Pryor, J.   168
Pugh, R. B. C.   260
Puissant, A.   53
Purtilo, D. T.   103
Pusztaszeri, G.   102

Rabinowitz, Y.   143
Raff, M. C.   142
Rager-Zisman, B.   53
Ramming, K. P.   170, 171, 189, 190, 249
Ramot, B.   168
Ran, M.   68
Ransom, L.   143
Rapp, H.   86
Rapp, H. J.   68, 157, 249
Rappaport, H.   110, 130, 143, 221
Rapson, N.   121
Rasmussen, B.   39
Redmond, C.   250
Reed, R.   221, 232, 249
Reed, R. C.   76, 233, 249
Rees, P. H.   53
Reeves, W. J.   86
Regelson, W.   157
Regnier, R.   17
Reich, F.   17
Reisfield, R. A.   86
Remington, J. S.   17, 28
Rempe, G. T.   68
Renoux, G.   168
Renoux, M.   168
Rensted, J.   28

Revesz, L.   28
Revesz, T.   115, 118, 121
Revillard, J. P.   39
Reynoso, G.   102
Rhines, F. N.   21, 28
Richman, S. P.   249
Riedwyl, H.   21, 28
Rigby, C. C.   260
Rilke, F.   250
Rimbaut, C.   100, 101, 103
Rios, A.   222
Robbins, D.   39
Roberts, M. M.   258
Roberts-Thomson, P.   53
Robins, R. A.   222
Robinson, E.   259
Robinson, M. R. G.   260
Robinson, N.   257
Rocklin, R.   86
Rodger, K. E.   76
Rodriguez, V.   221, 232, 249, 250
Rogentine, G. N.   109, 111
Rojas, A. F.   250
Romsdahl, M. M.   231
Ropartz, C.   103
Rosen, G.   45
Rosenberg, E. B.   46, 52, 231
Rosenberg, G. L.   68
Rosenfeld, C.   221
Ross, C. E.   69, 76, 86
Ross, G. D.   142
Rossen, R. D.   231
Roth, J. A.   189, 190
Rotter, V.   7
Rowland, G. F.   260
Rubellino, E. M.   142
Rümke, P.   254
Ruoslahti, E.   98, 103
Russ, S.   231
Russel, J.   262
Ryder, L. P.   111

Sabad, A.   143
Sabbadini, E.   189
Sabine, M. C.   101
Sachs, L.   265
Saffort, J. W.   102
Saiki, J. H.   143
Sakakitara, K.   103
Sakamoto, S.   103
Salsano, F.   130
Santoro, A.   131, 142
Saracino, R. T.   143
Savel, H.   86
Savi, N.   52
Saxen, L.   101
Schabel, F. M.   220
Scherle, W. F.   28
Schick, P. M.   190
Schiødt, T.   76, 86
Schlossman, S. F.   52
Schlumberger, J. R.   142, 143, 220, 221
Schmid, F. A.   157

Schneider, M.   142, 220, 221
Schneider, W. J.   204
Schrek, R.   143
Schuit, H. R. E.   263
Schwarz, R. S.   76
Schwarzenberg, L.   142, 220, 221, 222, 232, 249
Schweisguth, O.   103
Segall, A.   76, 86
Segerling, M.   261
Sehon, A. H.   189
Seibert, G. B.   249
Seligmann, M.   121, 123, 129, 130, 142, 143
Seljelid, R.   17
Seman, G.   231
Sen, L.   121
Sen, L. T.   143
Seppälä, M.   98, 103
Serrou, B.   261
Shearer, R. J.   260
Shevach, E. M.   130, 143
Shikata, T.   103
Shore, B.   86
Siegal, F. P.   142
Silva, J. S.   86
Silverstein, M. J.   190, 250
Simar, L. J.   19, 28
Simmler, M. C.   222
Simmons, R. L.   218, 222
Simone, J.   221, 232
Simone, J. V.   53, 221
Singh, S.   68
Siwarski, D. F.   46
Sjögren, H. O.   28, 68, 86
Skinner, D. G.   190
Skinner, J. M.   53
Skinner, M.   76
Skipper, H. E.   220
Skurzak, H. M.   28
Skvaril, F.   68
Slack, N. H.   168
Small, M.   7
Smart, C.   231
Smith, P. G.   111
Smith, R. T.   156
Smith, T.   221, 232, 249
Smith, T. J.   17
Søborg, M.   74, 75
Sokal   252
Solliday, S.   17
Sondel, P. M.   52
Sordat, B.   52
Sørensen, S. F.   68
Sorokin, J. J.   102
Soule, H. D.   86
Sparks, F. C.   249, 250
Speer, J. F.   249
Spilg, W. G. S.   75, 76, 86
Spitler, L. E.   39, 40, 204
Spreafico, F.   168
Sprecher-Goldberger, S.   168
Stadecker, M. J.   39
Staquet, M. J.   xi, xiii

Staub-Nielsen, L.   110, 111
Stecher, V. J.   17
Steiner, L.   68
Stejskal, V.   46
Sterescu, M.   142, 221
Stewart, T. N.   86
Stienon, J.   168
Stites, D. P.   204
Stjernswärd, J.   43, 55, 68, 76, 86
Stobo, J. D.   53
Stone, J. M.   232
Strander, N.   250
Stryckmans, P.   xiv, 262
Stupp, Y.   232, 250
Sturrock, R. F.   53
Sulit, H.   222
Sussman, E. H.   130
Svedmyr, E.   68
Svejgaard, A.   108, 110, 111
Sweet, R. G.   121
Symoens, J.   168

Tack, L.   168
Takahashi, A.   103
Takasugi, M.   41, 45, 53, 76
Talwar, G. P.   39
Taormina, V.   156
Tappeiner, G.   101
Tatarinov, Yu. S.   90, 98, 101
Taub, R. N.   121
Taylor, G. M.   255, 262
Terasaki, P. I.   53, 108, 109, 110
Terry, W. D.   39, 90, 101
Thierry, C.   261
Thiry, L.   168
Thivolet, J.   39, 252
Thomas, C. E.   75, 86
Thomas, L. B.   156
Thomsen, M.   111
Thomson, D. M. P.   93, 102
Thorbecke, G. J.   17
Thornes, R. D.   263
Thunold, S.   68
Till, M. M.   111
Tindle, B. H.   130
Ting, C. C.   46
Toben, T. R.   143
Todd, C. W.   91, 101
Todd, J.   17
Tokes, Z.   53
Tomita, J. T.   102
Tönder, O.   68
Touillon, C.   103
Touraine, J. L.   39
Trainin, N.   3, 5, 7
Trapani, R. J.   111
Trempe, G.   68
Trinchieri, G.   52, 53
Tripodi, D.   168
Trouillas, P.   101
Troupel, S.   102
Truelove, S. C.   53
Trujillo, J. M.   143

Tseng-Tong Kuo   97
Tsukada, Y.   102

Unanue, E.   18
Unkeless, J. C.   17
Unsgaard, B.   39, 76
Uotila, A.   257
Uriel, J.   103

Vadlamudi, S.   150, 156, 157
Vaillier, D.   28
Vaillier, J.   28
Väisänen, J.   257
Valentine, F. T.   204
Van Boxel, J. A.   53
Van Camp, B.   263
Van Hoegaerden, M.   265
Vánky, F.   55, 68, 86
Vasudevan, D. M.   42, 46
Vaughan, J. H.   76
Vaughan, L. C.   260
Vazquez, J.   86
Veltman, L. L.   189, 190
Venditti, J. M.   156, 157
Vennegoor, C.   264
Verbruggen, F.   168
Verhaegen, H.   168
Verhaegen-Declerq, M.   168
Verloes, R.   264
Veronesi, Y.   86
Verzosa, M.   221
Viac, J.   39, 252
Vidal, E.   231
Vieira, W.   156
Viza, D. C.   68, 231
Vogel, C. L.   250
Vogel, J.   38
Vogel, J. E.   265
Vogler, W. R.   213, 221, 232, 249
von Kleist, S.   89, 97, 101, 102
von Schreeb, T.   76

Wada, T.   103
Wadström, L. B.   76
Wagner, R. R.   17
Wahl, L. M.   17
Wahl, S. M.   17
Waksman, B. H.   17
Waldman, S. R.   17, 172, 189, 190
Waldron, J. A.   130
Waller, C.   51, 53
Waller, C. A.   53
Walzer, P. D.   130
Warner, G.   68
Warner, G. A.   86
Watabe, H.   102
Waters, M. F.   68
Watkins, E., Jr.   68
Watkins, E., III   68
Webb, D. R.   204
Wecker, E. E.   189

Weibel, E. R.   28
Weil, M.   221
Weiler, O.   76
Weiner, E.   17
Weiner, J.   28
Weiner, R.   221, 222
Weiser, R. S.   17, 28
Weiss, D. W.   232, 250
Welch, T.   202, 204, 205
Wernet, P.   130
Wetter, O.   265
Wetzel, B.   38
Whitaker, J.   249
White, A.   3, 7
White, G. S.   39
Whitehouse, J. M. A.   223, 224, 231, 262
Whiteside, M.   249
Whiteside, M. G.   232
Wiener, A. S.   107, 110
Wiernik, G.   53
Wigzell, H.   28, 39, 46, 52
Wikler, M.   265
Wilcox, W. S.   220
Wilcoxon, S.   70, 219
Wiler, O.   86
Williams, A.   51
Williams, E. A.   39
Williams, R.   18
Williams, R. C.   143
Wilson, D. B.   68, 189
Wilson, G. B.   198
Wilson, J. D.   142
Winchester, R. J.   130
Wiseman, B. K.   143
Withers, H. R.   249
Witz, P. I.   68
Woglam, W. H.   231
Wolberg, W. H.   86
Wolmark, N.   250
Wood, D.   17
Wood, J.   53
Wood, S. E.   76
Wortis, H. H.   39
Wrigley, P. F. M.   262
Wunderlich, J. R.   52
Wybran, J.   xi, xiii, 31, 38, 39, 40, 142, 193, 196, 204

Yachi, A.   103
Yang, J. P. S.   231
Yankee, R. A.   111
Yarbo, J. W.   222
Yee, K.   38
Yoffey, J. M.   191, 203
Young, J. D.   204
Young, R.   86
Yu, D. T.   39
Yu, V.   53
Yunis, E. J.   143

Zachrau, R. E.   86

Zamcheck, N.   102
Zawodnik, S. A.   52
Zbar, B.   68, 157, 249
Zelen, M.   250

Zetterlund, C. G.   39
Ziegler, J. L.   250
Zoschke, D.   17
Zuckerman, K. S.   205

SUBJECT INDEX

Acid eluted counts 66
Active E-rosettes 251, 253
Active immunotherapy *see* Immunotherapy
Active moiety 169
Adriamycin 236
Age, influence of 36
Allogenic grafts 20
Alpha-foeto-protein 97–100
Alpha-2H-ferroglobuline 100
Antibodies 64
    antimicrococcus 253
    membrane reactive 73
Antigen–antibody complexes 38
Antigen-induced capping 5
Antigens 196
    carcinoembryonic *see* Carcinoembryonic
        antigen
    HL-A 107–9
    solid tumour extracts as 60
    tumour-associated 19, 20, 77–86, 218
Anti-macrophage serum 117
Antimicrococcus antibodies 253
Antiserum, specificity of 264
Assay systems 41
Autologous tumour stimulation 55, 58, 59, 61, 67

B-cells 27, 31, 33, 47, 50, 51, 116–18, 123–5, 127, 128, 132, 136, 140, 191, 192
BCG 37, 38, 73, 75, 155, 207–9, 217, 218, 220, 225–30, 234–48, 251, 252, 260
Biclonal proliferations 127
1,3 bis-2-chlorethyl-1-nitrosourea (BCNU) 149, 155
Bladder carcinoma cells 257
Blastogenesis 55
Blood lymphoid cells 43
Blood T-rosettes-forming cells 34
B-lymphocytes 132, 136, 140, 141
Breast cancer 77–86, 236, 245, 247, 258
3'Bromo-5'chloromethotrexate (BCM) 147, 148
Bronchogenic carcinoma 159
Burkitt's lymphomas 129

cAMP synthesis 4
Carcinoembryonic antigen 89, 251, 256

characterization 90
    radioimmunoassay 93
Carcinofoetal antigens 89
Cell-mediated cytotoxicity 262
    in vitro 41–46
Cell-mediated immunity (CMI), detection of 77–86
Cell-separation techniques 42
Cell surface phenotyping 116
Cell volume 21
Cellular immunity in malignant melanoma, tumour-directed 69
Chang cells 48, 50, 51
Chemoimmunotherapy 235–48
Chemotherapeutic drugs 261
Chemotherapy 73, 217, 244, 251, 252, 259, 262
Chronic myelocytic 252
Colorectal carcinoma
    Duke's C 234, 242
    immunological studies 251
Concanavalin A 4
Cortisol 5
Corynebacterium parvum 155, 208, 225, 248
Cyclophosphamide 151, 152, 217, 233, 236, 245, 247
Cytolytic T-lymphocytes 42–43
Cytoplasmic membrane 23
Cytoplasmic staining 129
Cytostatic factor released by macrophages 12
Cytotoxic cells, quantitation of 48
Cytotoxic effects of lymphocytes 254
Cytotoxicity of human peripheral blood lymphocytes 257

Deoxyribonuclease 175
DIC 153, 154
DNA synthesis 55, 56, 202
Drug–antibody conjugate (DRAC) 260
Drug–carrier–immunoglobulin conjugates 260
Duke's C colorectal cancer 234, 242

Effector cells 42, 44
E-rosette-forming cells 132

Fluorescence microscopy in paraproteinaemia 263

6-Fluorouracil   235, 236
Folic acid, 3'5'-dichloromethotrexate   147–9

Golgi zone   22
Granulocytes   47
Guinea-pig complement   261

Hematosarcomas, classification of   131
Hemolytic plaque-forming cell (HPFC) test   219
HL-A antigens   107–9
Hodgkin's disease   140, 141
Host–tumour interaction   55
HuMA test   117
Human cancer   33

Idiopathic thrombopenic purpura   36
Imidazole carboxamide   235
Immune cells   33
    mechanisms   19–28
Immune cytolysis
    BT-20 tumour cells   177
    mediation of   171
    melanoma cells   177
    RI-H tumour cells   171, 175
Immune reactions   257
    against human tumours mediated by xeno-
        geneic-I-RNA   178
    breast cancer   258
Immune response   169, 223, 252
Immune RNA   169–90
    allogeneic   182
    clinical results   184–8
    concentration of   183
    duration of therapy   184
    immunotherapy with   181
    patients treated with   183, 184
    xenogeneic   170, 171, 178, 182
Immune system   33
Immunobacterial lectin   264
Immunoblastic acute lymphoid leukaemias   135
Immunoblastic lymphadenopathies   129
Immunoblasts   20, 21, 25–27
Immunochemotherapy   235–48
    combined modality   147
    preclinical approaches   147–57
Immunoglobulins   124, 126, 136
    detection test   65
    tumour-bound   64
Immunological response   20
Immunological studies on colorectal cancer
    251
Immunology   191
Immunomanipulation
    non-specific   218
    specific   218
Immunoresistance   210
Immunotherapy   37, 207–22, 262
    and chemotherapy interspersion   217
    clinical studies   209
    development   217

experimental studies   207
    in acute myeloblastic leukaemia   223, 226–30
    in acute myeloid leukaemia   255
    in chronic myelocytic leukaemia   252
    in prostate carcinoma   260
    of human solid tumours   233–50
        patients and methods   235–7
        results   237–47
    systemic active non-specific   234
    with immune RNA   181
Infiltrating cells   27
    population   25
Interferon   248
Irradiated tumour cells   218

K-cells   32, 45, 124, 141
    assays   49
    dissociation from other leukocytes   51–52
    function and evaluation of   47
    nature of   48, 51
    physical properties   51
Keyhole limpet hemocyanin   239, 242
Killer cells   27

Lectin, immunobacterial   264
Leucocyte adherence inhibition test   75
Leucocyte migration inhibition   69–76, 77–86
    frequency of   70, 71
Leucocytes, reactions induced by autologous and
        homologous combinations   71
Leukaemia   207
    acute   118
    acute lymphoblastic   118, 120, 121, 127,
        227, 251, 262
    acute lymphoid   134, 140, 209
    acute monoblastic   136
    acute myeloblastic   223–32, 234
        anti-tumour immunization studies in
            animals   225–6
        immunotherapy   226–30
    acute myeloid   118, 136, 212, 262
    advanced systemic, cure in mice   147
    associated cell surface antigens   119
    chronic   118
    chronic lymphatic   256
    chronic lymphocytic   118, 125, 126
    chronic lymphoid   136, 141
    chronic monocytoid   139
    chronic myelocytic, immunotherapy in   252
    classification of   131
    hairy cell   137, 141
    immunotherapy in acute myeloid   255
    lymphocyte populations in chronic lympho-
        cytic   254
    Moloney   151, 155
    myelo-monocytic   118
    reactivity with anti-macrophage serum   117
    specific   119
    treatment of   141
Leukaemic cells
    allogeneic   253

Leukaemic cells (*cont.*)
  FACS analysis of   119–21
  identification of   115
  normal or differentiation markers on   116
  surface phenotyping   116
Levamisole   115, 159–68
  actuarial analysis   164
  interim analysis   167–8
  methods used   160
  results   162
  side-effect   164
LSTRA   155
Lung cancer   259
Lupus erythematosus diffusis   32
Lymph nodes   140, 244
Lymphoblastic transformation tests   261
Lymphocyte functions in myeloma   265
Lymphocyte-mediated cytotoxicity   186
Lymphocyte membrane antigen   256
Lymphocyte membrane markers   123
Lymphocyte populations in chronic lympho-
    cytic leukaemia   254
Lymphocyte stimulation, suppression of
    in vitro   261
Lymphocyte-stimulation assays   77–86
Lymphocyte stimulation test   55–68
  dose–response relationships   57
  methodological considerations   55
  reproducibility   57
Lymphocytes   22, 25–27, 31, 52, 191
  bone marrow   265
  cytotoxic effects of   254
  cytotoxicity of human peripheral blood
    257
  DNA synthesis of   55, 56
  in vitro stimulation   57
  MMC-treated   56
  peripheral blood   265
  sensitized   193
  soluble   192, 193
Lymphocytotoxicity   74
Lymphoid cells   26, 42–44, 48, 169, 170
Lymphoid diseases of B-cell origin   123
Lymphoid system   253
Lymphokines   74
Lymphomas
  histiocytic   127, 128
  membrane markers in human non-Hodgkin's
    127
  non-leukaemic/non-Hodgkin's   139
  poorly differentiated   127
Lymphosarcomas   141
  leukaemic   137, 140
  prolymphocytic leukaemic   141
Lymphotoxin   258
Lysosomes   20
Lytic activity of normal peripheral blood   43

Macrophage electrophoretic mobility test   75
Macrophage inhibitory factor   74
Macrophage-mediated cell killing   74
Macrophage secretions   9, 18

factors affecting growth of other cells   10
Macrophages   22, 25, 26, 27, 45, 47
  cytostatic factor released by   12
  in tumour rejection   9
Mantoux conversion   73
Melanoma   37, 38, 69, 237, 247, 251, 252,
    254, 264
Membrane markers   127, 131–44
Membrane phenotypes   132
Membrane reactive antibodies   73
Memory cells   43
Methanol extract residues   228, 259
Microcytotoxicity assay   41, 43
Microphages   197
Migration inhibitory factor   193–6
Mitogen responses   4
Mixed lymphocyte reaction   74, 253
MLC test   63
Moloney leukaemia   151, 155
Moloney sarcoma   152, 153
Moloney sarcoma virus   42
MOLT-4 target cells   43
Monocytes   22, 25–27
Monocytic cells, identification of   125
Mononucleated cells   20, 21, 26
Myeloma, lymphocyte functions in   265

Nuclear volume   21
Nuclei, numerical density of   21
Nuclei acids   169

Osteosarcoma   198

Paraproteinaemia, fluorescence microscopy in
    263
Phagocytic cells   47
Phytohaemagglutinin (PHA)   51, 56, 63, 251
Plasma cells   20
Polyvinyl pyroidone   6
Prostate carcinoma, immunotherapy in   260
Proteolytic enzymes   263
Pyran copolymer   155

Radioimmunoassay of carcinoembryonic antigens
    93
Radioiodine labelled antibody elution test   65
Radiotherapy   73, 259, 261
Reactivity index   56, 59
Reed Sternberg cells   140, 141
Ribosomes   21, 22
Rosette-forming cells   3, 31–40, 132

Scanning electron microscopy   132, 139
Serum in macrophage culture   16
Sheep red blood cells   31, 32, 33, 34
Skin metastases   37
Skin tests   36, 60, 73, 194, 202, 203, 259
Sodium chloride   218

Solid tumours   215
Spleen cells   151, 152
Spontaneous cytotoxicity   49, 258
Statistical methods   237
Stereological methods   20
Steroid receptors   5
Suppressor T-cells   6, 192
Surface immunofluorescence   129
Syngeneic systems   19

Target cell of transfer factor   37
T-blasts   52
T-cell maturation   3
T-cell rosettes   31–40
T-cells   5, 6, 27, 31–35, 51, 116–18, 123,
        124, 128, 132, 191–5, 251
   immune   44
   suppressor   6, 192
TEa   34–38
TEt   34–38
Tetramisole   155
Theta conversion   4
Thymic factor   3, 6
Thymic hormone   3–7
Thymidine uptake   12
Thymocytes   5
Thymosin   3, 38
Thymus   37
Tilorone   155

T-lymphocytes   132, 140, 263
Transfer factor   37, 38, 191–205, 257
   and human cancer   198
   question of   194
   results of therapy   202
   specificity   202
   target cell of   37
Tumour-associated antigens   19, 20, 77–86,
      218
Tumour cells   23, 27, 42
   contacts with infiltrating cells   25
   qualitative study   21
   quantitative analysis   23
Tumour-directed cell-mediated immunity 73
Tumour-directed cellular immunity in
            malignant melanoma   69
Tumour immunity
   relevance of CMC reactions   44
   transfer of   170
Tumour rejection, macrophages in   9
Tumour specific immune response   55, 64
Tumour volume   21, 23

Waldenström's macroglobulinemia   126
Wiskott–Aldrich syndrome   35, 37, 195–7

X-irradiation   51